Practical Psychodermatology

For Arnold S. Coren (1922–1997) – for showing me the joy of medicine from the perspective of a patient. His memory continues to guide me.
J.S.R.

For Jeanette Magid (1947–2006) – a traditional mother who encouraged me to break tradition.
M.M.

For Anthony Downey (1963–1990).
A.P.B.

For my parents Alec and Elizabeth Taylor, husband Nicholas Moran, and children Hannah, Austin, and Mehetabel, with thanks for their love and support.
R.E.T

Practical Psychodermatology

Anthony Bewley BA (Hons), MBChB, FRCP
Consultant Dermatologist
The Royal London Hospital & Whipps Cross University Hospital
Barts Health NHS Trust
London, UK

Ruth E. Taylor BSc (Hons Psychology), MBChB, MRCPsych, MSc (Psych), MSc (Epid), PhD
Senior Lecturer and Honorary Consultant in Liaison Psychiatry
Centre for Psychiatry, Wolfson Institute of Preventive Medicine
Barts and the London School of Medicine and Dentistry, Queen Mary University of London, London, UK

Jason S. Reichenberg MD, FAAD
Associate Professor, Department of Dermatology
University of Texas Southwestern
Clinical Assistant Professor
University of Texas Medical Branch
Clinical Director for Dermatology
University Medical Center Brackenridge
Austin, TX, USA

Michelle Magid MD
Clinical Associate Professor, Department of Psychiatry
University of Texas Southwestern
Clinical Assistant Professor, University of Texas Medical Branch
Clinical Assistant Professor, Texas A&M Health Science Center
Austin, TX, USA

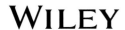

This edition first published 2014, © 2014 by John Wiley & Sons Ltd

Registered office: John Wiley & Sons, Ltd, The Atrium, Southern Gate, Chichester, West Sussex, PO19 8SQ, UK

Editorial offices: 9600 Garsington Road, Oxford, OX4 2DQ, UK
The Atrium, Southern Gate, Chichester, West Sussex, PO19 8SQ, UK
111 River Street, Hoboken, NJ 07030-5774, USA

For details of our global editorial offices, for customer services and for information about how to apply for permission to reuse the copyright material in this book please see our website at www.wiley.com/wiley-blackwell

Library of Congress Cataloging-in-Publication Data
Practical psychodermatology / [edited by] Anthony Bewley, Ruth E. Taylor, Jason S. Reichenberg, Michelle Magid ; foreword by Dr John Koo, Dr Christopher Brigett, and Dr Richard Staughton.   p. ; cm.
Includes bibliographical references and index.
ISBN 978-1-118-56068-6 (cloth)
I. Bewley, Anthony, editor of compilation.   II. Taylor, Ruth E., editor of compilation.   III. Reichenberg, Jason S., editor of compilation.   IV. Magid, Michelle, editor of compilation.
[DNLM: 1. Skin Diseases–psychology.   2. Mental Disorders–etiology.   3. Mental Disorders–therapy.   4. Psychophysiologic Disorders–therapy.   5. Skin Diseases–complications.   6. Skin Manifestations. WR 140]
RL96
616.5'0651–dc23

2013042712

A catalogue record for this book is available from the British Library.

Wiley also publishes its books in a variety of electronic formats. Some content that appears in print may not be available in electronic books.

Cover image: © Dreamstime/Ye Liew
Cover design by Meaden Creative

Set in 8.5/12 pt MeridienLTStd by Toppan Best-set Premedia Limited

1   2014

Contents

v

Contributors

Jonathan S. Abramowitz PhD
Professor of Psychology
Department of Psychology
University of North Carolina at Chapel Hill
Chapel Hill, NC, USA

Andrew G. Affleck BSc (Hons), MBChB, MRCP
(UK)
Consultant Dermatologist, Dermatological Surgeon
and Honorary Senior Clinical Teacher
Ninewells Hospital and Medical School
Dundee, UK

Christine S. Ahn BA
Dermatology Research Assistant
Center for Dermatology Research
Department of Dermatology
Wake Forest School of Medicine
Winston-Salem, NC, USA

Emma Baldock PhD, DClinPsy, PGDipCBT
Clinical Psychologist & Academic Tutor
Institute of Psychiatry, King's College London
and the South London & Maudsley NHS Foundation
Trust
London, UK

Susan Bradbrooke
Skin Camouflage Practitioner
Changing Faces
The Squire Centre
London, UK

Christopher Bridgett MA (Oxon), BM BCh,
FRCPsych
Consultant Psychiatrist
Chelsea & Westminster Hospital
Honorary Clinical Lecturer
Imperial College London
London, UK

Alison Bruce MBChB
Consultant Dermatologist and Associate Professor of
Dermatology
Mayo Clinic
Rochester, MN, USA

Christine Bundy PhD, AFBPsS, CPsychol, HCPC
registered practitioner
Senior Lecturer in Behavioural Medicine
Centre for Dermatology Research
Institute of Inflammation and Repair
University of Manchester
and Manchester Academic Health Sciences Centre
Manchester, UK

Anna Burnside MBChB, MRCPsych, MA
Consultant, Liaison Psychiatry Service
West London Mental Health NHS Trust
London, UK

Maureen Burrows MD, MPH
Forensic Psychiatrist
Central Texas Forensic Psychiatry Consultation
Service
Austin, TX, USA

Lis Cordingley PhD, AFBPsS, CPsychol, HCPC
registered practitioner
Senior Lecturer in Health Psychology
Centre for Dermatology Research
Institute of Inflammation and Repair
University of Manchester
and Manchester Academic Health Sciences Centre
Manchester, UK

Fiona Cowdell RN, DProf
Senior Research Fellow
Faculty of Health and Social Care
University of Hull, Hull, UK

Mark D.P. Davis MD
Professor of Dermatology
Chair, Division of Clinical Dermatology
Department of Dermatology
Mayo Clinic
Rochester, MN, USA

Wendy Eastwood
Changing Faces Practitioner
Changing Faces
The Squire Centre
London, UK

Libby Edwards MD
Chief of Dermatology
Carolinas Medical Center
Charlotte, NC, USA

Steven Ersser RGN, PhD
Professor of Nursing and Dermatology Care
and Dean, Faculty of Health and Social Care
University of Hull, Hull, UK

Paul Farrant BSc, MBBS, FRCP
Consultant Dermatologist
Brighton and Sussex University Hospitals (BSUH)
Trust
Brighton, UK

Steven R. Feldman MD, PhD
Professor of Dermatology, Pathology & Public Health
Sciences
Wake Forest School of Medicine
Winston-Salem, NC, USA

Roland Freudenmann PD Dr med
Associate Professor of Psychiatry
Department of Psychiatry
University of Ulm
Ulm, Germany

Tania M. Gonzalez Santiago MD, DTM&H
Dermatology Resident
Department of Dermatology
Mayo Clinic
Rochester, MN, USA

Chris Griffiths MD, FRCP, FMedSci
Professor of Dermatology, Centre for Dermatology
Research
Institute of Inflammation and Repair
University of Manchester
and Salford Royal NHS Foundation Trust
Manchester Academic Health Science Centre
Manchester, UK

Lesley Howells BA (Hons), MAppSci
(Psychological Medicine)
Maggie's Consultant Clinical Psychologist and
Research Lead (UK)
Maggie's Centre
Ninewells Hospital
Dundee, UK

Markus Huber MD
Specialist in Psychiatry, Consultant Psychiatrist and
Assistant Medical Director
Department of Psychiatry
General Hospital Bruneck
South Tyrol, Italy

Sara A. Hylwa MD
Dermatology Resident
Department of Dermatology
University of Minnesota
Minneapolis, MN, USA

Ryan J. Jacoby MA
Graduate Student
Department of Psychology
University of North Carolina at Chapel Hill
Chapel Hill, NC, USA

Simon Kirwin BEng (Hons), MSc(Eng), MBChB,
MRCPsych
Specialty Registrar in Liaison Psychiatry
East London NHS Foundation Trust
London, UK

Sussann Kotara MD
Psychosomatic Medicine Fellow
Department of Psychiatry
University of Texas Southwestern
Austin, TX, USA

Tillmann H.C. Kruger MD
Consultant Psychiatrist and Associate Professor
Department of Psychiatry, Social Psychiatry and
Psychotherapy
Center of Mental Health, Hannover Medical School
(MHH)
Hannover, Germany

Peter Lepping MRCPsych, MSc
Honorary Professor
School of Social Sciences and Centre for Mental
Health and Society
Bangor University
Consultant Psychiatrist and Associate Medical
Director
BCULHB, North Wales, UK

Peter J. Lynch MD
Professor Emeritus of Dermatology
UC Davis Medical Center
Sacramento, CA, USA

Osman Malik MBBS, MRCPsych
Consultant Child and Adolescent Psychiatrist
Newham Child and Family Consultation Service
London, UK

Sue McHale
Senior Lecturer in Psychology
Department of Psychology, Sociology and Politics
Sheffield Hallam University
Sheffield, UK

Jonathan Millard BSc(Hons), MMedSc,
MBChB, MRCPsych
Consultant Psychiatrist
South West Yorkshire Partnerships Foundation
Trust, UK

Leslie Millard MBChB, MD, FRCP(Lond),
FRCP(Edin)
Consultant Dermatologist
Hathersage, Derbyshire, UK

Audrey Ng MBChB, MRCPsych, MA
Consultant Liaison Psychiatrist
West London Mental Health NHS Trust
London, UK

Mark R. Pittelkow MD
Professor of Dermatology
Department of Dermatology and Biochemistry and
Molecular Biology
Mayo Clinic
Rochester, MN, USA

Steven Reid MBBS, PhD, MRCPsych
Clinical Director, Psychological Medicine
Central and North West London (CNWL) NHS
Foundation Trust
St Mary's Hospital
London, UK

William H. Reid MD, MPH, FACP, FRCP (Edin)
Clinical and Forensic Psychiatrist
Horseshoe Bay, TX
Clinical Professor, Texas Tech University Medical
Center, Lubbock
Adjunct Professor, University of Texas Medical
Center, San Antonio
Adjunct Professor, Texas Tech College of Medicine
University of Texas Southwestern Medical School
Austin, TX, USA

Angharad Ruttley MBBS, MRCPsych, LLM
Consultant Liaison Psychiatrist
Imperial College Healthcare NHS Trust
and West London Mental Health NHS Trust
London, UK

Laura F. Sandoval DO
Clinical Research Fellow
Center for Dermatology Research
Department of Dermatology
Wake Forest School of Medicine
Winston-Salem, NC, USA

Krysia Saul
User
Changing Faces
The Squire Centre
London, UK

Reena B. Shah BSc (Hons), MSc, DClin Psych,
CPsychol
Chartered Clinical Psychologist
Department of Dermatology
Whipps Cross University Hospital
London, UK

Henrietta Spalding
Head of Advocacy
Changing Faces
The Squire Centre
London, UK

Wei Sheng Tan MBBS
Senior Resident
National Skin Centre
Singapore

Mark B.Y. Tang MBBS (Singapore), FRCP (UK),
MMed Internal Medicine (Singapore), FAMS
(Dermatology)
Senior Consultant Dermatologist and Director of
Research
National Skin Centre
Singapore

Hong Liang Tey MBBS(S'pore), MRCP(UK),
FAMS
Consultant Dermatologist
National Skin Centre
Singapore

Andrew R. Thompson BA, DClinPsy, Dip.
Prac. Cognitive Analytic Therapy, C Psychol.,
AFBPss
Reader in Clinical Psychology & Practising Clinical
Health Psychologist
Department of Psychology
University of Sheffield
Sheffield, UK

Rochelle R. Torgerson MD, PhD
Assistant Professor of Dermatology
Department of Dermatology
Mayo Clinic
Rochester, MN, USA

David Veale FRCPsych, MD, BSc, MPhil
Visiting Senior Lecturer
Institute of Psychiatry, King's College London
and the South London and Maudsley NHS
Foundation Trust
London, UK

Alexander Verner BSc (Hons), MSc (Dist),
MBBCh (Hons), MRCPsych
Consultant in General Adult and Addictions
Psychiatry
Tower Hamlets Specialist Addictions Service (SAU)
East London Foundation NHS Trust
London, UK

Birgit Westphal MD, MRCPsych
Consultant Child and Adolescent Psychiatrist
Paediatric Liaison Team, Barts and The London
Children's Hospital
Royal London Hospital
London, UK

Wojtek Wojcik MD
Consultant Psychiatrist
Royal Edinburgh Hospital
Edinburgh, UK

M. Axel Wollmer MD
Head of Department, Asklepios Clinic North
– Ochsenzoll
Hamburg, Germany

Cooper C. Wriston MD
Dermatologist
Department of Dermatology
Mayo Clinic
Rochester, MN, USA

Foreword

From the US

"The dermatologist treats the disease; the psychodermatologist treats the patient who has the disease."

This new book on psychodermatology is extremely comprehensive. The content ranges from psychopharmacology to non-pharmacological approaches such as habit reversal therapy. It covers all age groups from pediatric to the elderly and is applicable to all providers including the nursing staff. This book is indeed a valuable addition to our specialty.

Psychodermatology is much more than delusions of parasitosis. Whereas dermatology has a tendency to focus more on minute details, psychodermatology encourages appreciating the patient as a whole. In fact, in the United States, a new book updating the entire field of psychodermatology is very timely. We are experiencing a radical change in reimbursement rates for physicians, whereby reimbursement becomes contingent on patient satisfaction. This new policy, "value based payment," increases or decreases compensation based on patient satisfaction as assessed by the Consumer Assessment of Healthcare Providers and Systems (CAHPS), a survey mandated by many insurance payers including the US government. As electronic consumer ratings become more prominent, physicians will be publicly rated, similar to how restaurants are rated on the website. Yelp! The reality that reimbursement rates are becoming contingent on how the dermatologist relates to and is perceived by his/her patient must be faced. Because this is a very subjective variable, it behooves all physicians to be familiar with psychodermatological aspects of their practice.

In short, psychodermatology is a subject matter most worthwhile learning about because of its relevance in our day-to-day practice. It is vital to investigate and appreciate aspects of our patients that are not visible, such as the intensity of emotional stress involved, the presence of depression, or the degree of support a patient needs to be adherent with his/her treatment regimen. As healthcare evolves, psychodermatology expertise will be of growing importance to the way we practice, above and beyond how to deal with a delusional patient.

John Koo
San Francisco, California
December 2013

From the UK

In the early 1970s at Addenbrooke's Hospital, Cambridge, we were fortunate enough to follow each other in the post of Senior House Officer in Psychiatry and Dermatology. The link between the two departments was part architectural, part financial: the Psychiatric Ward was next to the Dermatology Ward, and each service could only afford half a junior doctor. Arthur Rook was one of the dermatologists.

He drew the attention of one of us [CB] to the book *Psychocutaneous Medicine* by the American dermatologist Maximilian Obermayer. Arthur Rook suggested that this important book was to many UK dermatologists incomprehensible and off-putting. What was needed was an accessible and practically based volume that covered the important and fascinating clinical interface between psychiatry and dermatology.

After Addenbrooke's the two of us went our different ways, one to be a dermatologist, the other a psychiatrist, but 10 years later we found ourselves again working in the same hospital service in London. We decided to start a Psychodermatology Clinic together at the Daniel Turner Clinic, Westminster Hospital. Later at Chelsea & Westminster Hospital, we were fortunate to have working with us an energetic trainee dermatologist, Anthony Bewley.

In 2003 we inaugurated an annual meeting at the Medical Society of London for UK clinicians interested in psychodermatology. After 5 years we were delighted when Tony Bewley and Ruth Taylor agreed to continue to organize this regular event. We now have the pleasure

of writing this foreword to a book that we know will provide the resource that Arthur Rook saw the need for 40 years ago.

The editors have here brought together an important spectrum of topics, with authors from a range of disciplines, and many parts of the world. But most important is the attractive layout and practical, hands-on design of the book. Here psychodermatology is no longer an obscure and esoteric subspeciality. This book clearly demonstrates psychodermatology has come of age. It is on the curriculum. Now it is important that patients everywhere with skin complaints can benefit from the important holistic approach that psychodermatology represents.

Christopher Bridgett and Richard Staughton
London
December 2013

Preface

Psychodermatology is an emerging subspecialty of dermatology. It encompasses the management of patients with primary psychiatric disease presenting to dermatologists (e.g. delusional infestation, body dysmorphic disease and factitious diseases), together with patients who have primary dermatological disease (e.g. psoriasis, atopic eczema, hair disorders and others) where there is a large psychiatric or psychological co-morbidity.

There are a number of psychodermatology clinics starting out globally, and there has been provenance in the pioneering of psychodermatology by illustrious dermatological colleagues such as Dr John Koo from the US and Drs Richard Staughton, John Cotterell, Les Millard and John Wilkinson from the UK. But psychodermatology requires the input of a multidisciplinary team. In the UK, Dr Chris Bridgett, a consultant psychiatrist, helped found psychodermatology services. In mainland Europe, colleagues such as Dr John de Korte (The Netherlands), Françoise Poot (Belgium), Dennis Linder (Italy), Klaus-Michael Taube (Germany), Sylvie Consoli (France), Uwe Gieler (Germany), Gregor Jemec (Denmark), Andrey Lvov (Russia), Jacek Szepietowski (Poland) and Lucía Tomás (Spain) have provided inspiration and leadership in the field of psychodermatology for many years.

In *Practical Psychodermatology* two dermatologists (Drs Anthony Bewley and Jason Reichenberg) have combined forces with two psychiatrists (Drs Michelle Magid and Ruth Taylor) to edit a practical guide to the management of psychodermatological conditions. We aimed to emphasize the practicality of this book. Often, colleagues ask us *"How do you manage a patient with delusional infestation?"* or *"What's the best way to engage a patient with* *dermatitis artefacta?"* and so we wanted to produce a practical, hands-on approach to the management of patients with psychocutaneous disease. We are mindful that the management of patients with psychodermatological disease requires the input of a wide multidisciplinary team including dermatologists, psychiatrists, psychologists, primary care physicians, nurses, paediatricians, pain specialists and a whole range of other healthcare professionals HCPs. We have tried to include authorship of as wide a range of HCPs as possible, and we hope that *Practical Psychodermatology* will appeal to all those who are involved in the care and support of individuals with psychocutaneous disease. We have also tried to encompass the views of individuals who live with psychocutaneous disease, and we have specifically asked patient advocate groups such as Changing Faces to contribute to *Practical Psychodermatology*. In doing so, we aim to guide HCPs to useful resources that can be accessed either online or via other means of contact.

Just a note about the use of English in this book. We have kept the written English consistent with the author's origin, so where American English is used we have kept it as such and similarly for British English.

Finally we intend that *Practical Psychodermatology* is a text that trainees in dermatology, psychiatry, psychology, medicine, nursing and other HCP training programmes will find useful in their studies and clinical preparations. We are aware that colleagues are beginning to set up psychodermatology clinics across the globe and we hope that this practical guide will provide a helpful reference clinically and a source from which colleagues can access further research.

Anthony Bewley, July 2013

Over the past several months, as I began to review each of the submitted chapters for this textbook, I was struck by clear differences in the chapters written by authors from different countries. I was not surprised by variations in language or patient demographics , but instead by the large differences between the authors' concept of what it meant to offer a "practical" approach to patient care.

The chapters written by authors from the US are focused, precise guides to medication management, psychiatric care, or therapeutic techniques, varying by the disease type discussed. I found them very useful in my day-to-day practice and in teaching students who are new to psychodermatology. Just what I needed! The chapters written by authors from the UK, however, were not what I expected. They focused on patient resources, family education, and spoke about multidisciplinary care.

It was clear the authors had many years' experience in working on healthcare "teams" and shared a common vocabulary of acronyms such as "CPA" and "NICE." This information has helped me to greatly improve collaboration and patient care in my practice. Before I read these chapters, I did not know what I was missing.

In the UK, it is clear that the practitioners have spent their careers working within a system where patient-centered, evidence-based medicine was expected. In the US, there has been a recent shift toward coordination of care and quality of life measures, but these ideas have not been in play for very long. I hope that readers from outside of the UK (myself included) will take a cue from these authors and utilize all the "practical" approaches in this book.

Jason Reichenberg, July 2013

SECTION 1
Introduction

CHAPTER 1

Introduction

Anthony Bewley,[1] Michelle Magid,[2] Jason S. Reichenberg[3] and Ruth E. Taylor[4]

[1] *The Royal London Hospital & Whipps Cross University Hospital, Barts Health NHS Trust, London, UK*
[2] *Department of Psychiatry, University of Texas Southwestern, Austin, TX, USA*
[3] *Department of Dermatology, University of Texas Southwestern, Austin, TX, USA*
[4] *Centre for Psychiatry, Wolfson Institute of Preventive Medicine, Barts and the London School of Medicine and Dentistry, Queen Mary University of London, London, UK*

Psychodermatology: interfaces, definitions, morbidity and mortality

Psychodermatology or psychocutaneous medicine refers to the interface between psychiatry, psychology and dermatology. It involves the complex interaction of the brain, cutaneous nerves, cutaneous immune system and skin. Psychocutaneous conditions can be divided into three main categories, as illustrated in Figure 1.1.

Most patients attending psychodermatology clinics have either a primarily dermatological disease with secondary psychosocial co-morbidities or a primarily psychiatric disorder with a significant cutaneous symptomatology (Table 1.1). Clinical research has shown that there is an increasing burden of psychological distress and psychiatric disorder amongst dermatology patients [1]. In addition, stress is frequently reported as a precipitant or exacerbating factor of skin disease and is a major factor in the outcome of treatment [2]. Skin conditions may have a detrimental effect on most aspects of an individual's life, including relationships, work and social functioning. A national survey undertaken by the British Association of Dermatologists (BAD) in 2011 [3] to assess the availability of psychodermatology services, revealed poor provision despite dermatologists reporting:

- 17% of dermatology patients need psychological support to help them with the psychological distress secondary to a skin condition;
- 14% of dermatology patients have a psychological condition that exacerbates their skin disease;
- 8% of dermatology patients present with worsening psychiatric problems due to concomitant skin disorders;
- 3% of dermatology patients have a primary psychiatric disorder;
- 85% of patients have indicated that the psychosocial aspects of their skin disease are a major component of their illness;
- patients with psychocutaneous disease have a significant mortality from suicide and other causes.

These findings are not unusual and are mirrored throughout Europe, North America and globally.

The psychodermatology multidisciplinary team

Though patients often present to dermatologists, dermatologists are not usually able, in isolation, to manage patients with psychocutaneous disease. For these patients, there is increasing evidence that a psychodermatology

---

Practical Psychodermatology, First Edition. Anthony Bewley, Ruth E. Taylor, Jason S. Reichenberg and Michelle Magid.
© 2014 John Wiley & Sons, Ltd. Published 2014 by John Wiley & Sons, Ltd.

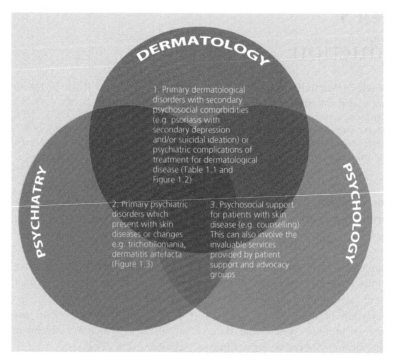

Figure 1.1 Psychodermatology interfaces (courtesy of Trevor Romain).

Table 1.1 Psychocutaneous disease

Primary dermatological disorders caused by or associated with psychiatric co-morbidity (Figure 1.2)	Primary psychiatric disorders that present with skin disease (Figure 1.3)
Psoriasis, eczema, alopecia areata, acne, rosacea, urticaria, vitiligo	Delusional infestation
Visible differences (disfigurements)	Body dysmorphic disorder
Inherited skin conditions (e.g. ichthyosis)	Dermatitis artefacta
	Obsessive-compulsive disorders
May be caused, exacerbated by or associated with:	Trichotillomania
Depression, anxiety, body image disorder, social anxiety, suicidal	Neurotic excoriation
ideation, somatization, psychosexual dysfunction, schema, alexithymia,	Dysaesthesias
changes in brain functioning	Somatic symptom disorders
	Substance abuse
	Factitious and induced injury
	Others

multidisciplinary team (pMDT) can improve outcomes [4]. Specialists who make up a pMDT require dedicated training in the management of patients with psychocutaneous disease, though such training is difficult to obtain (Box 1.1). This book, then, is aimed at being a practical, hands on guide to the *management* of psychodermatological diseases by *all* healthcare professionals. We are *not* saying that each patient with a psychocutaneous problem needs to be reviewed by a pMDT as that would be impractical and probably unnecessary. We *are* saying that for some

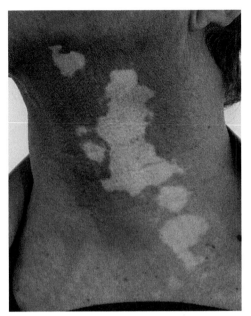

Figure 1.2 Patients with dermatological disease such as vitiligo may have psychological co-morbidities even if the condition is hidden or "milder". Such patients may feel out of control of their bodies, desperate and disempowered.

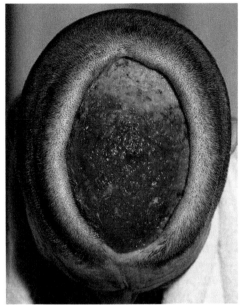

Figure 1.3 A patient with severe dermatitis artefacta (factitious and induced illness) of the scalp who required the careful input of a psychodermatology multidisciplinary team that included dermatologists, psychiatrists, plastic surgeons, nursing staff and psychologists in order to resolve her dermatological and psychosocial problems.

patients with psychocutaneous disease, a pMDT will be essential for their speedy, appropriate and effective management.

DSM-IV and DSM-5

The American Psychiatric Association (APA) has recently published the fifth edition of the *Diagnostic and Statistical Manual of Mental Health Disorders* (www.dsm5.org). The fourth version of the DSM (DSM-IV-TR, with a text revision) was published in 2000. The aim of the DSM manual is to provide general categorizations and diagnostic criteria for psychiatric disorders. These manuals are tools for healthcare professionals and do not represent a substitute for expert

Box 1.1 Possible members of the psychodermatology multidisciplinary team (pMDT)

- Dermatologists
- Psychiatrists
- Psychologists
- Dermatology and other nursing colleagues
- Child and adolescent mental health specialists (CAMHS)
- Paediatricians
- Geriatricians and older age psychiatrists
- Social workers
- Trichologists
- Primary care physicians
- Child and/or vulnerable adult protection teams
- Patient advocacy and support groups

clinical opinion. It is also important to note that categorization of psychodermatological disease is difficult and patients may exhibit symptoms of a variety of DSM diagnoses. For example, a patient with body dysmorphic disease (classified as an obsessive-compulsive related disorder) may have clear psychotic symptoms as well as being depressed at the same time; or a patient with psoriasis (a physical skin disease) may have symptoms of severe anxiety and depression as well as a substance use disorder.

The DSM-IV-TR consists of five axes (broad groups):

Axis I: Clinical psychiatric disorders (e.g. depression, schizophrenia)

Axis II: Personality disorders and mental retardation

Axis III: General medical conditions

Axis IV: Psychosocial and environmental problems

Axis V: Global assessment of functioning (0–100 scale of functioning level)

Of note, the DSM-5 work groups felt that there was no scientific basis for this separation and abandoned the axis system.

ICD-10

The tenth revision of the *International Statistical Classification of Diseases and Related Health Problems (ICD-10)* offers a general classification of all disease. As with the DSM-5, it does not include all psychodermatological conditions, but can be helpful in organizing psychodermatological conditions.

We have specifically designed *Practical Psychodermatology* to be as user friendly and hands on as possible. To this end, we have divided the chapters into the following sections:

1. *Introductory chapters* – introduction and psychodermatological history and examination.
2. *Management in psychodermatology* – these chapters aim to address psychological assessments as well as assessment of risk and management strategies for patients with psychocutaneous

disease. The chapters include psychopharmacology; adherence in the treatment of chronic skin disease; psychological assessment and interventions for people with skin disease; risk and risk management in psychodermatology; self-help for management of psychological distress associated with skin conditions; habit reversal therapy; and nursing interventions in psychodermatology.

3. *Skin disease with secondary psychiatric disorders* – including psychological impact of hair loss; psoriasis and psychodermatology; living well with a skin condition; and chronic skin disease and anxiety, depression and other affective disorders.
4. *Psychiatric disorders with secondary skin manifestations* – including delusional infestation; body dysmorphic disorder; obsessive-compulsive and related disorders; and dermatitis artefacta and other factitious skin disease.
5. *Cutaneous sensory (pain) disorders* – including medically unexplained symptoms and health anxieties: somatic symptom and related disorders; dysesthetic syndromes; chronic idiopathic mucocutaneous pain syndromes: (vulvodynia, penodynia and scrotodynia); burning mouth syndrome; and nodular prurigo.
6. *Special populations and situations* – including child and adolescent psychodermatology; psychodermato-oncology: psychological reactions to skin cancer; botulinum toxin treatment in depression; the Morgellons debate; and substance misuse and the dermatology patient.

By sectioning *Practical Psychodermatology* in this way we are intending that readers understand and logically access the broad sub-groups of psychocutaneous disease. We have where possible cross-referenced specific chapters to direct readers to further reading material.

Models of working psychodermatology services

There are several models of how psychodermatology services are delivered, all of which are compatible with a pMDT. These include:

- a dermatologist who refers a patient to a psychiatrist or psychologist who is in an adjacent room;
- a dermatologist who refers a patient to a psychiatrist or psychologist who is in a remote clinic;
- a dermatologist who has a psychiatrist sitting in clinic at the same time and a patient is seen by both specialists concurrently;
- a dermatologist who has a psychologist as a clinical adjacency (psychologists rarely sit in on clinics with dermatologist or psychiatrists).

Much of how a service is developed depends on local factors (availability of interested colleagues, finance) and there is little evidence that any one model is preferred over another. However, research makes it clear that at least regional psychodermatology services are essential [5] to cost- and clinically-effectively meeting the demands of psychodermatology patients [6].

Setting up a psychodermatology clinic

Many colleagues ask about how to set up a psychodermatology clinic in their area. The recommendations for setting up a psychodermatology service include [7]:

- *Financial investment* – managing psychodermatology patients in a general dermatology clinic is both frustrating and difficult. Dedicated psychodermatology services are mistakenly perceived as being expensive as there may be more than one healthcare professional (HCP) involved in the patient's care and because patients require longer consultations than routine dermatology patients and may need greater follow-up care. Joint delivery of care by dermatologists and psychiatrists can double the medical costs. So, it is important to cost psychodermatology services accordingly. This may require a specific psychodermatology tariff or reimbursement. Hospitals and managers

will expect a business case outlining the requirements of the service, especially for joint clinics. There is increasing evidence that psychodermatology services provide cost-effective use of resources (as otherwise psychodermatology patients will see a plethora of specialists without having their physical and psychological disease managed successfully) [6,7].

- *The team* – psychodermatology is a multidisciplinary sub-speciality. Developing expertise among nursing staff, psychiatrists and psychologists requires access to training.
- *Clinic templates* – consultations are often lengthy and appointments should be 45 minutes for new patients and 30 minutes for follow-up patients. Psychologists usually see patients for hour-long appointments.
- *Separate dedicated time* to coordinate care and to liaise with other healthcare providers.
- *Facilities* – counselling and consultation rooms are ideally situated within the dermatology unit and in a quiet, undisturbed area suitable for psychological interventions. For joint clinics, the consulting room will need to be of an appropriate size to accommodate two clinicians, the patient and a caregiver.

British Association of Dermatologists Psychodermatology Working Party Report

In 2012 the BAD reported the minimum standards required to support psychodermatology service provision in the UK [7], mindful of the UK Government's document *No Health Without Mental Health* [8]. The working party recommended:

- formalization of regional and national clinical networks to identify training needs of staff;
- development of at least regional dedicated psychodermatology service with a trained specialist psychodermatologist;

- development of at least regional dedicated clinical psychologist support;
- access to cognitive-behavioural therapy (CBT), delivered by a trained individual;
- that all dermatology units have a *named lead dermatologist* who has some experience and expertise in psychodermatology, and access to the Child and Adolescent Mental Health Service (CAMHS), integrated specialist adult psychiatric services, old age psychiatric services and community mental health teams.

Psychological interventions

Talk therapies such as CBT and habit reversal are backed by strong evidence, as discussed in subsequent chapters. Other treatment modalities that have begun to acquire a following include biofeedback, eye movement desensitization and reprocessing (EMDR), neuro-linguistic programming (NLP) and mindfulness relaxation therapy.

Psychopharmacology

Pharmacology relates to psychodermatology in that:
- medication may be necessary for the treatment of psychodermatological conditions;
- medication used in dermatology may have psychiatric and psychological sequelae;
- pharmacological treatment of psychiatric conditions may have dermatological side effects.

These issues will be discussed in Chapter 3.

Assessments tools for psychodermatology patients

Many HCPs are able to assess patients' psychosocial co-morbidities through a standard consultation/clinical interaction. However, simple well-validated tools do exist. For example:
- Dermatology specific:
  ○ Dermatology Life Quality Index (DLQI);
  ○ Skindex 29.
- Dermatological disease specific (usually validated for physical and psychosocial disease extent):
  ○ Cardiff Acne Disability Index;
  ○ Salford Psoriasis Index.
- Non-dermatology specific:
  ○ Hospital Anxiety and Depression Score (HADS);
  ○ Patient Health Questionnaire 9 (PHQ-9).

These indices are used extensively in research, but are becoming increasingly important in everyday dermatology practice as they offer a standardized snapshot of the patient's psychosocial well-being (some also include scores of disease extent). Some dermatology-specific indices may also be disease specific. Assessment tools are discussed in Chapter 5.

Global psychodermatology groups

Psychodermatology is a sub-specialty of dermatology that is gaining a voice and momentum within dermatological practice. There are a number of organizations that champion the clinical and academic excellence of psychocutaneous medicine (Table 1.2).

Medicolegal and ethical issues

Patients with psychocutaneous disease may be medicolegally challenging for a variety of reasons. Some may have personality disorders, which make negotiation with HCPs difficult; some may have forensic psychiatric problems; and some may have a delusional disorder, which may be difficult to manage. These issues will be discussed in Chapter 6.

Table 1.2 Organizations concerned with psychocutaneous medicine

	Organization/website	Meetings
PsychodermatologyUK	Psychodermatology UK www.psychodermatology.co.uk	Annually on fourth Thursday in January at the Royal Society of Medicine, London
ESDaP	The European Society for Dermatology and Psychiatry (ESDaP) www.psychodermatology.net	Biennial meeting which rotates throughout Europe, and a satellite meeting at the spring and autumn meetings of the European Academy of Dermatology and Venereology
APMNA	Association of Psycho-neuro-cutaneous Medicine of North America (APMNA) www.psychodermatology.us	Annual meetings on the Thursday before the American Academy of Dermatology meeting
JPSD	Japanese Society of Psychosomatic Dermatology www.jpsd-ac.org	Annual meetings

---

PRACTICAL TIPS

- Psychiatric and psychological factors are important in up to 85% of dermatology patients, and involve the complex interaction of the brain, cutaneous nerves, cutaneous immune system and skin.
- Dedicated training in psychocutaneous medicine is essential for healthcare professionals working in psychodermatology services, as psychocutaneous disease carries a substantial morbidity and a significant mortality.
- Psychodermatology multidisciplinary teams (pMDTs) are essential for the cost- and clinically-effective management of patients with complex psychocutaneous disease.
- Quality of life and level of disability in dermatology patients is influenced more by associated psychiatric morbidity than by severity of dermatological disease. Quality of life measures are useful verified standardized tools for assessing psychosocial burden of disease and progress with treatment.
- Therapeutics for psychodermatology patients include psychotherapies, psychopharmacological interventions, and support from family, social workers and patient advocacy groups.
- Globally, groups are emerging that champion the clinical and academic excellence of the study of psychodermatology.

References

1. Sampogna F *et al.* Living with psoriasis: prevalence of shame, anger, worry, and problems in daily activities and social life. *Acta Derm Venereol* 2012; 92(3): 299–303.
2. Fortune DG *et al.* Psychological distress impairs clearance of psoriasis in patients treated with photochemotherapy. *Arch Dermatol* 2003; 139: 752–756.
3. Bewley AP *et al.* Psychocutaneous medicine and its provision in the UK. *Br J Dermatol* 2012; 167(Suppl 1): 36–37.
4. Mohandas P *et al.* Dermatitis artefacta and artefactual skin disease: the need for a psychodermatology multidisciplinary team to treat a difficult condition. *Br J Dermatol* 2013; 169(3): 600–606.
5. http://www.bad.org.uk/site/1464/default.aspx
6. Akhtar R *et al.* The cost effectiveness of a dedicated psychodermatology service in managing patients with dermatitis artefacta. *Br J Dermatol* 2012; 167(Suppl 1): 43.
7. http://www.bad.org.uk/Portals/_Bad/Clinical%20Services/Psychoderm%20Working%20Party%20Doc%20Final%20Dec%202012.pdf
8. http://www.dh.gov.uk/prod_consum_dh/groups/dh_digitalassets/documents/digitalasset/dh_124058.pdf

CHAPTER 2

History and examination

Ruth E. Taylor,[1] Jason S. Reichenberg,[2] Michelle Magid[3] and Anthony Bewley[4]

[1] Centre for Psychiatry, Wolfson Institute of Preventive Medicine, Barts and the London School of Medicine and Dentistry, Queen Mary University of London, London, UK
[2] Department of Dermatology, University of Texas Southwestern, Austin, TX, USA
[3] Department of Psychiatry, University of Texas Southwestern, Austin, TX, USA
[4] The Royal London Hospital & Whipps Cross University Hospital, Barts Health NHS Trust, London, UK

A psychodermatological assessment requires both a comprehensive dermatological and psychiatric assessment. Most commonly, a dermatologist with an interest in psychodermatology will be the one to complete the initial assessment, with a psychiatrist brought in as the patient accepts the need to address the mind as well as the body. In a formal psychodermatology clinic, a dermatologist and psychiatrist may see the patient jointly.

The first visit

A patient with psychocutaneous disease will usually present to a dermatologist because he/she believes the problem is primarily related to the skin (even if this is not the case). The practitioner should approach a patient with a suspected psychocutaneous disease in the same way as he/she would approach any other patient with a dermatological complaint (i.e. on the first visit, the practitioner should begin with a comprehensive history and physical examination of the patient). Attentive listening and a willingness to "lay on hands" will serve to set the tone for a therapeutic relationship in the future.

Setting expectations

Patients with psychocutaneous disease will require more time than a routine dermatological visit. It is often this time pressure that causes the most strain during the patient–physician interaction. A dermatologist should book these patients at intervals of 30 minutes or more. In a joint clinic setting, an hour is allocated for each new patient assessment. When a patient is encountered during a general clinic and no additional time is immediately available, it can be helpful to point out to the patient that additional appointments may be required to complete the assessment.

The patient should be made aware that skin problems can have a big impact on a person's psychological well-being, and therefore it will be important to evaluate them both physically and psychologically. Patients may be concerned about who will have access to their psychiatric assessment. They should be informed that the conversation is confidential, but that information will be shared with other healthcare professionals (HCPs) as appropriate (e.g. letter to the referrer and to their primary care provider) and with their permission. When writing letters, the consultant should avoid sharing unnecessary details with other providers and make sure that all of the information in these letters has been discussed with the patient beforehand.

The setting

The unique challenges of seeing a patient with psychocutaneous disease require the consultation room to be chosen with an eye towards

Practical Psychodermatology, First Edition. Anthony Bewley, Ruth E. Taylor, Jason S. Reichenberg and Michelle Magid.
© 2014 John Wiley & Sons, Ltd. Published 2014 by John Wiley & Sons, Ltd.

safety and confidentiality. Though it is uncommon, patients with psychiatric disturbance may become very agitated or aggressive towards HCPs. The room needs an unobstructed exit with the physician sitting between the patient and the door. There should be a communication system to ensure rapid assistance from outside staff if the need arises.

It is common in standard dermatology clinics for there to be a lot of coming and going in the consultation room. This kind of disturbance needs to be minimized when seeing patients with psychocutaneous disease in order to help develop a setting in which patients will feel more able to discuss psychosocial issues that they may find embarrassing or stigmatizing.

Medical history

It is vital that every patient receives a comprehensive medical work-up, even if primary psychiatric disease is suspected. This will ensure that no medical conditions are left undetected and will serve to document and treat (if possible) any underlying disease, even if it is distinct from the patient's chief complaint. In addition, the patient is much more likely to share psychosocial concerns if he/she feels his/her skin and physical health concerns are being addressed.

Even those patients with a previously documented "delusional" disorder can be misdiagnosed; in one study of patients referred for a diagnosis of delusions of parasitosis, 11% were found to have an undiagnosed medical condition contributing to their disease, and 17% had obsessive-compulsive traits and no true delusions [1].

After the patient has received a thorough work-up (including laboratory testing and empiric treatments when warranted), it is important that the patient's other providers and the patient receive a copy of this work. This will prevent the patient from receiving the same work-up and treatment again, which can increase costs and impact on morbidity. It may be necessary on subsequent visits to repeat some investigations (such as examining specimens provided by a patient with delusional infestation) to maintain trust and rapport, but repeat testing should be limited.

The keystone of the first visit with a patient with suspected psychocutaneous disease is the patient interview. Many patients with psychocutaneous disease will have had the experience of being dismissed and rejected by medical professionals, so it is very important to let them ventilate any feelings of frustration and anger, and to fully hear their story.

For many patients, the most important question is: "*What do you think is going on?*" It is during this conversation that the healthcare provider can assess whether the patient has insight into the psychiatric aspect of his/her disease. Fears should be addressed; most dermatological patients have concerns of cancer or infection, and often will leave the visit not feeling that these issues have been specifically discussed [2].

If there are family members or friends available, it is helpful to ask them to corroborate the history of present illness, if any changes in behaviour have been observed (e.g. delirium or dementia) and what medications the patient is taking. They can also give useful information about the patient's premorbid personality and any changes in personality (see below).

The patient should be asked to provide a list of all the HCPs (including psychiatrists) who have cared for them in the past few years, and records should be obtained for a comprehensive review.

Psychiatric interview

If the patient is being seen in a joint clinic with appropriate time allotted, it is possible to complete a detailed psychiatric assessment at the initial visit. If the patient is being seen only by a dermatologist, the dermatologist should aim to start the psychiatric assessment and continue the discussion at subsequent visits. Some patients are keen to discuss the psychosocial impact of their disorder and are open to the idea of a psychiatric referral. Other patients (often those with delusional disorders or a body

Box 2.1 Psychocutaneous history

- Presenting complaint
- History of present illness:
  - Duration, previous episodes, known triggers?
  - Recent episodes of stress (physical or psychiatric) that may have precipitated psychiatric disease
  - Character of symptoms (burning, crawling, electric shock)
  - Distribution (dermatomal, sparing inaccessible areas)
- Previous medical history
- Previous psychiatric history
- History of substance abuse (see Chapter 27)
- Current medications:
  - Prescription and over-the-counter medications
  - Herbs/medications obtained from non-physician providers such as traditional healers
  - Look for polypharmacy
  - Look for medications that can especially affect the mental state (see Chapter 3):

- Medications with strong anticholinergic activity (e.g. antihistamines and loop diuretics)
- Narcotics
- Steroid-containing medications
- Family history (of both physical and mental health problems)
- Social history:
  - Childhood
  - Schooling
  - Occupation
  - Living arrangements
  - Relationship/marital history/children
  - Present social circumstances
  - Social support
- Forensic history:
  - History of legal difficulties
  - History of aggressive or violent behaviour
- Premorbid personality

dysmorphic disorder) may be hostile to such suggestions. In this latter group, pursuing the psychiatric assessment too soon can be detrimental to the therapeutic rapport to the extent that the patient may not return.

Even given time constraints, as a minimum the dermatologist should ask about the impact the problem is having on the patient's life and enquire about mood, and thoughts of harm to self or others should be assessed. If the patient expresses thoughts of harm, it is mandatory to explore them and make some assessment of how likely it is that the patient will act on these thoughts (see Chapter 5). If the dermatologist is concerned that the risk is high, he/she should seek further advice from psychiatric colleagues. It is therefore important that the dermatologist knows the route for urgent psychiatric referral. Where relevant, child protection issues should be assessed (see Chapter 6).

The dermatologist should aim to eventually cover all of the various areas of psychiatric history and mental state, as outlined in Boxes 2.1 and 2.2. For detailed information about how to conduct a mental state examination, the

Box 2.2 The mental state examination

- Appearance and behaviour
- Speech
- Mood: subjective and objective
- Thought: form and content
- Perception (e.g. auditory, visual, olfactory hallucinations)
- Cognitive assessment, including orientation, attention and concentration, registration and short term memory, recent memory, remote memory, intelligence, abstraction
- Insight

reader should refer to undergraduate psychiatry textbooks, any of which will cover this in detail.

Assessment of personality

Personality disorders are enduring patterns of behaviours that deviate from the expectations of the individual's culture. These patterns are persistent, inflexible and affect interpersonal functioning, emotional response, impulsivity and cognition (i.e. ways of perceiving the self and others). They usually begin in adolescence or early adulthood. In order to be diagnosed as

Table 2.1 Types of personality disorder

Cluster A	Paranoid	• Pattern of irrational suspicion and mistrust of others
	Schizoid	• Lack of interest in and detachment from social relationships, and restricted emotional expression
	Schizotypal	• Pattern of extreme discomfort interacting socially, distorted cognitions and perceptions
Cluster B	Antisocial	• Pervasive pattern of disregard for the rights of others, lack of empathy
	Borderline	• Pervasive pattern of instability in relationships, self-image, identity, behaviour and affect, often leading to self-harm and impulsivity
	Histrionic	• Pervasive pattern of attention-seeking behaviour and excessive emotions
	Narcissistic	• Pervasive pattern of grandiosity, need for admiration and a lack of empathy
Cluster C	Avoidant	• Pervasive feelings of social inhibition and inadequacy, extreme sensitivity to negative evaluation
	Dependent	• Pervasive psychological need to be cared for by other people
	Obsessive compulsive (personality)	• Characterized by rigid conformity to rules, perfectionism and control

Box 2.3 Personality disorders commonly encountered with dermatitis artefacta

Features of borderline personality disorder

- Frantic attempts to avoid abandonment
- Unstable and intense interpersonal relationships
- Unstable sense of self-image and identity
- Impulsiveness (e.g. in substance misuse, spending, bingeing or sex)
- Suicidal behaviour, gestures or threats
- Episodes of emotional instability over a period of hours
- Chronic feelings of emptiness
- Intense anger
- Stress-related symptoms that may superficially appear psychotic

Features of histrionic personality disorder

- Likes to be the centre of attention
- Inappropriately seductive or provocative
- Shallow and changeable displays of emotion
- Uses physical appearance to draw attention to self
- Speech that lacks detail and is excessively impressionistic
- Emotion that is exaggerated, theatrical and shows self-dramatization
- Easily influenced
- Over estimates degree of intimacy in relationships

Features of paranoid personality disorder

- Believes, without grounds, that they are being exploited, harmed or deceived
- Is preoccupied with doubts about loyalty and trustworthiness of associates
- Does not confide in others due to fear of information being misused against them
- Sees hidden, demeaning meanings in innocuous events or remarks
- Bears grudges
- Reacts angrily to perceived attacks not apparent to others
- Has recurrent suspicions, without justification, of fidelity of partner

a disorder, they must have a significant impact on the individual's social and occupational functioning. In assessing personality, it is important not just to rely on the patient, but to also elicit a description of patterns of behaviour from an informant (friend or relative) who knows the patient well.

DSM-5 lists ten main personality disorders, grouped into three clusters. ICD-10 lists nine of the same personality disorders, but classifies schizotypal disorder with schizophrenia and not with the personality disorders. Both ICD-10 and DSM-5 specify criteria that must be met to diagnose a particular personality disorder. The three "clusters" with their typical features are shown in Table 2.1.

In dermatology clinics, as anywhere in life, any of these disorders may be seen. However, there is a recognized association of dermatitis artefacta with borderline and histrionic personality disorder in females, and paranoid personality disorder in males (Box 2.3 and also Chapter 17).

Patients with personality disorders can be difficult to manage and dermatologists should be wary of trying to manage these patients alone. Assessment and advice should be sought from a psychiatrist.

Use of screening questionnaires in psychiatric assessment

There can be pros and cons to the use of questionnaires. When a brief questionnaire is given to all patients as a matter of routine (perhaps while in the waiting room), it can provide useful psychological information without patients feeling threatened. Even if these diagnoses are unrelated to the patient's presentation, if the patient shows signs of depression or anxiety, a questionnaire can allow the practitioner to explore psychiatric symptoms and to bring up the possibility of psychiatric referral in a less confrontational manner. A disadvantage may be that the screen may reveal more psychiatric morbidity than the doctor has time to evaluate. Commonly used questionnaires are listed in Table 2.2 and a few are included for convenience in this chapter (see also the Appendix).

Many questionnaires can be found free online (e.g. http://www.phqscreeners.com/). However, some questionnaires are copyrighted (e.g. Beck Depression Inventory-II, Mini Mental State Examination) and practitioners should be mindful of this issue before using them.

Some questionnaires are so brief that they can be worked into the course of conversation. The

Table 2.2 Focused psychiatric questionnaires for use in psychodermatology clinics

Name	Number of questions	Diagnoses screened
Patient Health Questionnaire-2 (PHQ-2) [3]	2	Depression
Patient Health Questionnaire-9 (PHQ-9) [3]	9	Depression
Patient Health Questionnaire-15 (PHQ-15)	15	Somatic symptom disorder
Patient Health Questionnaire (PHQ)	59	Depression, anxiety, somatic symptom disorder, alcohol, eating
CAGE questionnaire [4]	4	Substance use disorders
Hospital Anxiety and Depression Scale (HADS) [5]	14	Depression, anxiety
Mini Mental State Examination (MMSE) [6]	11	Cognitive impairment
Beck depression inventory-II (BDI-II) [7]	21	Depression

Box 2.4 Patient Health Questionnaire-2 for depression

Over the past 2 weeks, how often have you been bothered by any of the following problems?	Not at all	Several days	More than half the days	Nearly every day
1. Little interest or pleasure in doing things	0	1	2	3
2. Feeling down, depressed or hopeless	0	1	2	3
A score of 2 or more has a 86% sensitivity and a 78% specificity for depression [3]				

Box 2.5 SIG: E-CAPS mnemonic for the diagnosis of major depression (originally developed by Dr Carey Gross at Massachusetts General Hospital)

> Patient should have low mood plus four or more of the following for a minimum of 2 weeks:
> - **S**leep disorder (either increased or decreased sleep)
> - **I**nterest deficit (anhedonia)
> - **G**uilt (worthlessness, hopelessness, regret)
> - **E**nergy deficit
> - **C**oncentration deficit
> - **A**ppetite disorder (either decreased or increased)
> - **P**sychomotor retardation or agitation
> - **S**uicidality

Patient Health Questionnaire-2 (Box 2.4) for depression consists of just two questions. The SIG: E-CAPS (Box 2.5) mnemonic is only a little longer, but covers all of the symptoms needed to diagnose a major depressive disorder.

Physical examination and tissue evaluation

A full skin examination should be performed on all patients with psychocutaneous disease, unless this is likely to threaten the therapeutic relationship. This can often strengthen the therapeutic relationship as patients need to feel their skin condition is being taken seriously. All significant findings should be documented. Table 2.3 provides a guide to the skin examination.

Often, patients with psychocutaneous disease have not received a full skin examination because of hesitance on their part or on the part of their other practitioners. For this reason, during this full examination it is important for the practitioner to look for signs of skin cancer and the cutaneous manifestations of internal disease. If drug abuse is suspected, look for cutaneous signs of abuse, as outlined in Table 27.1.

Biopsy and laboratory evaluation

A biopsy may be indicated if primary skin lesions are visible. If time is limited during the

Table 2.3 Significant physical exam findings in psychodermatology

Finding	May indicate:
General appearance – dishevelled	Poor self-care
Lowered conscious level – disorientation	Delirium/dementia
Terra firma forme (brown spots)	Poor self-care
Bacterial superinfection of wounds	Secondary infection, not necessarily primary
Lice or parasitic infection	Poor self-care
Linear or geometric erosions/burns	Factitious lesions or signs of abuse
Stretch marks/skin atrophy	Overuse of steroids
Dermatitis/xerosis	Irritation from medications or caustic agents
Nail/cuticle fraying	Obsessive-compulsive tendencies
Nail or hair dystrophy	Nutritional disorder
Excoriation/excessive scratching	Skin picking disorder, delusional infestation

evaluation, it may be helpful to ask the patient to return for his/her biopsy on another day, and to ensure the area of concern has not been excoriated or treated with medication.

When patients provide the doctor with "samples", these should be approached in a methodical manner. A handheld dermatoscope can be used to perform an initial examination. It is helpful to provide the patient with a sample bottle or glass slide and ask him/her to return at the next visit with fresh specimens. Caution should be taken before submitting these samples to a commercial laboratory for evaluation. Speak to the pathologist/microbiologist in advance. They may find worms or bugs without biological significance to human skin disease, and may send a detailed report of their findings that can serve to validate patients' concerns, especially those of delusional patients, and

Box 2.6 Initial evaluation for delirium, confusion, dementia or changes in mental status (adapted from Magid M *et al.*, 2008 [8])

- Pulse oxygenation or other non-invasive measure of blood oxygenation (arterial blood gases should be obtained if any indication of a respiratory or metabolic derangement)
- Complete blood count
- Serum electrolytes: sodium, potassium, HCO, glucose
- Liver function tests (including bilirubin and ammonia if indicated)
- Thyroid function tests
- Urinalysis
- Iron (ferritin)
- B₁₂, folate
- Human immunodeficiency virus
- RPR with reflex FTA-Abs (tests for syphilis)
- Urine drug screen
- C-reactive protein and erythrocyte sedimentation rate (if indicated)
- Head MRI (if indicated)
- Complete listing of all medications/herbs taken, with an eye toward those that have psychiatric consequences (see Chapter 3, Table 3.8)

confuse future caregivers. In these cases, the laboratory may just want to write "*No human parasites identified*".

There are no "standard" tests for all patients with psychocutaneous disease; laboratory evaluation or other testing should be guided by the patient's presentation and examination findings. For patients with confusion or a change in mental status, it is helpful to perform a baseline evaluation for delirium and dementia (Box 2.6).

If drug use is suspected, a urine drug screen is more helpful than a blood screen.

Planning for follow-up

If there are signs of delirium or a change in mental status, ask the patient to stop all non-essential medications. If possible, enlist the help of the patient's significant others.

Quick follow-up should be scheduled when possible, and it may be necessary to admit the patient for full medical investigation. The

practitioner should allow time before the return visit to review outside records and liaise with other medical professionals.

Follow-up visits: shifting toward the psychiatric evaluation

During all subsequent visits, the practitioner should continue to ask about medications used by the patient and treat any signs of skin disease (infectious, inflammatory or malignant).

Where the patient has a primary skin disorder with secondary psychiatric disorder, the focus will be on treating the skin and reassessing the mental state at each visit. If the dermatologist has initiated any psychiatric medication, response to this must be assessed. Where referrals have been made to a mental health professional, enquiry must be made to ensure the appointment was attended.

In the case of primary psychiatric disorders presenting via the skin (e.g. delusional infestation), at initial assessment the focus will usually have been on the skin. The focus at follow-up is to continue to care for the patient's skin and at the same time build up a trusting relationship. This can take several subsequent visits.

Psychiatrist's approach to a patient with psychocutaneous disease

Unfortunately many of the dermatology patients most in need of psychiatric input will not make an appointment with a psychiatrist. In these circumstances, the psychiatrist may become involved in managing the patient through "curbside discussions" with the dermatologist.

The assessment and management of patients with a psychiatric disorder secondary to a primary skin condition (e.g. anxiety, depression or body image difficulties) will be very straightforward for any psychiatrist. Particular attention needs to be paid to medication which may either affect mental state adversely (e.g. steroids and isotretinoin), or may interact with psychotropic medications (see Chapter 3).

Patients with primary psychiatric disorders presenting via dermatology (e.g. delusional infestation, body dysmorphic disorder or dermatitis artefacta) can be challenging even for experienced psychiatrists, as they are often rather unfamiliar territory. These patients rarely see psychiatrists! In these patients, it is useful to focus on the psychological distress caused by the skin symptoms rather than being drawn into the patients' need to find a cause for their difficulties. The psychiatrist should focus on the impact the patient's condition is having on his/her well-being and ability to function. Diary keeping can be another useful technique to engage patients psychologically, with a focus on tracking skin changes as they relate to stressful life events. Examining this information together can increase insight and help develop a psychotherapeutic rapport, especially in patients with dermatitis artefacta. Where the psychiatrist sees the patient alone, it is best to avoid performing a physical exam or rendering dermatological opinions during the visit, to prevent the patient from "splitting" the providers or playing them against one another. Close working is vital to ensure the patient does not lead his/her psychiatrist into an erroneous view of the nature of the skin problem.

PRACTICAL TIPS

- During the initial visit, it is very important to set patient expectations appropriately and to adjust the setting of the consultation for a psychiatric assessment.

- Every patient deserves *one* thorough work-up to rule out organic causes for symptoms. Proceed with caution regarding subsequent diagnostic testing, as this often does not reassure the patient, but rather perpetuates the idea that an organic cause is there, but has not been found.

- It is vital to convey to the patient that the physical and psychosocial aspects of his/her disease are equally important and should both be evaluated.

- Developing a trusting relationship with the patient is crucial so that the patient feels able to share psychosocial information and engage with psychiatric assessment and management. This will often take several visits to establish.

- Treatment of the skin with topical and oral medications (when appropriate) is an important part of the overall process of caring for the patient and helps develop trust and therapeutic rapport.

- Dermatologists, psychiatrists and primary care providers should work closely in caring for patients with psychocutaneous disease.

References

1. Reichenberg JS *et al.* Patients labeled with delusions of parasitosis compose a heterogenous group: a retrospective study from a referral center. *J Am Acad Dermatol* 2013; 68(1): 41–46, 46.e1–2.
2. Ahmad K, Ramsay B. Patients' fears and expectations: exploring the hidden agenda in our consultation. *Arch Dermatol* 2009; 145(6): 722–723.
3. Arroll B *et al.* Validation of PHQ-2 and PHQ-9 to screen for major depression in the primary care population. *Ann Fam Med* 2010; 8(4): 348–353.
4. O'Brien CP. The CAGE questionnaire for detection of alcoholism: a remarkably useful but simple tool. *JAMA* 2008; 300(17): 2054–2056.
5. Zigmond AS, Snaith RP. The hospital anxiety and depression scale. *Acta Psychiatr Scand* 1983; 67(6): 361–370.
6. Folstein MF *et al.* "Mini-mental state". A practical method for grading the cognitive state of patients for the clinician. *J Psychiatr Res* 1975; 12(3): 189–198.
7. Beck AT *et al.* Comparison of Beck Depression Inventories-IA and -II in psychiatric outpatients. *J Personal Assess* 1996; 67(3): 588–597.
8. Magid M *et al.* Management of psychodermatologic disorders. In: *US Dermatology*, vol 3, 2008. Published online Touch Briefings.

Management in psychodermatology

CHAPTER 3

Psychopharmacology in psychodermatology

Sussann Kotara,[1] Michelle Magid[1] and Maureen Burrows[2]

[1] Department of Psychiatry, University of Texas Southwestern, Austin, TX, USA
[2] Central Texas Forensic Psychiatry Consultation Service, Austin, TX, USA

This chapter describes pharmacologic treatments used in psychodermatology.

Pharmacology relates to psychodermatology in three ways:
- medication may be necessary for the treatment of psychodermatologic conditions;
- medication used in dermatologic conditions may have psychiatric and psychological sequelae;
- medication used in psychiatric conditions may lead to the dermatologic side effects.

Introduction to prescribing antidepressant medications

Antidepressant medications have proven efficacy in managing depression, anxiety and panic disorders, obsessive-compulsive spectrum disorders, as well as pain and somatic symptom disorders. In general, 3–6 weeks of treatment with an antidepressant at a therapeutic dose is required before improvement of symptoms is seen. If there is minimal improvement after 3–4 weeks, consider increasing the dose. If there continues to be a lack of response or if the medication is not tolerated, consider switching to a different medication. It is important to monitor for the development of suicidal ideation (black box warning) at the initiation of treatment, especially for patients under 25 years old. Antidepressant medications are not addictive, but the dose should be gradually tapered over several weeks prior to discontinuation, as there can be an uncomfortable discontinuation syndrome if stopped abruptly.

Five major classes of antidepressants are mentioned here. The selective serotonin reuptake inhibitor (SSRI) class works primarily by affecting serotonin. SSRI medications include citalopram, escitalopram, fluoxetine, and sertraline. This class is generally the first line for treating depression, anxiety, panic, and obsessive-compulsive disorder due to its favorable tolerability profile. Common side effects include gastrointestinal symptoms (nausea, vomiting, dyspepsia), sweating, headache, and changes in sexual functioning such as anorgasmia, decreased libido, or delayed ejaculation. There can be an activating effect, with patients feeling increased anxiety when they are first taken but this usually settles in a few days. Hyponatremia and increased risk of bleeding can rarely occur. The serotonin and norepinephrine reuptake inhibitor (SNRI) class acts on both serotonin and norepinephrine. Many of the side effects of the SNRIs overlap with those of the SSRIs, but generally their sexual side effects are less. The norepinephrine component can be activating, which can improve energy, but may sometimes worsen insomnia and anxiety. Duloxetine and venlafaxine fall into this class. The tricyclic antidepressants (TCAs) are an older class of medication that also acts on serotonin

Practical Psychodermatology, First Edition. Anthony Bewley, Ruth E. Taylor, Jason S. Reichenberg and Michelle Magid.
© 2014 John Wiley & Sons, Ltd. Published 2014 by John Wiley & Sons, Ltd.

and norepinephrine. TCAs are more sedative than SSRIs or SNRIs and also have strong anti-histaminic properties, which help with pruritic complaints and insomnia, and anticholinergic properties that can cause dry mouth and blurry vision. TCAs are contraindicated in patients with pre-existing heart conditions and have the potential to be lethal in overdose, so avoid in patients at risk of overdose. Medications in this class include amitriptyline, clomipramine, dothiepin, and doxepin. Mirtazapine belongs to the class called noradrenergic and specific serotonergic antidepressant (NaSSA) and the unique properties of this medication may cause sedation and excessive weight gain. It is best avoided in patients who are overweight, but it can be a helpful medication in patients suffering from insomnia and weight loss, which is commonly seen in the geriatric population. Mirtazapine has minimal sexual side effects. Bupropion belongs to the norepinephrine–dopamine reuptake inhibitor (NDRI) class and is well known for its minimal sexual side effects and activating properties, which are helpful in patients with poor energy and poor concentration. This same activating effect may be problematic for anxious patients. In the UK, buproprion is not used as an antidepressant but is used in smoking cessation (marketed as Zyban).

Treatment of depression

Depression may be a co-occurring condition in patients presenting for dermatologic care, either as a factor contributing to skin complaints or as a result of the psychosocial burden from dermatologic illness [1]. The skin is a target for stress hormones, and it is well known that emotional distress can result in flares of many conditions, including psoriasis, eczema, urticaria, alopecia areata, and herpes [2].

For patients who are resistant to referral for psychiatric services or who have limited availability to these services, pharmacologic treatment may be managed within the dermatology practice. Antidepressants are the appropriate pharmacologic treatment for depression (Table 3.1). The dermatologist should be familiar with at least one agent. Citalopram is a common choice due to its low cost, good efficacy, and tolerability. Antidepressants should be continued for 6–9 months after the patient has responded, and then tapered gradually. Some patients may require longer periods of treatment. Psychotherapy is helpful for patients suffering from depression and should be considered in addition to pharmacologic treatments [2].

Treatment of anxiety disorders

Management of anxiety symptoms has particular benefits for patients suffering from dermatologic conditions where illness flares are exacerbated by emotional distress [3,4]. It is important to screen for depression in patients who are expressing anxiety symptoms, as anxiety may be a symptom of underlying depression [5].

Anxiety symptoms can be acute or chronic. As a general guideline, acute anxiety is defined as time limited exacerbations of anxiety, generally lasting 2 months or less, or intermittent brief exacerbations associated with stressful situations such as flying or public speaking. Chronic anxiety is defined as excessive worry that is difficult to control and has lasted for greater than 6 months [6]. Anxiety can produce a variety of somatic symptoms, including muscle tension, digestive complaints, and headaches. Panic attacks may occur in the context of anxiety and often respond well to treatment with SSRIs. Both acute and chronic anxiety can respond to psychotherapy in addition to medication treatments. Several medication options for acute anxiety are outlined in Table 3.2.

Side effects for benzodiazepines, commonly used in acute anxiety, include sedation, confusion, respiratory depression, and impaired ability to safely operate a motor vehicle or machinery. The maximum dosages listed in Table 3.2 are not ordinarily prescribed due to associated risks. Use low doses when initiating treatment and increase gradually. If a patient requires the maximum dosage of these medications, or if these medications are prescribed for longer than 1 month, consider switching to a

Table 3.1 Treatment of depression

Medication*	Activating	Sedating	Sexual side effects	Weight gain	Starting dose	Target dose	Max dose	Monitoring/ interactions*	Notes
Escitalopram	−	+	++	−	5–10 mg daily	10 mg daily	20 mg daily	No routine monitoring labs	Tends to have few side effects and few drug interactions. Good for patients with anxiety. Expensive so use in the UK NHS is restricted
Citalopram	−	+	++	−	10–20 mg daily	40 mg daily	40 mg daily	Consider ECG for higher doses	Evidence of increased cardiac risks for certain populations in doses >40 mg
Sertraline	−	+	++	−	25–50 mg daily	100 mg daily	200 mg daily	No routine monitoring labs	Tends to have few side effects and few drug interactions. Good for patients with anxiety
Fluoxetine	+	−	++	−	10–20 mg daily	40 mg daily	80 mg daily	No routine monitoring labs.	Longest half-life of SSRI class, good for patients with poor compliance who may miss doses. Does not cause discontinuation syndrome if abruptly stopped
Venlafaxine ER	++	−	+	−	37.5–75 mg daily	150 mg daily	225 mg daily	Consider monitoring blood pressure	Has norepinephrine component which causes activation. Good for patients with fatigue, pain, or poor energy
Duloxetine	++	−	+	−	20–30 mg daily	60 mg daily	120 mg daily	Consider monitoring blood pressure	Has norepinephrine component which causes activation. Good for patients with fatigue, pain, or poor energy

(Continued)

Table 3.1 (*Continued*)

Medication*	Activating	Sedating	Sexual side effects	Weight gain	Starting dose	Target dose	Max dose	Monitoring/ interactions*	Notes
Amitriptyline	–	+++	++	++	10–25 mg at bedtime	100 mg at bedtime	150 mg at bedtime	Pre-treatment ECG in elderly or those with pre-existing cardiac disease. May prolong QT interval	Very sedating, helpful for patients with insomnia. Do not use in patients at high risk of overdose as excessive use can be lethal due to cardiotoxicity
Doxepin (US) /dothiepine (UK)	–	+++	++	++	25–50 mg at bedtime	150 mg at bedtime	300 mg at bedtime	Pre-treatment ECG in elderly or those with pre-existing cardiac disease. May prolong QT interval	Helpful for itching. Good for patients with insomnia due to strong sedation. Do not use in patients at high risk of overdose as excessive use can be lethal due to cardiotoxicity
Buproprion HCl XL	+++	–	–	–	150 mg in the morning	300 mg	450 mg in the morning	No routine monitoring labs. Do not use in patients with active eating disorder or history of seizure	Does not have sexual side effects. Activating properties are good for patients with poor energy. Can increase anxiety. Used for smoking cessation. Not labeled for depression in the UK
Mirtazapine	–	+++	–	++	7.5–15 mg at bedtime	30 mg	45 mg at bedtime	Monitor weight	Good for patients with weight loss and insomnia. Widely used for geriatric patients. Avoid in overweight patients. Warn patients about weight gain and monitor weight

*This brief summary is not all inclusive. Reference a comprehensive source for complete prescriber information.

–, none; +, mild; ++, moderate; +++, severe

Table 3.2 Treatment of acute anxiety

Medication*	Onset of action	Elimination half-life	Daily dosing	Max dosing	Notes
Clonazepam	Slow	30–40 hours	0.25–2 mg daily or bid	4 mg daily	Long duration of effect and less risk of rebound anxiety
Diazepam	Slow	30–100 hours	2–10 mg bid or tid	40 mg daily	Long duration of effect and less risk of rebound anxiety
Lorazepam	Intermediate	10–20 hours	0.5–1 mg bid or tid	6 mg daily	Safe in hepatic impairment, no hepatic metabolism
Alprazolam	Fast	12–15 hours	0.25–0.5 mg bid or tid	4 mg daily	Highest potential for abuse, dependence, and rebound anxiety. Use with extreme caution
Hydroxyzine	Intermediate	20 hours	25–50 mg tid or qid	600 mg daily	Used mostly in the US. No potential for dependence or withdrawal. Anti-itch benefit

*This brief summary is not all inclusive. Reference a comprehensive source for complete prescriber information.

treatment strategy for chronic anxiety and referral to a psychiatrist.

Psychiatrists view alprazolam as a less favorable option due to its greater potential for abuse relative to other medications in that class (i.e. longer-acting benzodiazepines); however, for the reliable patient it can be a useful tool for relief of brief or intermittent anxiety symptoms or before anxiety-provoking surgical procedures. Before prescribing a benzodiazepine, it is important to screen for current alcohol abuse, as these medications can potentiate the effects of alcohol and result in life-threatening respiratory depression. Avoid prescribing this class of medication to patients with chemical dependency due to the potential for addiction. Also, avoid this class of medication in patients with severe pulmonary impairment due to the risk of respiratory depression. Prolonged use of these medications can result in physiologic dependence and abrupt discontinuation after prolonged use will result in withdrawal. Intermittent use (i.e. not daily) may reduce problems of addiction and tolerance.

The first-line treatment for chronic anxiety symptoms is with SSRI antidepressants. As SSRIs may cause an initial increase in anxiety and take 3–6 weeks to work, consider providing short-term treatment with a benzodiazepine or hydroxyzine while initiating treatment with an SSRI. Table 3.3 outlines four commonly used agents in the treatment of chronic anxiety disorders (e.g. generalized anxiety disorder, social anxiety disorder, and persistent panic disorder).

Treatment of obsessive-compulsive and related disorders

Obsessive-compulsive and related disorders (OCRDs) involve repetitive and compulsive behaviors, such as skin picking, hair pulling, and nail biting, which can complicate primary dermatologic conditions [7,8] (see Chapter 19). Symptoms of OCRDs can benefit from habit reversal therapies (see Chapter 8 and Chapter 16) as well as pharmacologic treatment with SSRIs and TCAs [8]. Table 3.4 outlines several of these first-line treatment options.

Table 3.3 Treatment of chronic anxiety

Medication*	Activating	Sedating	Sexual side effects	Weight gain	Starting dose	Target dose	Max dose	Notes
Escitalopram	-	+	++	-	5–10mg daily	10mg daily	20mg daily	Few side effects and few drug interactions
Citalopram	-	+	++	-	10–20mg daily	40mg daily	40mg daily	Consider ECG. Evidence of increased cardiac risks in certain populations with doses >40mg daily
Sertraline	-	+	++	-	25–50mg daily	100mg daily	200mg daily	Few side effects and few drug interactions
Fluoxetine	+	-	++	-	10–20mg daily	40mg daily	80mg daily	Longest half-life, good for patients with poor compliance who may miss doses

*This brief summary is not all inclusive. Reference a comprehensive source for complete prescriber information.
–, none; +, mild; ++, moderate; +++, severe

Table 3.4 Treatment of obsessive-compulsive (OCD) and related disorders

Medication*	Activating	Sedating	Sexual side effects	Weight gain	Starting dose	Max dose	Notes
Clomipramine	-	+++	++	++	25mg at bedtime	250mg daily	Well studied in OCD. High efficacy, but more side effects than SSRIs. Lethal in overdose so avoid if high risk of overdose
Doxepin (US)/ dothiepin (UK)	-	+++	++	++	25–50mg at bedtime	300mg at bedtime	Pre-treatment ECG in elderly or those with pre-existing cardiac disease. Do not use in patients at high risk of overdose
Escitalopram	-	+	++	-	5–10mg daily	20mg daily	Few side effects and few drug interactions
Citalopram	-	+	++	-	10–20mg daily	40mg daily	Consider ECG. Evidence of increased cardiac risks in certain populations with doses >40mg daily
Sertraline	-	+	++	-	25–50mg daily	200mg daily	Few side effects and few drug interactions
Fluoxetine	+	-	++	-	10–20mg daily	80mg daily	Longest half-life; good for patients with poor compliance who may miss doses

*This brief summary is not all inclusive. Reference a comprehensive source for complete prescriber information.
–, none; +, mild; ++, moderate; +++, severe; ECG, electrocardiography

Effective treatment of OCRD symptoms often requires higher doses of SSRIs, and dose should be increased to the maximum effective dose that is tolerated. Lack of response to one SSRI for OCRD does not predict failure to another: after a 10-week trial at therapeutic dosing, a switch to another SSRI agent may be helpful [9]. Pharmacologic treatment should be continued for 6 months or longer following therapeutic response.

Treatment of somatic symptom and related disorders

Somatic symptom and related disorders are a cluster of psychiatric conditions in which patients present with pain or physical complaints above and beyond what is expected from diagnostic work-up and physical exams. The patient does not create or produce these symptoms intentionally and no general medical condition accounts for the extent of symptoms [6]. Many disorders encountered in dermatologic practice fall into this category, including vulvar pain syndrome and penile dysaesthetic syndrome (see Chapter 20). Many classes of psychiatric medications have been used to treat these conditions (Table 3.5). The SSRI antidepressants seem to show particular efficacy when there are overlapping anxiety and OCD symptoms, and the SNRIs, TCAs, and pregabablin appear to be more helpful when pain is the prominent symptom [10].

Introduction to prescribing antipsychotic medications

When prescribing an antipsychotic for delusional symptoms (Table 3.6 and Table 3.7), it is best to start with a very low dose to decrease the risk of side effects such as dizziness, sedation, and hypotension. Increase the dose gradually and in small increments to help with tolerability. In patients suffering from delusional infestation, relatively small antipsychotic doses can be effective.

It is important to monitor for the development of involuntary movements in patients taking these medications, as these can become permanent and may be profoundly disabling. These movement disorders are sometimes referred to as extrapyramidal symptoms and include akathisia, dystonia, parkinsonian symptoms, and tardive dyskinesia. There is an increased risk of developing metabolic syndrome when taking antipsychotics. Metabolic syndrome includes three or more of the following: weight gain, increased blood sugar, increased cholesterol, and increased blood pressure, which can lead to heart disease, stroke, and diabetes. In addition, elderly patients who were treated with antipsychotics (vs. placebo) for dementia-related psychosis had a 1.7-fold increased risk of death from cardiac events and infection. In elderly patients with dementia, antipsychotics increase the risk of stroke and transient ischemic attacks. Caution should be exercised and the risks considered before prescribing antipsychotics in the elderly, and patients should be warned of these risks and monitored accordingly (Table 3.7). The risk of cerebrovascular accident (CVA) is about the same for all antipsychotics except quetiapine, which has a slightly lower risk than the others and also uniquely a dose–risk relationship (the higher the dose, the higher the risk). There is also a suggestion that aripiprazole has a lower risk of CVA.

Many antipsychotics increase the QT interval and this is particularly pronounced with haloperidol and pimozide; sudden cardiac death has been reported. Antipsychotics should be used with caution in patients with cardiac disease, the formulary should be consulted, and potential interactions with other drugs should be considered.

Treatment of delusional disorders

Patients may present with a fixed, false belief of a perceived disorder [6] and lack insight. Delusional disorders of the somatic type often

Table 3.5 Treatment of somatic symptom and related disorders

Medication*	Activating	Sedating	Sexual side effects	Weight gain	Starting dose	Target dose	Max dose	Notes
Escitalopram	–	+	++	–	5–10 mg daily	10 mg daily	20 mg daily	Few side effects and few drug interactions
Citalopram	–	+	++	–	10–20 mg daily	40 mg daily	40 mg daily	Consider ECG. Evidence of increased cardiac risks for certain populations in doses >40 mg daily
Sertraline	–	+	++	–	25–50 mg daily	100 mg daily	200 mg daily	Few side effects and few drug interactions
Fluoxetine	+	–	++	–	10–20 mg daily	40 mg daily	80 mg daily	Longest half-life, good for patients with poor compliance who may miss doses
Venlafaxine ER	++	–	+	–	37.5–75 mg daily	150 mg daily	225 mg daily	Consider monitoring blood pressure
Duloxetine	++	–	+	–	20–30 mg daily	60 mg daily	120 mg daily	Consider monitoring blood pressure. Helpful for patients with chronic pain
Amitriptyline	–	+++	++	++	10–25 mg at bedtime	100 mg at bedtime	150 mg at bedtime	Consider pre-treatment ECG in elderly or those with pre-existing cardiac disease. Sedating, helpful for insomnia. Do not use in patients with high risk of overdose
Pregabalin	–	++	+	+	50 mg bid or tid	300 mg total daily dose	600 mg total daily dose	Used for a variety of pain syndromes including post-herpetic neuralgia and neuropathic pain
Gabapentin	–	++	+	+	300 mg at bedtime	300 mg tid	3600 mg total daily dose	Used for a variety of pain syndromes including neuropathic pain and post-herpetic neuralgia

*This brief summary is not all-inclusive. Please reference a comprehensive source for complete prescriber information.

–, none; +, mild; ++, moderate; +++, severe; ECG, electrocardiography

Table 3.6 Treatment of delusional disorders

Medication	Efficacy	Tolerability	Risk of EPS	Weight gain and sedation	Starting dose	Max dose	Notes*
Risperidone	+++	++	++	++	0.5 mg at bedtime	6 mg daily	May increase prolactin levels
Olanzapine	+++	++	+	+++	2.5–5 mg at bedtime	20 mg daily	Very effective but increased weight gain and sedation, significant risk of metabolic syndrome
Aripiprazole	++	+++	+	+	5 mg daily	30 mg daily	Slightly less effective but decreased risk of weight gain and less sedating. Can be used as augmentation agent in depression. Suggestion that it may have less risk than other antipsychotics of CVA in the elderly
Quetiapine	++	++	+	+++	50 mg at bedtime	600 mg at bedtime	Increased weight gain and very sedating. Can be helpful in small doses for insomnia. Like aripiprazole, less risk of CVA in the elderly and risk is dose related
Amisulpide	+++	++	++	++	200 mg at bedtime	1200 mg daily	Commonly used in Europe. Category B for pregnancy
Pimozide	+++	+	+++	++	1 mg twice daily	10 mg daily	Baseline and periodic ECG. Higher risk of EPS, more anticholinergic side effects. Due to risk of prolonged QT and risk of sudden cardiac death, rarely used in Europe

*This brief summary of monitoring/interactions is not all inclusive. Reference a comprehensive source for complete prescriber information.

–, none; +, mild; ++, moderate; +++, severe; EPS, extrapyramidal symptoms; CVA, cerebrovascular accident

Table 3.7 Monitoring for patients on antipsychotic medications

Side effect	Monitoring parameter
Electrocardiography (ECG)	Baseline ECG for patients starting on pimozide. For other agents, consider ECG in patients with cardiac history, strong family history of cardiac disease, or who develop symptoms such as syncope or dizziness while taking antipsychotics
Tardive dyskinesia	Every 6 months
Lipids	Consider baseline and every 5 years
Body mass index (BMI) or weight	Monthly for 3 months, then every 3 months
Glucose (fasting blood glucose or HbA1$_c$)	Baseline, at 3 months, then annually
Blood pressure	As clinically indicated
Waist circumference	Consider at baseline and annually. Most patients refuse this

involve the person's belief that they emit a foul odor; that there is infestation with insects or parasites (see Chapter 14); or that parts of the body are ugly or misshapen (i.e. body dysmorphic disorder psychotic subtype without insight, see Chapter 15) [6]. If the delusional beliefs occur as part of another primary psychiatric condition such as schizophrenia, bipolar mania, or severe depression with psychotic features, the patient should be referred to a psychiatrist. If there is concern that the patient is at acute risk of suicide or harm to others due to their psychiatric condition, prompt referral to emergency services is indicated (see Chapter 6).

Clinical management of patients with delusional disorders presents unique challenges. Due to the delusional nature of their complaints, these patients may be extremely resistant to psychiatric referral. Encouraging treatment with antipsychotic agents can be presented as a means of decreasing distress. The patient may never be completely "cured" – the goal of treatment should be to decrease preoccupation with the belief and improve social and occupational functioning.

Some commonly used antipsychotic agents and a brief outline of monitoring parameters for them are outlined in Table 3.6 and Table 3.7. The dermatologist should familiarize himself/herself with at least one agent. Risperidone is a common choice due to its low cost, good efficacy, and tolerability.

Psychiatric and dermatologic side effects

Certain medications commonly prescribed in dermatologic practice can produce psychiatric side effects. Table 3.8 highlights the most common culprits.

Table 3.8 Medications prescribed in dermatologic practice with possible psychiatric consequences

Medication	Possible psychiatric consequences
Antihistamines	Depression, extrapyramidal symptoms, confusion
Antimalarials (e.g. hydroxychloroquine)	Affective disorders, psychosis (rare)
Dapsone	Psychotic disorders (rare)
Dianette (for acne)	Depression, anxiety
Isotretinoin	Affective disorders (especially depression), suicidal ideation
Methotrexate	Mood changes, affective disorders
Minocycline	Lupus erythematosus-like syndrome which may include psychiatric features
PUVA and UVB	Affect changes (e.g. euphoria)
Systemic steroids	Depression, confusion in elderly (common), mania, psychosis (rare)

Table 3.9 Medications prescribed in psychiatric practice with possible dermatologic consequences

Psychotropic medication	Dermatologic side effects
Mood stabilizers	
Lithium	Hair loss, folliculitis, acne, nail pigmentation, precipitation or exacerbation of psoriasis
Valproic acid	Hair loss, lupus, hair color change, scleroderma, cutaneous vasculitis
Lamotrigine	Stevens–Johnson syndrome (Figure 3.1), toxic epidermal necrolysis, angioedema
Carbamazepine	Pruritic rash, hypersensitivity reaction (Figure 3.2) (e.g. rash, lymphadenopathy, fever), hair loss, Stevens–Johnson syndrome
Antidepressants	
General	Allergic reactions (e.g. hives, urticaria), excessive sweating, pruritus
Fluoxetine	Hair loss
TCAs	Photosensitivity
Antipsychotics	
General	Photosensitivity, urticaria, maculopapular rash, petechiae, edema
Phenothiazines, haloperidol, clozapine	Skin pigmentation (blue–gray discoloration)
Haloperidol, fluphenazine, thioridazine	Contact dermatitis
Anxiolytics	
Alprazolam	Photosensitivity

TCA, tricyclic antidepressant

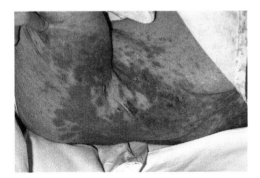

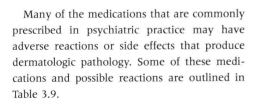

Figure 3.1 Stevens–Johnson syndrome can be secondary to a range of psychotropic medications, in this case haloperidol (courtesy of Dr A. Bewley).

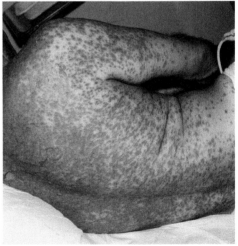

Figure 3.2 Hypersensitive reactions (in this case an acute generalized exanthematous pustulosis) secondary to carbamazepine (courtesy of Dr A. Bewley).

Many of the medications that are commonly prescribed in psychiatric practice may have adverse reactions or side effects that produce dermatologic pathology. Some of these medications and possible reactions are outlined in Table 3.9.

PRACTICAL TIPS

- As some patients refuse psychiatric referral, the dermatologist may need to manage psychiatric conditions.

- Consider antidepressants such as citalopram, sertraline, and fluoxetine for the treatment of depressive disorders, chronic anxiety disorders, and somatic symptom disorders.

- Consider short-term use (no more than 1 month) of anxiolytics such as lorazepam, clonazepam, and diazepam for the treatment of acute anxiety, but avoid in those who have a history of substance misuse.

- Consider prescribing antipsychotics such as risperidone and amisulpiride for the treatment of delusional disorders.

- Be aware that some dermatologic medications may have psychiatric side effects, and that some psychiatric medications may have dermatologic side effects.

References

1. Lee CS, Koo J. Psychopharmacologic therapies in dermatology: an update. *Dermatol Clin* 2005; 23: 735–744.

2. Locala JA. Current concepts in psychodermatology. *Curr Psychiatry Rep* 2009; 11: 211–218.

3. Lee CS *et al.* Psychopharmacology in dermatology. *Dermatol Ther* 2008; 21: 69–82.

4. Poot F *et al.* Basic knowledge in psychodermatology. *J Eur Acad Dermatol Venereol* 2007; 21: 227–234.

5. Gupta MA, Gupta AK. The use of psychotropic drugs in dermatology. *Dermatol Clin* 2000; 18: 711–725.

6. American Psychiatric Association. *Diagnostic and Statistical Manual of Mental Disorders*, 4th edn, text revision. Washington, DC: American Psychiatric Association, 2000.

7. Gupta MA, Gupta AK. A practical approach to the assessment of psychosocial and psychiatric comorbidity in the dermatology patient. *Clin Dermatol* 2013; 31: 57–61.

8. Folks DG, Warnock JK. Psychocutaneous disorders. *Curr Psych Rep* 2001; 3: 219–225.

9. Rasmussen SA, Eisen JL. Treatment strategies for chronic and refractory obsessive-compulsive disorder. *J Clin Psychiatry* 1997; 58 (Suppl 13): 9–13.

10. Somashekar B *et al.* Psychopharmacotherapy of somatic symptoms disorders. *Int Rev Psychiatry* 2013; 25: 107–115.

CHAPTER 4

Adherence in the treatment of chronic skin diseases

Laura F. Sandoval,[1] Christine S. Ahn[1] and Steven R. Feldman[2]

[1] Center for Dermatology Research, Department of Dermatology, Wake Forest School of Medicine, Winston-Salem, NC, USA

[2] Pathology & Public Health Sciences, Wake Forest School of Medicine, Winston-Salem, NC, USA

Adherence refers to the extent to which a patient's behavior (whether it is taking a medication or modifying a behavior) is consistent with medical advice (Box 4.1) [1]. Adherence is not a single entity, but a series of events that contributes to treatment outcome. First, a patient must seek medical advice, be evaluated, and receive a diagnosis, followed by being prescribed a medication, filling that prescription, and then taking the drug (well or poorly). Non-adherence to an early step results in a cascade effect of non-adherence to later steps. Small declines in adherence at each step can lead to failure to achieve desirable treatment outcomes; in dermatology, the role of poor adherence as a cause of poor treatment outcomes has gone unrecognized for too long.

Methods of assessing adherence

Adherence to medication can be measured in several ways (Box 4.2). Most commonly, clinicians have relied on patient self-reporting; research studies may rely on patient logs as a measurement of medication adherence. These methods are limited by reliance on patients' ability and honesty, limitations that, given patients' psychological propensities, make these poor measures of true adherence behavior. Self-reported methods such as diary entries are often completed some time after the actual medication usage, which may result in recall bias, inaccuracies, and overestimated adherence. Other common and inadequate methods of measuring adherence involve pill counts, pharmacy records, or tube weights. The unreliability of traditional methods of measuring adherence has been demonstrated repeatedly.

The medication electronic monitoring system (MEMS) is one of the most common and widely studied adherence monitoring systems. It involves a medication bottle cap containing a microprocessor that detects and records each time the bottle is opened (Figure 4.1). The opening of a bottle is assumed to be equivalent to taking a single dose of medication. This system has been largely applied to studies of adherence to oral medications; however, it has also been demonstrated to be feasible and accurate in studies of adherence to topical therapies.

Carroll *et al.* measured adherence to topical treatment in psoriasis by multiple methods, including electronic monitoring caps, medication logs, and medication usage by weight [2]. The average overall MEMS adherence rate was 55% compared to 87% according to self-reported medication logs, providing evidence that patients overestimate their medication use. Adherence rates based on the medication weight showed wide variation (27–458%),

Practical Psychodermatology, First Edition. Anthony Bewley, Ruth E. Taylor, Jason S. Reichenberg and Michelle Magid.
© 2014 John Wiley & Sons, Ltd. Published 2014 by John Wiley & Sons, Ltd.

Box 4.1 Definitions

- **Adherence** – the extent to which a patient's behavior (whether it is taking a medication or modifying a behavior) is consistent with medical advice
- **Concordance** – a collaboration between the patient and the provider where negotiation takes place and an agreement is reached that respects the patient's needs and beliefs concerning taking (or not taking) a medication
- **Compliance** – the extent a patient's behavior matches the prescriber's recommendation. This term has negative connotation, placing blame on the patient for not following advice, and has been largely replaced by the term adherence.

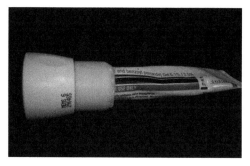

Figure 4.1 Example of a topical acne medication with a medication electronic monitoring system (MEMS) cap attached.

Box 4.2 Methods of measuring adherence

- Subjective (patient's reported adherence, diaries) – unreliable, patients consistently over-report adherence
- Semi-objective (weight of used treatments/pill counts) – variable and often unreliable; subject to patient manipulation. Do not provide details such as timing and frequency of use
- Objective (MEMS) – reliable, but not always a practical means of measuring adherence. Provide details on timing and frequency of use, allowing patterns of adherence to be established

which indicated that medication weight was also not a reliable method of measuring adherence to topical mediations.

In addition to providing a more accurate measure of adherence, electronic monitoring systems collect dosing times and dosing intervals, providing a means of identifying adherence patterns (Figure 4.2). The use of MEMS caps to monitor adherence to topical treatment of acne, atopic dermatitis, and psoriasis has been shown to improve adherence around the time of scheduled physician visits [2–4]; the

psychological underpinnings of the consistent and powerful effect of return visits on patients' adherence is not well characterized. Additionally, a decline in adherence was observed over the course of one study, with an increasing number and length of treatment gaps throughout the study [2].

Adherence in chronic skin diseases

About a third of prescriptions to treat dermatologic conditions never get filled [5]. This is primary non-adherence; secondary non-adherence is not using a medication as recommended. Non-adherence, both primary and secondary, in the treatment of chronic skin diseases such as atopic dermatitis and psoriasis is higher compared to that in treatment of acute dermatologic conditions [5]. Furthermore, adherence to treatment with topical agents is worse than that to treatment with other options such as systemic treatment [1,5]. Perhaps surprisingly, worse disease severity tends to be associated with worse adherence; the psychology of this is not well characterized. In general, dissatisfaction with the treatment of chronic skin diseases is common, and this dissatisfaction is associated with poor adherence [6].

AARDEX▸Ltd   **PowerView**   **Compliance Report**

| Patient number: | **018** | Patient initials: | |
| Patient name: | | Monitor number: | |

| Investigator: | | Drug name: | |
| Regimen: | **Once a day** | | |

Results:	**8/7/2012 3:00: to 9/26/2012 2:59: (1)**	Number of monitored days:	**50**
Number of doses taken:	**40**	Shortest interval (hrs):	**0.4**
Longest interval (hrs):	**117.4**	% Prescribed number of doses taken:	**80.0%**
% Days correct nbr of doses taken:	**60.0%**	% Prescribed doses taken on schedule:	**46.9%**
Therapeutic coverage:	**81.7%**	Drug duration of action (in hours):	**36.0**
Number of prescribed doses:	**50**		

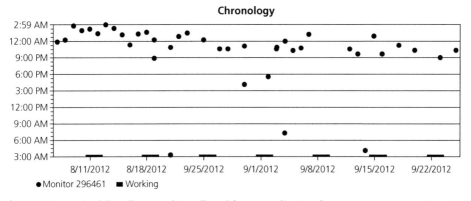

Chronology

Figure 4.2 Example of the adherence data collected from a medication electronic monitoring system (MEMS). Data from the MEMS cap are downloaded and analyzed using PowerView software (Aardex Group Ltd., Switzerland).

Table 4.1 Factors affecting adherence to the treatment of chronic skin diseases

Disease characteristics	Patient characteristics	Medication characteristics	Physician characteristics
• Disease severity • Longevity of disease experience	• Smoking • Being unmarried • Patient education • Forgetfulness • Frustration	• Lack of efficacy • Side effects • Fear of side effects • Cost • Too complicated (e.g. multiple vs. once-daily dosing) • Too time consuming • Too messy	• Frequency of visits • Patient–physician relations

Factors affecting adherence

Multiple factors affect adherence to treatment of chronic skin diseases (Table 4.1). Lack of efficacy is often cited by patients as a significant barrier to adherence [6,7]. Patients' perception of ineffective treatment is likely multifactorial, including lack of education on the chronicity of their disease and unrealistic expectations of a cure, or it is possible that patients just do not use the medication or use it too infrequently for it to be effective. Frustration with treatment is common [6,7]. In fact, a third of patients with atopic dermatitis and nearly 50% of those with psoriasis did not fill a new prescription for a medication they had not previously used [5].

Side effects such as dryness and irritation are common factors leading to non-adherence to topical acne treatment. Newer, more tolerable agents are available. Since cost is cited as a reason for non-adherence [7], the benefits of better tolerability need to be weighed against the risk of increased cost.

Patients often admit to simply forgetting to take their medications [7]. While the psychology behind this forgetfulness may be extensive, including patients' perceptions of their illness, which are influenced by their beliefs and cultures, or lack of motivation. Patients are human and even highly motivated patients may forget to take their medication. Patients also forget how they were told to take their medication, resulting in non-adherence. Many patients cannot recall medication instructions immediately after a visit, either because clear instructions were not given in the first place or because the patient quickly forgets the details amongst the overwhelming amount of information they often receive.

Additional factors that patients cite for non-adherence to topical agents are that they are too messy, unpleasant and time consuming to apply [6,7].

Ethnicity or culture, health beliefs, and socioeconomic status also play a role in adherence [1]. Cultural beliefs with regards to healthcare need to be identified and addressed when they are a barrier to adherence. Similarly, socioeconomic status may need to be addressed to ensure appropriate treatment options are considered; one way to make certain a patient will be non-adherent is to recommend treatment regimens he/she cannot afford.

Interventions to improve adherence

More frequent interactions

Based on data from MEMS adherence studies, there is a distinct pattern of improved adherence around the times of follow-up visits. This "white coat compliance" phenomenon has been well described in the treatment of non-dermatologic diseases, and occurs in patient populations using topical medications for psoriasis, acne vulgaris, and atopic dermatitis [2–4]. More frequent visits provide the opportunity to address medication issues, including efficacy and side effects, and give physicians the chance to provide the encouragement that many patients need. Psychologically, patients may feel a reduced burden of treatment if short-term treatment goals are set (having to take a medication for 1 or 2 weeks seems much more achievable than having to take a medication for months or a lifetime). Although there may be concern that more frequent visits are not practical, moving the first return visit from 8 or 12 weeks to 1 week does not increase the number of visits. If the early return visit causes patients to use their treatment and improve, the number of future visits for follow-up of poor responses may be reduced.

Patient–physician relationship

The quality of the patient–physician relationship is a considerable factor in influencing adherence to treatment. Good communication, including taking the time to adequately educate the patient about his/her disease, treatment options, expectations, and potential side effects, contributes to establishing a good relationship. Patient trust is a significant predictor of adherence and satisfaction, with 62% of patients in the highest quartile of trust reporting that they always took medication and followed their doctor's recommendation, compared with just 14% of patients in the lowest trust quartile [8]. All patients differ in their beliefs and perceptions, and by acknowledging these differences physicians have the opportunity to strengthen their relationship with their patient.

Education

Educating patients can be empowering and provide patients with the autonomy they desire. Additionally, patients are often forgetful or con-fused about what they have been instructed to do and education through demonstrations, pamphlets, or videos provides an opportunity to reinforce physician instructions. Recognizing the time constraints on typical office visits with a physician, these education interventions can be conducted by nurses. Nurse-led eczema educational sessions (videos, demonstrations, discussions) have resulted in greater adherence and greater improvement in atopic dermatitis. A decrease in severity of disease, by as much as 89%, was reported after education interventions in patients with atopic dermatitis [9]. Nursing assessment of patients' educational needs and nursing-specific interventions are discussed further in Chapter 9.

Written action plans (WAPs), which are formal written guides to help manage a chronic disease, have been used with success in pediatric patients with asthma and have potential to be of benefit in the treatment of atopic dermatitis [10]. WAPs could potentially improve adherence and outcomes by providing clearly written guidelines for treatment and a daily reminder to use medications, and aiding in the communication between healthcare providers and patients.

Support groups may also educate patients and improve adherence. These groups allow patients to share experiences and keep patients informed of treatment options. For chronic skin diseases such as psoriasis that are known to affect patients' quality of life, support groups can address psychosocial needs and help patients feel less isolated. Similarly, psoriasis patients should be encouraged to join the National Psoriasis Foundation, or a similar advocacy group, which can also provide some of these same support services, as well as encouraging adherence to treatment recommendations.

Reminders

One of the common hurdles to good adherence is forgetfulness. Telephone reminder systems or text messages to remind patients to use their medication have resulted in significant improvement in adherence and treatment outcomes [1]. In fact, some pharmaceutical websites, specifically those of manufacturers of biologic agents, have implemented reminder programs that utilize phone calls, emails, or texts message to remind patients to use their medication. Reminders, however, are not a universally effective means to enhance adherence. Given some patients' tendencies toward oppositional-defiant behavior, a reminder may be unwelcome and may reduce adherence. In a study of adolescents with acne vulgaris, patients were randomized to one of four different groups: a standard care group that did not receive any additional intervention, a group with frequent office visits (weeks 1, 2, 4, 6, 8, and 12), a group receiving daily phone call reminders, and a group where parents received daily phone call reminders. The strategy with the highest median adherence (82%) was the frequent office visits. The groups that received daily reminders either directly by phone or through phone calls to their parents had the lowest levels of adherence, with adherence in the parent reminder group being significantly lower than that in all the other groups [4].

The use of sticker charts may be beneficial in improving adherence in children with chronic skin conditions like atopic dermatitis. While the goal of these charts is positive reinforcement, hanging the chart in a visible area like the bathroom or kitchen can serve as a reminder for children to take their medications.

Simplifying treatment regimens

Simplifying treatment regimens is a psychologically rational approach to improving adherence and treatment outcomes. Patients with once-daily chronic dosing regimens are more likely to adhere than those with more frequent dosing regimens [1]. Once-daily formulations of oral antibiotics are available, as are topical combination products for psoriasis or acne.

Other psychological tools to promote adherence (see also Chapter 5 and Chapter 9)

Humans have a strong psychological tendency to weigh losses greater than they do gains. This can be used by presenting the impact of poor adherence as a loss rather than good adherence as a gain. For example, you might say, *"If you don't use sunscreen, you will lose your youthful complexion,"* rather than saying, *"You can keep your youthful look longer if you protect yourself from the sun."*

Saliency also affects patients' perceptions and can be used to modify their perceptions of risks of side effects. The more descriptive picture seems more likely to affect change. You might use this phenomenon to encourage better adherence to sunscreen. Instead of telling patients, *"If you don't use sunscreen, you may get skin cancer,"* you might say, *"If you don't use sunscreen, you could end up with an ulcerating, crusty, golf ball-sized skin cancer on your nose, resulting in surgery requiring removal of your nose and placement of a removable rubber prosthesis over the resulting defect."*

PRACTICAL TIPS

- Adherence in the treatment of chronic skin diseases is poor and is often responsible for treatment failure.
- Factors that contribute to non-adherence include lack of efficacy, frustration, side effects, cost, forgetfulness, and the messiness and time it takes to apply topical treatment.
- Establishing a good patient–physician relationship that promotes good communication, including acknowledging patients' beliefs about their disease and treatment, and providing education and caring support, plays a significant role in adherence.
- Interventions such as increasing frequency of visits, simplifying treatment regimens, promoting educational resources, and providing reminders all may help improve adherence in the treatment of chronic skin diseases.

References

1. Gupta G *et al.* Adherence to topical dermatological therapy: lessons from oral drug treatment. *Br J Dermatol* 2009; 161(2): 221–227.
2. Carroll CL *et al.* Adherence to topical therapy decreases during the course of an 8-week psoriasis clinical trial: commonly used methods of measuring adherence to topical therapy overestimate actual use. *J Am Acad Dermatol* 2004; 51(2): 212–216.
3. Krejci-Manwaring J *et al.* Stealth monitoring of adherence to topical medication: adherence is very poor in children with atopic dermatitis. *J Am Acad Dermatol* 2007; 56(2): 211–216.
4. Feldman SR *et al.* Adherence to topical therapy increases around the time of office visits. *J Am Acad Dermatol* 2007; 57(1): 81–83.
5. Storm A *et al.* One in 3 prescriptions are never redeemed: primary nonadherence in an outpatient clinic. *J Am Acad Dermatol* 2008; 59: 27–33.
6. Krejci-Manwaring J *et al.* Adherence with topical treatment is poor compared with adherence with oral agents: implications for effective clinical use of topical agents. *J Am Acad Dermatol* 2006; 54(5 Suppl): S235–S236.
7. Brown KK *et al.* Determining the relative importance of patient motivations for nonadherence to topical corticosteroid therapy in psoriasis. *J Am Acad Dermatol* 2006; 55(4): 607–613.
8. Thom DH *et al.* Further validation and reliability testing of the Trust in Physician Scale. The Stanford Trust Study Physicians. *Med Care* 1999; 37(5): 510–517.
9. Cork MJ *et al.* Comparison of parent knowledge, therapy utilization and severity of atopic eczema before and after explanation and demonstration of topical therapies by a specialist dermatology nurse. *Br J Dermatol* 2003; 149(3): 582–589.
10. Chisolm SS *et al.* Written action plans: potential for improving outcomes in children with atopic dermatitis. *J Am Acad Dermatol* 2008; 59(4): 677–683.

CHAPTER 5

Psychological assessment and interventions for people with skin disease

Reena B. Shah

Department of Dermatology, Whipps Cross University Hospital, London, UK

The link between dermatological conditions and psychological problems has long been recognized, with some studies indicating that 30% of those with dermatological conditions have clinically significant levels of psychological distress [1]. Stigmatization of imperfect skin is a huge problem within our society and being visibly different can cause and perpetuate psychological difficulties, impacting a patient's quality of life (QoL). Rates of suicidal ideation in those with skin disease have been reported at 8.6%, which is higher than in general medical patients [2]. This chapter will outline the approach to a dermatology patient from the perspective of a psychologist, from initial assessment to treatment modalities.

There is significant research looking at the psychological impact of skin disease, with the majority being on psoriasis, eczema, acne and vitiligo. The most widely cited difficulties are those around social anxiety, poor social skills and self-concept due to body image concerns. These patients can have relationship difficulties and often avoid any activities where their skin might be on display, from sporting activities to intimate relationships. This may be due to the fear of stigmatization or rejection, or from embarrassment and/or feelings of shame and low-esteem (Figure 5.1). There is also a strong link between stress and the exacerbation of skin disorders.

It is important to note the variability in distress for dermatology patients, with the severity of the psychological distress experienced not necessarily correlated with the severity of the skin condition. This may stem from differences in social support, illness perceptions, beliefs and coping skills. It is also key to remember that those with non-visual skin conditions (such as vulvodynia) also show high levels of psychological distress and negative personal evaluation [3].

Race, gender and culture all influence how skin disorders affect QoL. For example, clients with vitiligo may note that losing their pigmentation has affected their racial identity, or they may have the cultural belief that their pigmentation is a manifestation of a "wrongdoing" in a previous life.

Psychologist's initial approach to dermatology clients

When working with clients, the most important aspect is to develop a therapeutic relationship, as this is the vehicle through which change occurs. It has been shown that clients get

---

Practical Psychodermatology, First Edition. Anthony Bewley, Ruth E. Taylor, Jason S. Reichenberg and Michelle Magid.
© 2014 John Wiley & Sons, Ltd. Published 2014 by John Wiley & Sons, Ltd.

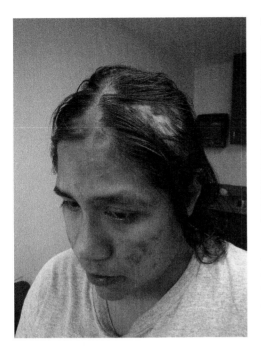

Figure 5.1 Patient is a 21-year-old female with a new diagnosis of systemic lupus erythematosus. She suffers from hair loss and facial lesions. Though the systemic aspects of her disease are well controlled, it is important to assess her dermatological and psychosocial co-morbidities.

Box 5.1 What is Socratic questioning?

Socratic questioning involves asking the client questions which:
- The client has the knowledge to answer
- Draw the client's attention to information which is relevant to the issue being discussed, but which may be outside the client's current focus
- Generally move from the concrete to the more abstract, so that
- The client can, in the end, apply the new information to either re-evaluate a previous conclusion or construct a new idea [4]

better quicker and better adhere to treatment when a positive therapeutic relationship has been developed. This therapeutic alliance can be secured by being empathic, genuine, and respectful, maintaining eye contact, showing support, and building trust.

Socratic questioning

During consultations, using Socratic questioning can be an effective way to engage clients and to learn about the client's perspective (Box 5.1 and Box 5.2). Socrates, the Greek philosopher, used this systematic questioning to come to a "truth" to engage in a thoughtful dialogue to *change* a person's viewpoint. Padesky [4] argued that it can also be helpful to use this questioning technique to *learn* about the client's view of

their presenting problems and to *explore* alternatives together to make positive changes. It has been used extensively within cognitive-behavioural therapy (CBT) as a form of "guided discovery."

There are four main stages to the process of Socratic questioning:
- *Asking informational questions*: this helps the client explore his/her difficulties and make them more concrete and understandable to both clinician and client.
- *Listening:* noticing and reflecting back on the non-verbal cues, idiosyncratic words and emotional reactions can intensify the dynamic and dialogue.
- *Summarizing what you have heard:* this can help the client feel he/she is being listened to and that his/her concerns have been understood.
- *Asking analytical and synthesizing questions:* this should be done every few minutes, after new information has been heard and explored, by applying the new information to the client's original concern. For example, *"How does all this information fit with the idea that you feel you are a failure?"* [4].

Psychological assessment

It is important to recognize that conducting an assessment can be therapeutic in itself, and can

Box 5.2 Examples of Socratic questioning

Clarification questions

- What do you think is the main issue?
- What is your experience of having psoriasis/how does it impact you day-to-day?
- What do you mean by X?
- What are you most worried about?
- What would you like to change?

Gaining assumptions

- Why do you think that?
- How did you get to that belief/what influenced your thinking?

Gaining reasons and evidence

- What led you to that belief?
- What has changed in your life since you developed these difficulties?
- What things have you stopped/started doing since you have experienced these difficulties?
- How has the problem worsened?
- What thoughts go through your mind when you are feeling like this/get into this situation?
- Have you noticed any changes in your body/what does your body feel like when you experience this problem?
- What do you do to cope in these situations?

Gaining viewpoint/different perspectives

- What would your partner/caregiver think about X?
- What is an alternative/another way to look at it?
- What are your strengths and weaknesses in dealing with the skin condition?

Gaining implications and consequences

- What effect would that have?
- How would your eczema be different if this problem went away?
- How does X affect Y?

---

improve treatment outcomes. In an ideal world, you would have an hour (or more) to conduct a psychological assessment. Given short consultation times, an initial screening assessment should assess whether a referral to psychiatry and/or psychology is warranted before conducting a "fuller" assessment. When exploring psychological distress, "normalizing" is crucial, together with explaining the link between the mind and the skin. Figure 5.2 and Box 5.3 suggest what areas should be covered in a brief psychological assessment (the inner circle) and in a further psychological assessment (outer circle).

Standardized measures

Standardized measures and subjective ratings can be used during the assessment period (for baseline scores), throughout therapy and for follow-up (e.g. every 3 months) to track the client's progress. Subjective ratings (e.g. *"rating how anxious you feel from 0–10, where 10 = 'bad'"*) can be taken at every appointment and reflected upon. Table 5.1 outlines some useful, widely-used standardized measures, including both those that are generic and specific to dermatology. Any medical professional can use the measurements suggested, without further training, as long as he/she follows the instructions for administering and grading the measurement.

Risk assessment

There is a high rate of suicidal ideation amongst those with skin conditions and a risk assessment for self-harm should always be conducted. Men are four times more likely to kill themselves, but women attempt suicide three times more often than men [5]. If a patient is a suicidal risk, it is important to take time to genuinely listen to his/her concerns. Asking about suicide will not put ideas into his/her head; the patient is likely to have been experiencing such thoughts and will feel relief from sharing them. Stay with the client and engage him/her to help you in the process of helping him/her. Know your resources and referral options and make a safety plan/contract with the client. Create hope and

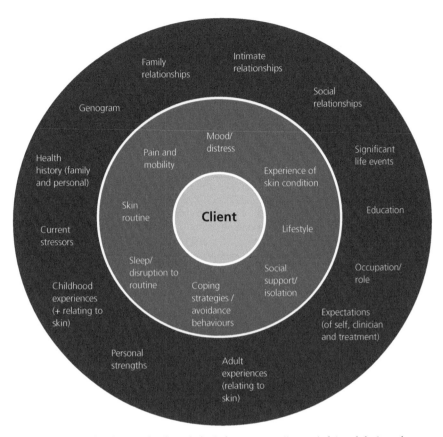

Figure 5.2 Areas to consider during a brief psychological assessment (inner circle) and during a longer psychological assessment (outer circle) for people with skin disease.

Box 5.3 Initial psychological assessment of dermatology patients

- Ask how the client experiences the skin condition (rated on a severity scale of 0–10)
- Ask how the skin condition impacts their daily life (disruption of daily routine, elicit coping strategies and avoidance behaviours)
- Ask about their lifestyle and sleep (note the impact on their life)
- If they scratch, ask when (particular times of the day/situations/when alone) and "how" (whether they use instruments)
- Ask about the details of their skin routine (i.e. the ease and difficulties)
- Ask about symptoms of pain from the condition or when applying creams (i.e. stinging)

- If/when the client uses creams, how are these used (thickly or thinly, consistently or only when dry), and what stops the client from applying cream/taking medication(s)?

Questions for further psychological assessment

- If worried about cognitive functioning, perform a Mini Mental State Examination
- If the client is over 50–55 years old, consider the possibility of dementia

Table 5.1 Examples of general standardized measures used in psychodermatology – divided into dermatology-specific, disease-specific and non–dermatology-measures

Dermatology-specific measures	Domain	Age range
Dermatology Life Quality Index (DLQI)	QoL	15 years +
Skindex-29	QoL	18 years +
Skindex-16	QoL	18 years +
Children's DLQI	QoL	4–16 years
Family DLQI	QoL of family member/client's caregiver	16 years +
EQ-5D-5L (www.euroqol.org)	Qol	18 year +
Dermatology disease-specific measures		
Skin Cancer Index	QoL of people with non-melanoma skin cancer	21 years +
Skin Cancer QoL Impact Tool (SCQOLIT)	QoL for clients with non-metastatic skin cancer	–
Psoriasis Disability Index (PDI)	QoL for people with psoriasis	16 years +
Vitiligo Specific health related QoL (VitiQoL)	QoL for people with vitiligo	18 years +
Cardiff Acne Disability Index (CADI)	QoL for teenagers with acne	Teenagers–young adults
Patient Orientated Eczema Measure (two versions, according to age)	QoL for people with eczema	Children (by parents) Adults
Dermatitis Family Impact Questionnaire (DFI)	QoL of family members/client's caregiver	16 years +
The Infant's Dermatitis Quality of Life (IDQOL)	QoL (completed by parents/caregiver)	4 years +
Non–dermatology-specific measures		
General Health Questionnaire (GHQ)	Current mental health	16 years +
Hospital Anxiety and Depression Scale (HADS)	Anxiety and depression	16 years +
Brief – Derriford Appearance Scale (DAS-24)	Appearance-related concerns	18 years +
Brief Fear of Negative Evaluation Scale (Brief–FNE)	Social anxiety	16 years +
Illness Perception Questionnaire (IPQ)	Health beliefs	18 years +
Patient Health Questionnaire (PHQ)	Depression, anxiety, somatic concerns, alcohol and eating.	18 years +
Patient Health Questionnaire 9 (PHQ-9)	Depression	18 years +
Patient Health Questionnaire 15 (PHQ-15)	Somatic concerns	18 years +
Generalized Anxiety Disorder (GAD-7)	Anxiety	18 years +
The Holmes and Rahe Stress Scale	Risk of illness due to stress	–

QoL, quality of life

work together towards something that the client is realistically able to do. Find out who else can help or who the client can contact (e.g. family members, teacher, friends, religious leader) and make sure he/she has contact details for immediate help such as a suicide help line or emergency mental health services. If you believe that a client is at immediate risk of suicide, then a psychiatry referral is warranted and detention under the Mental Health Act may need to be considered. See Chapter 6 for a more detailed discussion of suicidality.

Special situations

When treating "difficult" clients (e.g. clients with dermatitis artefacta or delusional infestation), the current dogma is not to confront them for fear of breaking the relationship. It is hypothesized that the lesions are created to satisfy an unconscious psychological need, and if this need could be met, the disease may remit. This further emphasizes the importance of developing a therapeutic relationship before exploring the client's psychological burden. Emphasizing the connection between the mind and the skin helps when discussing psychological distress related to having a skin condition and the impact it can have.

For clients who may be ambivalent about treatment, motivational interviewing is a method that can help explore and resolve ambivalence. It centres on the motivational processes in the client that facilitate change. For further information on this, see www.motivationalinterview.org.

Psychological interventions

Both psychiatry and psychology input may be required for the care of dermatology patients, and in the ideal setting of having these services embedded within dermatology, can reduce stigma and enhance treatment. Psychodermatology nurses (see Chapter 9) within this group

can offer guided self-help, which has been shown to be more effective than self-help alone for those with mild difficulties (Figure 5.3).

There is plethora of basic and complex therapies that could help people with skin conditions (for individuals, groups, couples or families), but currently there is no clear evidence base as to which is the most effective.

Basic therapies
Psychoeducation

Within clinical practice, providing psychoeducation, including explanation and leaflets, has proven to be useful in terms of increasing client's understanding and treatment adherence, and reducing anxiety. The provision of leaflets reinforces the link between the mind and the skin, increases the client's insight and normalizes the situation, reducing feelings of shame and fear.

Self-help

Self-administered treatments are simple techniques (often based on CBT) that minimize contact with a therapist and maximize self-help. Self-help (computer or literature based) can be cost and resource effective, as well as providing positive outcomes for the client when matched with appropriate levels of need. In addition, providing self-help (including a plan of when to use it) can reduce psychological distress in relation to the skin disease [6] (see Chapter 7).

Relaxation

There are numerous studies highlighting the relationship between stress and flare ups of skin conditions, such as psoriasis, eczema and acne [7]. Stress can cause exacerbation of disease and this in turn can cause more stress, leading to a vicious cycle. Relaxation can be effective in reducing arousal levels and hence feelings of anxiety and stress. There are many types of relaxation techniques, such as imagery, progressive muscle relaxation, colour breathing,

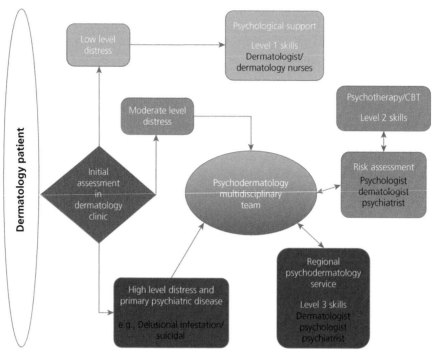

Figure 5.3 Stepped provision of psychodermatology services (BAD Working Party report, 2012; http://www .bad.org.uk/Portals/_Bad/Clinical%20Services/Psychoderm%20Working%20Party%20Doc%20Final%20 Dec%202012.pdf). NB: Level of distress ascertained using the HADS and DLQI. CBT, cognitive-behavioural therapy.

external focusing, yoga and meditation. Self-help leaflets containing basic relaxation techniques have also been found to be helpful within clinical practice. Relaxation and shifting attentional focus are techniques that have been found to be user friendly and effective. Free hand-outs can be accessed on the internet (e.g. http://www.getselfhelp.co.uk/docs/Relaxation .pdf).

Teaching clients simple breathing techniques (e.g. breathing slowly in through the nose and out through the mouth for counts of 3 and practising this every day for a few minutes before bed) is very effective and practising these during the session can help clients to understand the process. Practising a technique yourself may help you to appreciate and explain the effect. A single relaxation session with an "imagery" component can greatly reduce states of anxiety and subjective ratings of itchiness, and increase mental relaxation levels in those with eczema

[8]. Free imagery hand-outs can be accessed on the internet (e.g. http://www.getselfhelp.co.uk/ docs/ImagerySelfHelp.pdf).

Social skills training

Social skills training has been shown to be effective for those with skin disorders, helping them to deal with the reactions of others and learn about social interactions. Social skills training can also lead to a positive adjustment; social distress and anxiety are reduced by facilitating individuals to elicit more positive feedback from others in social interactions, and thus they develop a more positive sense-of-self [9]. See Chapter 12 for more details on social skills training.

More complex therapies

For more complex therapies, specific training is required and, when facilitating the therapy, supervision must be sought.

Habit reversal therapy

Habit reversal therapy (a behavioural therapy) can help to reduce the desire to scratch, which exacerbates some conditions (see Chapter 8).

Cognitive-behavioural therapy

CBT is a treatment grounded in the idea that our perception influences how we think and behave, and that psychological problems are acquired and altered through learning processes. Clients are active collaborators in their therapy and are helped to identify, challenge and modify the problematic thoughts and behaviour patterns that maintain their symptoms. CBT works on the "here and now" in reducing signs and symptoms of psychological difficulties [10]. The basic model in Figure 5.4 shows the relationship between our thoughts, physical feelings, emotions and behaviours, and how this is influenced by the environment, stressors and early experiences.

CBT must be adapted for each individual/couple and their specific problem(s). For example, social anxiety has been shown to be associated with vitiligo [6]. It is thought that avoidance is the main reason for the maintenance of these fears. People with social anxiety develop a series of assumptions about themselves and their social world, based on early experiences. Such assumptions lead the individual to appraise the situation as dangerous and to predict that they will fail to achieve their desired level of performance. They also interpret often benign or ambiguous social cues as signs of negative evaluation by others [11]. It is also important to consider the client's coping strategies, given that the way in which clients cope with their skin condition influences the way they deal with feelings of social anxiety.

During therapy the trained therapist tailors sessions and chooses techniques based on their

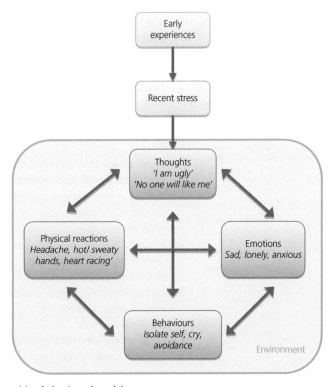

Figure 5.4 Basic cognitive-behavioural model.

ongoing conceptualization of the client and their problem(s) and in relation to their specific goals. Table 5.2 shows examples of the techniques most commonly used within CBT; the notion of homework is important between sessions.

Research, particularly in patients with psoriasis, eczema and pruritus, has shown that CBT is an effective treatment. This psychological intervention can be effective in reducing symptom severity, decreasing the reliance on medication, reducing psychological distress and increasing the ability to control and adjust to the skin condition [12].

There are particular CBT models adapted for body dysmorphic disorder [13]. The approach assumes that for those who have body image concerns, the psychological difficulties are mediated primarily by fear and avoidance, and are perpetuated by dysfunctional thoughts [13].

Introductory self-help courses on CBT are available online (e.g. http://www.getselfhelp.co.uk/docs/SelfHelpCourse.pdf). For moderate to severe patients, clinician-guided CBT is recommended.

Table 5.2 Cognitive and behavioural techniques used in cognitive-behavioural therapy

Behavioural	Cognitive
Weekly diary	Beliefs survey
Behavioural experiments	Exploring types of thinking
Safety behaviour experiments	Challenging thoughts
Distraction	Cost–benefit analysis
Relaxation/physical activity	Positive affirmations
Balance of event scheduling	Thought diary
Graded challenges	Positive thought, feeling, behaviour diary
Self-reward	

Other therapies based on clinical practice

For some clients, psychological difficulties predate the onset of the skin condition; the skin condition could be viewed as an expression of psychosocial stressors, such as trauma, abuse, retirement or bereavement. When working with these clients, concentrating on the psychological problem rather than the skin condition can help reduce the skin condition and resolve psychological distress. Various therapies have been shown to be helpful, such as CBT, systemic family therapy, acceptance and commitment therapy, schema therapy, mindfulness and narrative therapy.

Within clinical practice, use of the principles of systemic family therapy has been effective in reducing psychological distress, increasing positive relationships and reducing severity of the skin condition, particularly in those with psoriasis, skin picking and dermatitis artefacta. The key to this approach is the understanding that the problem is based in the context of family and social relationships and how reciprocal dynamics influence the problem. The problem is thus jointly constructed; it does not exist within individuals but rather is a product of interactions between people and wider systems, such as communities and cultures [14]. Empirical research is warranted to confirm the efficacy of this therapy for those with skin disorders.

How does the dermatologist access psychological therapies?

An ideal psychodermatology service would consist of a multidisciplinary team with input from a dermatologist, liaison psychiatry, psychology and nurse specialists. In reality the dermatologist will often be working alone and will need to learn local routes for referring clients for psychological help. Dermatologists should make contact with the hospital liaison psychiatry service, clinical health psychology departments or teaching programme via the hospital switchboard, and familiarize themselves with referral routes. Psychological services can be searched for by postcode via Internet resources; in the UK, refer to the Improving Access to Psychological Services (IAPT) website (www.iapt.nhs.uk), and in the US, to www.psychologytoday.com.

PRACTICAL TIPS

- Developing a therapeutic relationship is key as this is the vehicle for change.
- Using Socratic questioning is beneficial to engage the client, learn about your client and explore options together.
- Using resources such as DLQI, Skindex-16 and HADS will help to speed up consultations.
- Psychoeducation and self-help are useful basic psychological interventions.
- Understanding when, why and how to refer to a mental health specialist is vital in the management of psychodermatology patients.

References

1. Gupta MA, Gupta AK. Psychiatric and psychological co-morbidity in patients with dermatologic disorders. *Am J Clin Dermatol* 2003; 4(1): 833–842.
2. Picardi A *et al.* Prevalence and correlates of suicidal ideation among patients with skin disease. *J Am Acad Dermatol* 2006; 54: 420–426.
3. Wylie K *et al.* Psychological difficulties within a group of patients with vulvodynia. *J Psychosom Obstet Gynecol* 2004; 25: 257–265.
4. Padesky CA. *Socratic Questioning: Changing Minds or Guided Discovery?* Keynote address delivered at the European Congress of Behavioural and Cognitive Therapies, London, September 24, 1993. Available at www.padesky.com.
5. American Psychiatric Association. *Dimensions Proposed for Suicide Risk Assessment in DSM-V*, 2010. Available at www.DSM5.org. Accessed 12.01.13.
6. Shah R *et al.* Enhancing self-help for social anxiety associated with vitiligo. Oral presentation at The Division of Clinical Psychology Annual Conference, Birmingham, December 2011. *Clinical Psychology Proceedings*.
7. Al'Abadie M *et al.* The relationship between stress and the onset and exacerbation of psoriasis and other skin conditions. *Br J Dermatol* 1994; 130: 199–203.
8. Horne D *et al.* The effects of relaxation with and without imagery in reducing anxiety and itchy skin in patients with eczema. *Beh Cog Psychotherapy.* 1999; 27: 143–151.
9. Robinson E *et al.* The evaluation of the impact of social interaction skills training for facially disfigured people. *Br J Plast Surg* 1996; 49: 281–289.
10. Roth A, Fonagy P. *What Works for Whom? A Critical Review of Psychotherapy Research.* New York: Guildford Press, 1996.
11. Clarke *et al.* A cognitive model of social phobia. In Heimberg R *et al.* (eds) *Social Phobia: Diagnosis, Assessment and Treatment.* New York: Guilford Press, 1995, pp. 69–93.
12. Shenefelt P. Psychodermatological disorders: recognition and treatment. *Int J Dermatol* 2011; 50: 1309–1322.
13. Veale D. Cognitive-behavioural therapy for body dysmorphic disorder. *Ad Psych Treat.* 2001; 7: 125–132.
14. Dallos R, Stedmon J. Systemic formulation: mapping the family dance. In: Johnstone L, Dallos R (eds). *Formulation in Psychology and Psychotherapy.* Hove: Routledge, 2006.

CHAPTER 6

Risk and risk management in psychodermatology

William H. Reid[1] and Simon Kirwin[2]

[1] Texas Tech University Medical Center, Lubbock, TX, USA
[2] East London NHS Foundation Trust, London, UK

Psychiatric risk and the dermatology patient

This chapter addresses the three kinds of psychiatric or psychosocial risk that dermatology healthcare providers should be aware of, and be prepared to recognize and manage until consultation or referral can be obtained. They are *risk of suicide* or other self-injury, *risk to others* (including clinicians, staff, and family), and *risk of child or other abuse or neglect* (which may or may not involve a psychiatric condition). The chapter also refers to some co-morbid psychiatric conditions that affect either the dermatologic presentation or the patient generally.

Some settings, such as psychodermatology clinics and specialty units, are well-suited for detailed psychiatric evaluations and some clinical interventions. For most others, the goal is recognition of potentially dangerous or complicating conditions, better understanding of their effects on the dermatologic tasks at hand, and appropriate interim management when indicated. We do not expect general dermatologists to perform detailed mental assessments of all their patients, nor do we advocate comprehensive risk management in the usual dermatology clinic.

The principles of clinical risk, risk management, and protecting patients are universal, but the laws relating to them vary by location.

Matters such as clinician liability (e.g. malpractice liability) are treated quite differently in different countries. This chapter discusses universal clinical and safety principles using examples from the US and UK. It does not purport to cover the laws and cultures of all countries, nor should it be considered any form of legal advice.

Suicide, suicidal thoughts, and suicide risk

Suicide, although an uncommon cause of death in the general population (8–12 people/100 000/year in the UK and US) [1], is an important consideration in dermatology for at least two reasons. First, patients seen in dermatology clinics sometimes have significant suicide risk factors. Second, suicide is very often preventable given adequate risk recognition and psychiatric care. In general, patients with chronic medical illness are at statistically increased suicide risk [2]. That risk may become a practical concern with increasing symptoms, patient frustration, physical stigmata, debilitation, and/or psychiatric vulnerability.

Dermatologic conditions rarely "cause" marked increases in suicide risk. It is much more likely that an emotionally vulnerable patient who presents with a skin issue, whether

Practical Psychodermatology, First Edition. Anthony Bewley, Ruth E. Taylor, Jason S. Reichenberg and Michelle Magid.
© 2014 John Wiley & Sons, Ltd. Published 2014 by John Wiley & Sons, Ltd.

associated with the psychiatric disorder or independent of it, already has risk that can be made worse by the addition of a severe (or perceived severe) dermatologic problem such as disfiguring psoriasis.

Suicide risk assessment and recognition

Comprehensive risk assessment is beyond the scope of most dermatologists' practices, but there are several principles for discriminating and prioritizing important risk factors. Understanding them should substantially decrease the likelihood of patient suicide.

Most suicides occur in the context of a psychiatric disorder, usually depression, severe anxiety, psychosis, substance misuse, or some combination of these. Thus, *screening for psychiatric disorders and significant symptoms*, such as during initial patient evaluation or review of symptoms, *is highly recommended*.

- *Assess the emotional impact of the patient's dermatologic condition.* Asking frankly about the psychological and psychosocial effects of, for example, a patient's severe acne is important. Try to recognize odd or exaggerated emotional affects, moods, or reactions (such as expression of fears, hopelessness, or other concerns that seem out of context for the patient's situation), then follow-up with direct questions about what they mean to that patient.
- *Be direct when asking about suicide and other psychiatric issues*, while trying not to put patients off with excessive bluntness. Contrary to some lay anecdotes, there is very little risk that concerned inquiry will make things worse, and far more risk that insufficient inquiry will miss something important.
- *Do not believe reassurances from patients with substantial risk factors.* Patients very often lie about suicidal thoughts and impulses, and doctors are very poor at determining when patients are telling the truth. Get as much corroborating information as possible from others and available medical records.

- *Major risk factors are rarely counter-balanced by the presence of so-called "protective factors"* (contrary to what is stated in some risk assessment protocols). Most people with substantial suicide risk are driven by factors that overwhelm their insight, logic, and judgment, causing a sort of "tunnel vision" toward death in which "positive factors" such as family, religion, or good clinical prognosis become irrelevant to their immediate risk.
- *It is important that practitioners understand the concept of "suicide attempt."* For our purposes, any intentional behavior that harmed, or could have harmed, the patient should be considered an "attempt." *Do not try to differentiate suicidal "gestures" from "attempts."* Non-lethal attempts, "rehearsals," and "para-suicidal" behavior (such as loading and unloading a gun, making nooses in ropes, or cutting or burning the skin) are common predecessors of suicide.

Important additional risk factors for suicide are summarized in Box 6.1.

Generally speaking, the more recent the worrisome behavior, the more seriously it should be taken. Attempts within the past several days or weeks virtually always necessitate immediate psychiatric consultation or referral (and protecting the patient until the referral is completed).

Some other factors listed in many risk assessment protocols (such as age or marital status) are not very predictive in practice, and actually muddy the waters of accurate risk assessment (e.g. by creating a false sense of confidence when a patient is not in a target age or gender group). When deciding whether or not a patient's risk level warrants further steps, the major factors discussed in Box 6.1 deserve top priority.

Specific dermatologic risk issues

Many dermatologic disorders can increase suicide risk in psychiatrically vulnerable patients, and some (such as intractable pruritus) can be sufficiently intolerable to lead to suicidal thoughts in otherwise emotionally healthy

Box 6.1 Risk factors for suicide

- Prior suicide *attempts* (see text)
- Suicide *plans*
- Thinking seriously or obsessively of suicide (take increased fleeting thoughts seriously, but they are common and do not always substantially increase risk)
- *Acute depression or anxiety*
- *Psychiatric instability* (including unstable mood and waxing and waning of suicidal thoughts)
- *Psychosis*, particularly in a context of perceived persecution, disfigurement, danger, or significant loss
- *Hopelessness* (whether associated with mental illness, physical issues such as terminal illness or severe disfigurement, or other life conditions)
- *Substance misuse* (including intoxication, addiction, misuse of prescription drugs, and some forms of substance withdrawal)
- *Isolation* (either living alone or recently isolating oneself)
- Substantial *loss* (including loss of an important relationship or job, amputation, recent arrest or conviction, significant financial loss, disfigurement, and significant humiliation). Suicide risk is more affected by recent *change* in social or relational condition than by chronic situations, but both are important
- *Impaired insight, judgment, or self-control* in the context of any of the above

persons. Their specific links to suicidality have not been well studied.

It goes without saying that potentially terminal dermatologic disorders, and serious systemic diseases with dermatologic presentations, are associated with significant psychological distress. Patients facing death from malignant melanoma, for example, and particularly those who *believe* their condition will lead to death or prolonged suffering, may be at substantial risk of suicide. Screening for risk using the above factors, clear and realistic discussion of prognosis and treatment options, and liberal consideration of psychiatric referral are all important.

Many patients with seemingly ominous diagnoses do not realize that medical progress

has improved their prognoses. Others overestimate the seriousness of diagnoses like squamous or basal cell carcinoma (which imply the frightening word "cancer"). Patients who are not adequately informed often suffer unnecessary dismay, and a few become suicidal (see Chapter 24).

Disfigurement from skin disease can cause measurable decrease in self-esteem in even psychiatrically healthy patients. Those with co-morbid psychiatric illness (Chapter 13), especially depression, severe anxiety, psychosis, and disorders of body image, should receive extra attention.

The face is particularly important to body image (Chapter 12). Most practitioners know that severe acne can precipitate or worsen depression, particularly in adolescents. It has been estimated that 15% of psoriasis patients seen by dermatologists have had suicidal thoughts associated with poor self-esteem and disturbance of body image [3]. Those with atopic eczema have similar levels of psychological distress.

Severe acne and similarly disfiguring conditions may be a factor in humiliation (by others or as a result of an internal feeling) or bullying (including so-called "cyberbullying"), especially among adolescents. Bullying is probably rare as a cause of suicide in such patients, but those with pre-existing emotional vulnerability deserve additional assessment, support, and sometimes psychiatric referral.

Significant alopecia (see Chapter 10) is often associated with depression and concern about self-image. Women and psychiatrically vulnerable patients may suffer more serious emotional symptoms, including hopelessness to the point of suicidal thoughts.

Psychiatric disorders that may first present as dermatologic complaints

Dermatologists and primary care physicians may be the first clinicians to see patients with body dysmorphic disorder (see Chapter 15), an often serious psychiatric condition in which the patient has an obsessive, intractable perception of a significant physical defect or flaw where none exists (or there is marked exaggeration of a minor flaw). Depression and anxiety are common in such patients; thoughts of suicide are often entertained when the exaggeration is substantial; and at least one paper suggests a suicide rate higher than that associated with clinical depression [4].

A complete discussion of all the psychiatric disorders that may simply exist in patients who seek dermatologic care is beyond the scope of this chapter. The dermatologist, like all clinicians, should be alert for untreated or inadequately treated psychiatric disorders, aware of potential interactions between dermatologic and psychiatric diagnoses and treatments, and generally cautious about altering a patient's psychiatric treatments without discussing the matter with the clinician who prescribed them.

For dermatologists who frequently see patients with psychiatric co-morbidities, a change in office layout may reduce agitation and improve staff safety (Box 6.2).

Non-suicidal harm in dermatologic presentations

Many patients with delusional infestation (see Chapter 14) have attempted to treat or clean themselves in harmful ways (e.g. using gasoline, electricity, burning, or gouging). Some of these methods, like some forms of suicide attempt, are dangerous to others as well (e.g. fire danger from using gasoline).

Patients with factitious skin disorder (see Chapter 17) may seriously injure themselves when trying to create believable lesions. Children and disabled proxies are particularly at risk, since they are not in control of the perpetrator's damaging behavior and usually cannot complain or provide adequate history (see Abuse and neglect section).

Risk management

The primary principle of risk management, whether for suicide risk or some other kind, is *protect the patient*. For the situations anticipated

in this chapter, this implies reducing the risk as promptly as is feasible, and seeking specialized help.

The first step in reducing severe suicide risk is often some form of *containment and monitoring*. This usually means asking the patient to remain in the office or clinic, *with an appropriate chaperone*, until psychiatric consultation or other appropriate help arrives. Clinicians are not policemen, but every reasonable, non-physical, attempt should be made to keep the patient safe and prevent him/her from leaving. At-risk patients sometimes demand to leave, and occasionally become quite agitated; do *not* attempt to restrain the patient physically unless he/she or others are in immediate danger (in which case moving out of the way is often a safer alternative than approaching the patient). Do not place yourself, staff, or others in unnecessary danger.

Do not overestimate your ability to predict or control physical agitation or violence. Most staff injuries at the hands of patients occur in a context of unpredictability and surprise. With the exception of an acute emergency, leave techniques such as "talking the patient down" to trained personnel.

Avoid attempts to restrain the patient. Dermatology and primary care staff are rarely trained in safe patient restraint. In addition, local laws may have strict guidelines regarding restraining and detaining patients against their will (e.g. Box 6.3). If the patient leaves, try to observe his/her direction but do not attempt to apprehend him/her; that is a job for emergency responders.

- *Seek help.* Most of the time this means obtaining an emergency psychiatric consultation, often in an emergency department or psychiatric hospital. If a patient refuses emergency psychiatric evaluation (e.g. the patient walks out of the clinic before you are able to stop them), strongly consider calling the police or a close relative.
- *Do not rely on the patient's family to do the job of a clinician or hospital.* Spouses and others cannot be expected to watch the patient around the clock, or to make good decisions

Box 6.2 Minimizing risk in outpatient clinics (see Chapter 2)

Layout

- Minimize corners in corridors so that reception can easily observe the waiting area
- Quiet, calm atmosphere
- Consultation and counseling rooms in quiet areas, conducive to psychological work-up
- If running a joint clinic, space to accommodate two clinicians, the patient and his/her caregiver
- Doors in clinical rooms, lockable from outside, but not inside, or easily unlocked from outside, to prevent a patient from locking himself/ herself in
- Shatter-proof windows. If on a high floor, windows that are not easily opened
- Clinic room free of breakable furniture or sharp objects
- Safe routes of entry and exit (ideally two separate exits) from clinic room should patient become violent or aggressive
- If one exit, layout situated in such a way that the physician is always closest to the door (e.g. exam bed positioned on the wall furthest from the door)
- Panic alarm system – either on person or in room. Make sure all staff know how to use/ respond

Clinical

- Reception staff training to enable understanding of patients' needs
- Do not assess on own if patient risk is high
- Consider chaperone use when assessing a patient of the opposite gender. Every patient has a right to a chaperone
- Staff (nurses or reception) should be discouraged from entering the room during a consultation.

Box 6.3 Mental Health Act (MHA) 1983 (amended 2007), England & Wales [8]

A section under the UK's MHA requires three people to agree that the person must be detained: Two doctors, one of whom must be registered under Section 12 of the MHA, and an Approved Mental Health Professional (AMHP). The two doctors must first agree. The AMHP then decides whether to make the application for compulsory admission. The exception is S4, which is an emergency section for use in a crisis, and is allowed if the criteria for S2 have been met, but there is no time to wait for a second recommendation (which must then be gained within 72 hours). The AMHP will consult or inform the nearest relative (NR) about the person's detention. The NR cannot stop S2, but can stop S3, and can also apply for his/her relative's discharge from detention. In some circumstances the powers of the NR can be displaced.

If police think a person needs immediate care, S136 allows them to take someone from a public place to a place of safety. S136 lasts for 72 hours, during which time the person must be assessed as above, for S2, S3, or discharged.

S2 can last for up to 28 days; S3 can last for up to 6 months and can be renewed. S4 and S136 last for up to 72 hours, during which time arrangements must be made to assess for S2 or S3.

Detained patients are able to appeal their section, and their appeal will go to tribunal.

Criteria for S2

- The person is suffering from a mental disorder of a nature or degree that warrants his/her detention in hospital for assessment (or for assessment followed by treatment) for at least a limited period, and
- Detention is necessary in the interest of the person's own health, safety, or protection of others.

Criteria for S3

- The person is suffering from a mental disorder of a nature or degree that makes it appropriate for him/her to receive medical treatment in hospital, and
- Necessary that he/she is treated for the health and safety or for protection of others, and
- Appropriate medical treatment is available.

about whether, for example, the patient can safely go to the bathroom alone. They cannot be expected to remove all potential implements of suicide from the environment.

- *Never rely on a "contract for safety."* Having a patient "promise" or "contract" not to commit suicide does *not* measurably decrease suicide risk. This technique was popular a couple of decades ago, but it is now very clear that so-called no-suicide "contracts" must not be relied upon. ("Safety contracts" are not the same as careful "risk management plans" in which potentially suicidal patients and mental health treatment staff collaborate in the patient's psychiatric care.)
- *Err on the side of safety.* When in doubt, protect the patient and seek competent help.
- *Once you have made a protection decision, stick to it.* A patient who does not want to go to an emergency room or wait in the office for a psychiatric consultation frequently tries to talk the doctor into changing his/her mind. Sometimes he/she brings new "facts" into the conversation, or makes promises to go to the emergency room on his/her own. Remember the first principle: *protect the patient.*

Risk management principles are summarized in Box 6.4.

Risk to others

We will briefly address three kinds of risk to other persons: danger from direct, intentional violence; danger from undirected patient vio-

Box 6.4 Risk management principles

- Protect the patient
- Seek specialized help
- Do not expect a patient's family to be a substitute for hospital monitoring and care
- Never rely on patient promises or "safety contracts"
- Err on the side of safety
- Once you have made a safety decision, stick to it

lence; and danger from accidental patient behavior. Dermatologic presentations of patient abuse and neglect are addressed in the next section.

Direct, intentional violence

The incidence of intentional violence toward dermatologists and office staff, like that for most other specialties, is very low. From time to time reports are heard of people with delusional disorders, such as delusional infestation, whose delusional systems expand to include their physicians, occasionally with dangerous behavior [5].

Most assaults by patients come without warning; many are simply the result of being in the wrong place at the wrong time. Sometimes clinicians', including dermatologists', actions are misperceived as threatening to mentally ill patients and they react violently out of fear or anger. Sensitivity to patients who behave oddly, and particularly to those who appear frightened or suspicious, should make you cautious about seeing them alone, and encourage a measured, deliberate technique, explaining your actions and avoiding surprising the patient.

When threatened or faced with an assaultive patient, the first principle is safety for yourself and your staff. Get people out of danger. Do not attempt to de-escalate the situation or physically engage the patient unless there is no alternative (see the similar, more detailed discussion in the Suicide risk section).

It is important to try to protect others whom you believe are in danger (e.g. if you become aware of threats or instability that may cause injury to others). In the context of this chapter, that usually means notifying facility security or the police, calling a facility risk manager, discussing safety with treatment staff, or letting a patient's family know that you are concerned, depending on the situation. Do not be shy about good-faith notification regarding danger. *Confidentiality is not an issue when safety is a genuine concern.*

Undirected or collateral danger, including danger from accidents

Although not highly relevant to dermatology, clinicians in many countries have some obligation to mitigate danger from patients whose conditions (or treatment effects) make them unsafe. Patients are cautioned about medications that affect their ability to drive; seizure patients are reported to driver licensing agencies; and warnings or even quarantine are required for certain communicable diseases.

Part of the importance of recognizing suicide risk and getting help is that the patient is not always the only person at risk. Those who attempt suicide with firearms often injure or kill others, as do those who try to kill themselves in automobile accidents or fires. Self-inflicted carbon monoxide poisoning can kill unintended victims (e.g. when fumes from an automobile running in a closed garage seep into a room where others are sleeping).

Even if others are not physically injured, the emotional damage to family members (and sometimes others) from suicide by a spouse, parent, or offspring cannot be overstated. Those left behind feel loss, guilt, blame, and often the expectation that "it will happen to me, too" for years and decades into the future.

Abuse and neglect of children and other vulnerable people

Child abuse is a well-known social and clinical pandemic. Abuse of the elderly and disabled is perhaps just as common, particularly if malevolent neglect in homes and in institutions is included.

There are a number of dermatologic presentations of abuse and neglect (Figure 6.1, Figure 6.2a,b, Figure 6.3, and Figure 6.4) . If dermatologists recognize abuse or neglect, they are usually in a position to stop it.

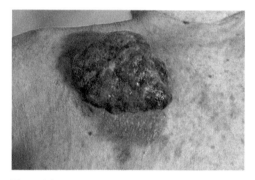

Figure 6.1 A patient with a neglected malignant melanoma. This patient was elderly and socially isolated. He presented with very late malignant disease when the skin cancer became extremely malodorous (courtesy of Dr A. Bewley).

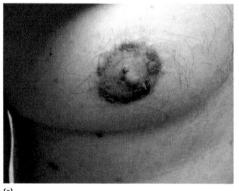

(a)

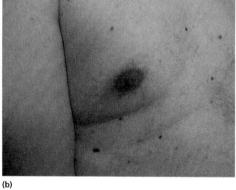

(b)

Figure 6.2 (a) Terra firma forme (a form of dermatitis neglecta) in an isolated older man who showered infrequently and who did not have an adequate caretaker. (b) The crust was removed with vigorous scrubbing with an alcohol swab (courtesy of Dr J. Reichenberg).

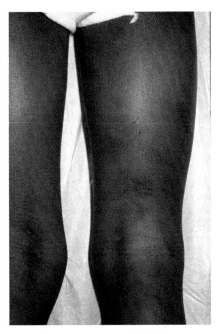

Figure 6.3 Young child with geometric brown patches and crusted erosions on posterior thighs from a belt injury (courtesy of Dr Moise Levy).

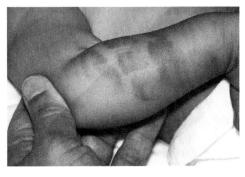

Figure 6.4 Bruising on the forearm of a toddler from forceful gripping (courtesy of Dr Moise Levy).

Some dermatologic conditions are difficult for others to tolerate, sometimes, in part, because of the emotional reactions they elicit (e.g. guilt, anxiety, repulsion, disappointment). The combination of such "imperfection" and/or need for care with immature, unstable, psychotic, antisocial, or sadistic caregivers can be very dangerous.

Risk recognition and index of suspicion

Being sensitive to the possibility of abuse or neglect, and a constant level of suspicion, are necessary components of any clinical practice.

It is logical to think about abuse or neglect when evaluating such things as stasis ulcers, rashes, and skin sensitivities, especially if they recur repeatedly or fail to heal as expected. Avoid unfair criticism and realize that poor caregiving is sometimes a result of lack of education, training or experience, but be vigilant and place the patient's safety first. Do not hesitate to report good-faith suspicions to appropriate investigators.

Do *not* attempt to investigate possible neglect or abuse by yourself. Recognition and reporting of suspicious lesions or symptoms is a crucial role for clinicians, but social service authorities in most western countries prefer to carry out their own abuse/neglect assessment protocols using trained investigators. Failure to report suspected abuse or neglect is a crime in many states and countries.

Perpetrators often try to control the information the clinician receives. Information from collateral sources is important, but try to spend some time talking privately with the patient. Be suspicious if a relative or caregiver refuses to leave the room. (A chaperone from your own staff is often a good idea.) Review records from the patient's nursing home, clinicians, hospital, and even school nurses as feasible and appropriate.

Sometimes a non-abusing person brings the patient to the clinician's attention, and sometimes the perpetrator presents him/herself when symptoms become too severe to ignore (such as when others notice them). A perpetrator may also injure patients as part of (proxy) factitious behavior, psychosis, or malingering.

In factitious disorder (Munchausen's) "by proxy," the perpetrator intentionally creates signs and/or symptoms in the vulnerable person and disguises the real etiology, all for psychological reasons rather than obvious personal gain. Although stemming from a genuine psychiatric disorder, factitious behavior by proxy does not absolve the perpetrator of responsibility, and is abuse.

In so-called "malingering by proxy," an unscrupulous person intentionally creates symptoms in someone else in order to gain money or something else of value. The behavior may be murderous (as when slowly poisoning someone to gain an inheritance) or non–life-threatening (as when creating a fake chronic condition to obtain disability income for the family or, in a few cultures, mutilating a child so that he/she is a more effective beggar).

The issue for the dermatologist or other clinician must be the safety and protection of the vulnerable person, regardless of intent; suspected abuse or neglect should be reported at once.

Situations in which a parent or other caregiver refuses treatment for a child or other vulnerable person should be carefully examined for signs of abuse or neglect, and often referred to an appropriate agency for investigation. Competent adults can refuse most kinds of medical care for themselves, but most countries, including the US, Canada, and UK, do not allow them to refuse needed care for their children or incompetent wards (Box 6.5).

A clinician's decision about "needed" care is not always as straightforward as in the case presentation in Box 6.5. Does a mother's refusal to give her son dermatologist-prescribed antibiotics for severe acne constitute neglect? Are the current and future consequences of facial disfigurement, assuming a very favorable benefit-to-risk ratio for the treatment, a matter for parental choice? Is the child being damaged by the parent's seemingly irrational refusal?

Although the doctor is not usually the person who makes final decisions about abuse/neglect, he/she should be prepared to:
• recognize signs of abuse or neglect;
• provide immediate protection when necessary and appropriate (including hospitalization at times);

Box 6.5 Case presentation

Malignant melanoma was diagnosed in a 12-year-old child. Several weeks after the initial wide excision, new melanotic cells were found at the borders of the excision site. Additional, more aggressive surgery was strongly recommended by both her oncologist and her dermatologist, but the parents refused, saying that their religion had preached against the first surgery and the recurrence was a punishment for their lack of faith. The matter was referred to a court, alleging, in part, parental neglect. An attorney was appointed specifically to oversee the rights of the child.

The risks and benefits of the surgery were reviewed in detail by an independent medical expert. The court noted the child's own wish not to have the surgery, but chose not to view her as a competent, refusing adult. The court also noted that although the proposed surgery would be somewhat disfiguring, the potential benefits far outweighed the risks, and cosmetic measures could minimize the scarring. The court found that, given no substantial risk of a severely adverse outcome, the parents did not have a right to keep their daughter from a potentially life-saving treatment.

• report findings and suspicions;
• advocate for the victim during investigations, court hearings, and the like.

Many of the principles for dealing with suspected abused or neglected patients are similar to those for acutely suicidal patients, including protecting the patient, seeking consultation, erring on the side of patient safety, and being resolute once a safety decision has been made.

Dermatologists and psychiatric risk assessment

In spite of the common association between some skin disease and psychiatric illness, many dermatologists are uncomfortable diagnosing and treating psychodermatologic conditions. Although physicians of all kinds are expected to have some acquaintance with the interface between psychiatry and their practices, and although the UK Department of Health expects all clinical staff to be able to assess and manage self-harm (and has issued guidelines on risk assessment and management) [6,7], *we do not recommend that dermatologists undertake secondary roles as psychiatric clinicians, primary assessors of suicide risk, violence risk evaluators, or abuse and neglect investigators.*

The dermatologist's roles, given his/her lack of comprehensive psychiatric training and experience, are awareness, relevant screening, and recognition of signs and symptoms that indicate

that complications may arise when dermatology patients have co-morbid psychiatric disorders/ symptoms (and *vice versa*). Further, we must advise clinicians (in the UK and US at least) that non-psychiatrists who choose to manage or treat psychiatric conditions are expected to meet the standard of care for psychiatrists (e.g. for purposes of avoiding malpractice liability), not some imaginary lesser standard for "dermatologists practicing psychiatry." The clinician's choices are to reasonably recognize the need to call for consultative or referral help, or to continue care and meet the psychiatric standard of care.

PRACTICAL TIPS

- The dermatologist's role is awareness, relevant screening, and recognition of signs and symptoms that indicate a need for psychiatric consultation or referral.
- If a patient is at high risk for suicide, seek immediate help from emergency psychiatric services.
- The primary principle of risk management, whether for suicide risk or some other kind, is *protect the patient*.
- Confidentiality is not an issue when safety is a genuine concern.
- The dermatologist should be familiar with signs of child or vulnerable adult abuse or neglect. Suspected abuse or neglect should be reported to the appropriate authorities.

References

1. Royal College of Psychiatrists. Self-harm, suicide, and risk: helping people who self-harm. RCP Report CR158, 2010. Available at www.rcpsych .ac.uk/files/pdfversion/cr158.pdf. Accessed 13.8 .2013.
2. Gupta MA, Gupta AK. A practical approach to the assessment of psychosocial and psychiatric comorbidity in the dermatology patient. *Clin Dermatol* 2013; 31(1): 57–61.
3. Gupta MA *et al.* Suicidal ideation in psoriasis. *Int J Dermatol* 1993;32(3): 188–190.
4. Phillips KA (2007). Suicidality in body dysmorphic disorder. *Primary Psychiatry* 2007; 14(12): 58–66.
5. Bourgeois ML *et al.* Delusional parasitosis: folie à deux and attempted murder of a family doctor. *Br J Psychiatry* 1992; 161: 709–711.
6. NICE Clinical Guidelines for Self Harm (the short-term physical and psychological management). 2004. Available at http://www.nice.org.uk/CG16.
7. NICE Clinical Guidelines for Self-harm (longer term management). 2011. Available at http:// www.nice.org.uk/CG133.
8. Department of Health. *Code of Practice Mental Health Act 1983*: 24. London: The Stationery Office, 2008.

CHAPTER 7

Self-help for management of psychological distress associated with skin conditions

Andrew R. Thompson

Department of Psychology, University of Sheffield, Sheffield, UK

It is widely acknowledged that skin conditions can cause distress associated with living with a condition that may be unpredictable in its course, causes pain or irritation and/or is simply noticeable to others. Visibility is the only objective variable that has been persistently identified as being predictive of psychological distress. Certainly, managing the reactions of other people can be burdensome and cause distress in its own right. People with a range of conditions have reported being subjected to discrimination and the risk of stigmatization may be particularly high for those whose condition is highly visible and/or misunderstood [1].

Conservative estimates suggest that around a third of those attending dermatology clinics experience significant psychological co-morbidity [2]. Anxiety tends to be the predominant presenting problem and avoidant coping styles are frequently seen to negatively affect quality of life. While people living with a skin condition may well have to manage the reactions of others, increasing evidence suggests that the psychological impact is more significantly influenced by individual psychological factors, such as the degree of fear of negative evaluation, and these factors are amenable to psychological intervention.

This chapter is concerned with introducing one type of psychological intervention, self-help, which is a highly cost-efficient approach that also has the potential to increase patient self-efficacy.

It should be noted that self-help is not suitable for the treatment of all forms of psychological disturbance that might be associated with the skin. For example, people with a severe primary psychological condition (such as body dysmorphic disorder, dermatitis artefacta or delusional disorder) or with severe secondary psychological distress (such as severe depression) usually require "higher intensity" psychiatric or psychological intervention and would be unlikely to benefit from stand-alone self-help.

What is self-help?

Self-help covers a variety of interventions ranging from stand-alone psychoeducational information and guidance on the use of specific coping techniques (this might be thought of as "pure self-help"), to guided support using similar materials. Self-help is increasingly being built into wider mental healthcare delivery care pathways and provided via a range of media including:

- internet;
- bibliotherapy;

Practical Psychodermatology, First Edition. Anthony Bewley, Ruth E. Taylor, Jason S. Reichenberg and Michelle Magid.

- leaflets;
- apps.

There is some evidence that the use of multimedia forms of self-help is linked to effects in establishing behavioural change, but this has not been examined in the dermatology field [3].

Surprisingly, few mental health studies have critically reviewed the efficacy of self-help and little is known about using self-help specifically for intervening with psychological distress associated with skin conditions. Reviews of self-help for treating anxiety in the general population typically show that such interventions, compared to controlled conditions, are effective, with a medium to large effect size that is maintained at follow-up [3]. Self-help in the wider anxiety literature has typically included the following techniques:

- psychoeducation as to what maintains anxiety;
- relaxation;
- exposure (to feared stimuli or situations);
- self-monitoring (via, for example, diary keeping);
- guidance on recognizing and restructuring unhelpful thoughts;
- reintroducing activity or behavioural activation.

Box 7.1 directs the reader to some general self-help resources for further reading.

The majority of existing psychological interventions targeting skin conditions have used collections of techniques rather than evaluated formal psychotherapy interventions, and there are a handful of trials of specifically developed self-help interventions in this context. Lavda *et al.* [4] conducted a meta-analysis of trials of psychological interventions that have targeted skin conditions and, promisingly, found that existing interventions have a medium effect size on psychosocial outcomes. They identified seven types of psychological interventions as having been used to treat skin conditions: habit reversal, interventions informed by cognitive-behavioural therapy (CBT), relaxation, group therapy, psychoanalytical or psychodynamic

Box 7.1 Self-help materials and resources for further independent learning

- An excellent collection of self-help leaflets for free download written by NHS staff in Northumberland: http://www.ntw.nhs.uk/pic/selfhelp
- Free downloads of CBT self-help resources from a well-respected independent site: http://www.getselfhelp.co.uk/freedownloads.htm
- Information about self-help from NHS Choices: http://www.nhs.uk/Conditions/stress-anxiety-depression/Pages/self-help-therapies.aspx
- Mood Gym is a free self-help computer programme to teach CBT skills to anyone vulnerable to depression and anxiety: https://moodgym.anu.edu.au/welcome
- The overcoming series of CBT self-help books is used within healthcare book prescription services: http://www.overcoming.co.uk/single.htm?ipg=4795
- Atopic Skin Disease, the online community for practitioners and patients, contains useful information, particularly on habit reversal: http://www.atopicskindisease.com/categories/about-us

The evidence suggests that many of these resources work better if an individual is supported and monitored by a healthcare professional.

approaches, emotional disclosure (therapeutic writing) and combined interventions (i.e. those including a mixture of the other techniques). Relaxation techniques were one of the most commonly tested interventions and formed the basis of five studies that were found to have a medium effect size [4]. Relaxation seems to be one particular form of self-help technique that can be easy to use and learn, and so further details of this technique are described below.

Relaxation techniques include progressive muscle relaxation, mindfulness meditation and guided imagery (scripts and MP3 downloads for relaxation can be found on some of the websites listed in Box 7.1). Self-help containing mindfulness-based meditation has been examined in at least three studies in people living with psoriasis, with positive findings in terms of accelerated rate of skin clearing [5] and improvements in levels of anxiety [6]. However, the findings remain equivocal, with the first study not finding any statistically significant improvement in anxiety and the second having significant methodological problems, most notably lack of power. Recently, a randomized controlled feasibility trial was conducted that involved 130 participants with psoriasis. Participants were allocated to either compassion-based self-help or mindfulness-based self-help over a 4-week period. Both interventions were found to be acceptable, with over 70% of study completers reporting finding the materials helpful. Both interventions also showed modest yet statistically significant reductions in shame and improvements in quality of life [7]. These findings need to be replicated, but suggest that people distressed by their psoriasis might benefit from engaging in self-help that facilitates relaxation and targets self-criticism.

Stepped care

In the UK, the National Institute for Health and Care Excellence guidelines [8] for treating "common mental health disorders", such as anxiety and depression, advocate the delivery of self-help within a stepped-care model of service provision. Essentially, a stepped-care model seeks to ensure that patients have access to the most easily available, least costly, least restrictive and most effective form of intervention relevant to their specific level of need. For example, a first step might be providing a mildly distressed patient with advice and monitoring, with the patient then being "stepped up" to more intensive forms of intervention when and if required. Thompson [9] reviewed the psychosocial impact associated with skin conditions and provided an outline of a stepped-care model of psychosocial interventions (Figure 7.1). More recently, this model of care has been advocated

by a British Association of Dermatologists (BAD) psychodermatology working party [10].

While patient perception of stepped care and self-help has generally been reported to be positive, there are some studies suggesting patients mistrust such approaches [3]. Implementing stepped care into psychodermatology services will need careful planning and a clear evaluation strategy.

The number of steps required in a pathway has been debated; however, four steps appear sufficient in mental healthcare provision [3]. The first step, for those experiencing mild psychological distress, typically includes directing patients to the appropriate educational resources and active monitoring; the second includes guided self-help and psychoeducational groups, which may address stress management, relaxation and habit reversal training; the third includes psychotropic medication and practitioner-guided psychodynamic therapy or CBT; and the fourth, reserved for severely distressed patients, involves a tertiary level of care (i.e. hospitalization) and a multidiscilplinary approach from dermatologists, psychiatrists and psychologists. The model shown in Figure 7.1 is deliberately confined to the three steps that could be contained within dermatology services, with a fourth step probably best involving referral to highly specialist mental health services.

Implications of stepped care and self-help for assessment

This author has previously suggested:

> "that there is a thin line separating assessment from intervention and that an empathetic and sensitive dermatology assessment can provide patients with an important opportunity for emotional disclosure, normalisation of symptoms and provision of self-help information." [9, p.46].

Conducting a detailed mental health assessment is a clinical skill gained through specific postgraduate training; however, all healthcare practitioners can, with support and limited

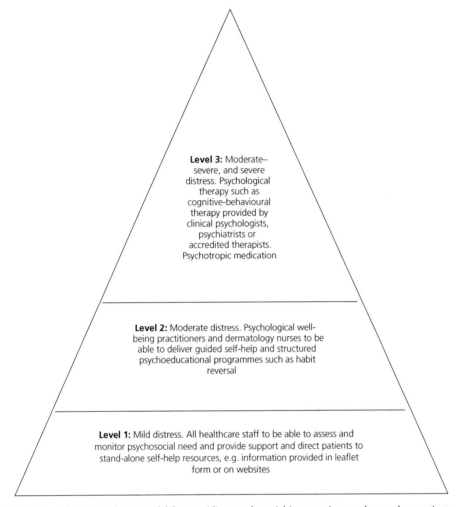

Level 3: Moderate–severe, and severe distress. Psychological therapy such as cognitive-behavioural therapy provided by clinical psychologists, psychiatrists or accredited therapists. Psychotropic medication

Level 2: Moderate distress. Psychological well-being practitioners and dermatology nurses to be able to deliver guided self-help and structured psychoeducational programmes such as habit reversal

Level 1: Mild distress. All healthcare staff to be able to assess and monitor psychosocial need and provide support and direct patients to stand-alone self-help resources, e.g. information provided in leaflet form or on websites

Figure 7.1 Simplified stepped care model for providing psychosocial interventions to dermatology patients (source: Thompson, 2009).

further training, ask questions to cover all of the domains shown in Box 7.2. Further training should also be available to enable core clinic staff to be able to conduct a suicide risk assessment where this is indicated. Box 7.2 is not an exhaustive list of assessment areas, but provides a useful starting point to taking a wider approach to dermatology assessment.

As well as examining people's concerns in the areas outlined in Box 7.2, consideration should also be given to measuring some of these concerns using simple subjective ratings of

distress (1–7 scales). Such scales can be made up on the spot and thus be tailored to the specific presenting problems. In addition, as there is consistent evidence that the clinically rated severity of the condition does not correlate well with levels of psychological distress, it is important to ask the patient about perceived severity rather than to rely solely on objective measures. Exploring patients' *expectations* of their physical treatments (topicals, phototherapy, etc.) may also provide important information in relation to the presence of psychological vulnerability

Box 7.2 General areas to explore during assessment of psychosocial distress in dermatology patients

Emotion

The central question here is *"How are you feeling?"* Ask specific questions around the following areas:

- Nervousness
- Low mood (and suicidal ideation)
- Embarrassment and shame
- Anger

Behaviour and coping strategies

The central question here is *"How does the condition affect your behaviour and how do you cope?"* Ask specific questions around the following areas:

- Avoidance
- Over use of concealment
- Irritability
- Scratching
- Substance use

Cognitive factors (thinking styles and content)

The central question here is *"What thoughts do you have about your skin condition, and how do these affect your view of yourself and what you think other people will think?"* Ask specific questions around the following areas:

- Worries
- Self-esteem
- Self-critical tendencies
- Unhelpful expectations as to what others will think, perceptions of coping

Social and relational impact

The central question here is *"What effect is your skin condition having on your life and relationships?"* Ask specific questions around the following areas:

- Current stresses
- Perception of support
- Incidents of specific discrimination
- Intimacy and sexual functioning

Perceptions of the condition and of treatment

The central question here is *"How do you feel your treatment is going?"* Ask specific questions around the following areas:

- Perception of change
- Perception of severity of the condition
- Perception of side effects
- Feedback on care

(e.g. when treatment is *perceived* to be unsuccessful).

One model of stepped care is to assess people and step them up if necessary to more intensive forms of psychological intervention. This requires a measure or measures of severity; psychometric tools may be useful for this, as well as providing a measure to evaluate practice and outcomes. The British Association of Dermatology (BAD) working party [10] suggested a number of measures that might be used in this context, including the Dermatology Life Quality Index (DLQI; see Appendix A2) and the Hospital Anxiety and Depression Scale (see Appendix A4). This author would also suggest the Patient Health Questionnaire-9 (PHQ-9; see Appendix A7) and the Generalized Anxiety Disorder-7

(GAD-7), as these are freely available and widely used in primary care mental health services [11].

Future research

Relatively few studies have examined the effectiveness of self-help in dermatology; however, there is promising evidence for the use of fairly simple techniques such as relaxation and mindfulness-based stress reduction.

Further development of self-help specific for dermatology patients is needed. The BAD (www.bad.org.uk) is seeking to provide a one-stop shop for patients that will link to existing disease-specific resources, support groups, forums and help lines. Researchers and clinicians should also be prepared to develop and test further self-help interventions, and to make their materials available for replication and further development.

PRACTICAL TIPS

• Be aware of the nature and importance of the psychosocial impacts associated with living with skin conditions and actively seek to assess these.

• Consider routinely asking patients about their subjective perception of the severity of their skin condition as this is highly associated with psychological distress. Simple 1–7 subjective scales can be easily woven into the consultation.

• Consider routinely using psychometric measures to assess psychosocial distress and quality of life. Measures such as the GAD-7, PHQ-9 and DLQI are particularly useful.

• Understand what self-help is available and build up your awareness of where you might direct patients for resources.

• Practise some of the techniques yourself so as to build confidence in recommending them.

• Understand under what circumstances people should have their care "stepped-up" and be prepared to strongly advocate further assessment where necessary.

References

1. Thompson AR. Skin conditions. In: Cash T (ed) *The Encyclopaedia of Body Image and Human Appearance*, vol 2. San Diego: Academic Press, 2012, pp. 738–743.

2. Gupta MA, Gupta AK. Psychiatric and psychological co-morbidity in patients with dermatologic disorders – epidemiology and management. *Am J Clin Dermatol* 2003; 4: 833– 842.

3. Webster R *et al.* Self-help treatments and stepped-care. In Emmelkamp P, Ehring T (eds). *Handbook of Anxiety Disorders: Theory, Research and Practice*, Vol II. Oxford: Wiley Blackwell, in press.

4. Lavda A *et al.* The effectiveness of psychological interventions for adults with skin conditions: A meta-analysis. *Br J Dermatol* 2012; 167: 970–979

5. Kabat-Zinn J *et al.* Influence of a mindfulness meditation-based stress reduction intervention on rates of skin clearing in patients with moderate to severe psoriasis undergoing phototherapy (UVB) and photochemotherapy (PUVA). *Psychosom Med* 1998; 60: 625–632

6. Jackson K. Undertaking nurse-led research in stress and psoriasis. *Dermatol Nurs* 2006; 5: 11–12.

7. Muftin Z. A randomised controlled feasibility trial of online compassion-focused self-help for psoriasis. *Body Image (Dissertation Abstracts and Summaries)* 2013; 10: 1.13

8. National Institute for Health and Care Excellence. Anxiety: management of anxiety (panic disorder, with or without agoraphobia, and generalised anxiety disorder) in adults in primary, secondary and community care. Clinical Guideline 22 (amended). London: NICE. Available at http://www.nice.org.uk/nicemedia/pdf/cg022niceguidelineamended.pdf

9. Thompson AR. Psychosocial impact of skin conditions. *Dermatol Nurs* 2009; 8: 43–48

10. Bewley A *et al. Working Party Report on Minimum Standards for Psycho-dermatology Services.* British Association of Dermatologists, 2012. Available at http://www.bad.org.uk/Portals/_Bad/Clinical%20Services/Psychoderm%20Working%20Party%20Doc%20Final%20Dec%202012.pdf. Accessed 22.06.2013

11. Spitzer RL *et al.* Validation and utility of a self-report version of PRIME-MD: the PHQ Primary Care Study. *JAMA* 1999; 282: 1737–1744.

CHAPTER 8

Habit reversal therapy: a behavioural approach to atopic eczema and other skin conditions

Christopher Bridgett

Chelsea & Westminster Hospital, London, UK

Behavioural medicine links medicine with human behaviour to improve our understanding of physical illness, and therefore improve its treatment. The behaviour of everyone involved can be taken into account: practitioners, patients and significant others. The term behaviour refers to not only overt actions, but also to thoughts and feelings, including attitudes and beliefs and necessarily links with important social and cultural influences.

Understanding and taking account of the presentation of illness and the response given by a health service, all generally influenced by the attitudes, motivation, and expectations of those involved, is very much part of behavioural medicine.

In dermatology a behavioural approach seems particularly useful for a number of conditions, especially atopic eczema [1]. This chapter begins with an account of habit reversal training in the management of atopic eczema in adults and older children. The treatment of younger children using the same principles is then described. In conclusion, there is a brief account of other skin conditions that may especially benefit from a behavioural approach.

Adults and older children with atopic eczema

In the 1980s Dr Peter Norén and his colleagues in Sweden introduced the behaviour modification technique called habit reversal into the management of atopic eczema, recognizing that the lichenification of the skin seen in chronic eczema is caused by habitual scratching. Habit reversal combined with optimal topical treatment – The Combined Approach – successfully treats chronic atopic eczema in 4–6 weeks [2,3]. The treatment programme is suitable for patients from the age of 8 years upwards and can be offered by practitioners in secondary or primary care. A self-help version is also available [4].

Patients with chronic eczema can be demoralized and dispirited. Some have in the past sought advice from many sources; their expectations are coloured by this previous experience. Many report their condition as both sensitive to stress and stressful in itself.

The programme for The Combined Approach is educational. It is supported by the use of a patient handbook, and necessarily involves the

---

Practical Psychodermatology, First Edition. Anthony Bewley, Ruth E. Taylor, Jason S. Reichenberg and Michelle Magid.
© 2014 John Wiley & Sons, Ltd. Published 2014 by John Wiley & Sons, Ltd.

Box 8.1 Appointment schedule

1. Assessment – 1 week homework
2. Treatment – 2 weeks homework
3. Reinforcement – 2 weeks homework
4. Follow-up

patient in homework tasks, as well as several clinic appointments.

In the programme, there is a focus on three levels of treatment:

- level 1 – emollients;
- level 2 – topical steroids;
- level 3 – habit reversal,

Attention is also paid to three further dimensions of behaviour:

- attitudes of self;
- attitudes of others;
- stress management.

The suggested schema for clinic appointments shown in Box 8.1 can be adapted to suit those involved.

Assessment

The Combined Approach tackles enduring atopic eczema that seems resistant to topical treatment. As the eczema is longstanding, at the first assessment appointment asking *"Why now is a new treatment approach being considered?"* can reveal the relevant attitudes, expectations and motivation. Understanding the part played by significant others may be important. It is useful to assess the quality of life effects of chronic eczema, and to discuss the improvement that will be achieved by following the programme. The difference between previous treatments and this programme needs emphasis. Thus, the series of appointments is important, to ensure the treatment programme is followed successfully; emphasis is placed on the patient learning how to manage his/her own condition successfully, rather than depending on the expertise of the practitioner.

Chronic eczema is described as fluctuating; relapsing and remitting, but never clearing up altogether with topical treatment. The chronicity is discussed and linked to habitual scratching. It is necessary to distinguish itching, a sensation, from scratching, an action. Scratching includes rubbing and picking, and when asked what percentage of their scratching is due to itch, patients with chronic eczema usually admit that a significant amount is habitual; it is not due to itch. The automatic, relatively unconscious nature of habitual behaviour is reviewed, and the principles of habit reversal introduced. In order to change things, it is first necessary to make this behaviour as conscious as possible.

A hand tally counter is given to the patient with the patient handbook. The first week of homework requires counting the daily frequency of scratching episodes with totals recorded in the handbook, together with a list of the main associated circumstances for scratching. Habitual scratching in adults tends to occur first thing in the morning, first thing in the evening and last thing at night. Otherwise it is triggered by boredom, frustration and stress. During this week no attempt is made to stop scratching. Others can be asked to give appropriate help; this involves avoiding saying anything like *"Stop scratching!"*, but rather saying, for example, *"Click!"* – if this is acceptable to the patient. Scratching during sleep is not counted.

Treatment

At the second appointment importance is attached to optimizing topical treatment. The rationale for emollients and topical steroids is reviewed. The handbook is used to ensure the principles of effective treatment are understood. Thus, with emollients it is important to explain that they do not add water to the skin from the outside, but act as an insulation to water loss from the inside. It is also important to ensure that emollients are applied thinly, frequently and gently, without rubbing. The anti-inflammatory effect of topical steroids is

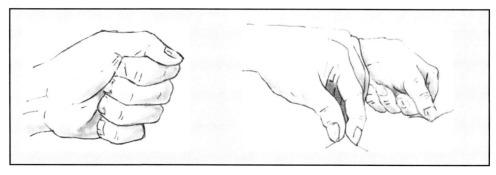

Figure 8.1 Fists, followed by pinch or pressure (reproduced with permission of Peter Norén).

explained and worries about possible long-term side effects discussed; the risk of early relapse through stopping the use of topical steroids too soon needs special mention.

The simple instructions for habit reversal are then given; these are also detailed in the handbook and on the programme's website (http:// www.atopicskindisease.com). Brief closing of the hands into fists, followed by either light skin pinching or finger pressure on itchy skin, is from now on to replace all scratching (Figure 8.1).

Otherwise difficult circumstances associated with scratching (e.g. changing clothes) are planned for, with tactics agreed in advance. Examples are listed in the handbook. Each patient is encouraged to draw up his/her own list of tactics to use.

With adults and older children, scratching during sleep can be ignored; sufficient healing quickly occurs with The Combined Approach during the hours of wakefulness.

Use of the hand tally counter is continued to show the effect of habit reversal, with daily totals recorded in the handbook. Before leaving the appointment, topical treatments are recorded in the handbook, and the opportunity is taken to ensure that their method of use has been understood. It is often useful to suggest that the treatment programme is explained by the patient to significant others, and their help enlisted in prompting habit reversal practice.

Reinforcement

Two weeks later at the third appointment, it is typical to hear that significant improvement has occurred. Often sleep is the first aspect of life to improve, both for the patient and for anyone who sleeps with them. Each level of treatment is reviewed to ensure advice has been understood and is being followed. Frequency of scratching is now reduced. A focus on particular times each day for habit reversal can be encouraged to ensure successful outcome.

The relationship between stress and atopic eczema can often be best explored at this third appointment. The experience of chronic atopic eczema is stressful in itself. The effectiveness of The Combined Approach over 2 weeks relieves stress significantly for many patients. If other measures need to be considered, a simple stress reduction programme can be discussed, as detailed in the practitioner's manual [3].

Follow-up

By the fourth appointment the great majority, if not all, of the chronic eczema has cleared. The future management of episodes of acute eczema is discussed, with an emphasis on early recognition and firm response with appropriate use of topical treatment. It may be useful to arrange further follow-up appointments to monitor progress.

Results

Clinical audit of the use of The Combined Approach has shown that the good results reported from the original research [2] are easy to achieve in the clinic without any specialist expertise in psychological therapies.

Why some do not do well?

Clinical experience suggests there are three main reasons for failure with The Combined Approach. First, it can be a matter of timing. The programme requires 5 weeks of commitment to achieve success. If this clashes with a major life event or similar distracting experience, the results can be understandably disappointing. Trying again when things are back to normal is worth considering. Second, a few patients unfortunately seem relatively unable to grasp what is involved, even when allowances are made and extra time allocated. Finally, there are those whose attitude towards and expectation regarding their condition seem to make failure inevitable. They may say they feel they are being blamed for their condition, but also are not motivated to learning how to cope successfully by using a new treatment approach.

Younger children with atopic eczema [5]

For children the programme necessarily involves their parents, and the younger the child the more the parents need to be involved. This is especially so for children younger than 4 years, for whom the following programme is appropriate. It may be important when considering the use of this programme to first ask if either of the parents have troublesome atopic eczema. If this is the case, he/she should consider first tackling his/her own condition with The Combined Approach, before following the approach with his/her child. Discovering the effectiveness of the programme for him/herself can be an important preliminary to embarking on the approach with his/her child.

Assessment

As with adults, The Combined Approach may be indicated for a child when atopic eczema seems not to be responding to topical treatment; it relapses and remits without clearing up altogether. At the first appointment the link between chronic eczema and habitual scratching is explained. The nature of habitual behaviour is reviewed and habit reversal introduced with the patient handbook. No hand tally counter is used. Instead, the parents and others who can be recruited need to be involved in making a plan. Over a few days three lists are made. The first is of all the trigger factors that seem to make the child's eczema worse (e.g. house dust, cats, getting too hot, woolen clothing). The second is of all the things that the child enjoys doing, especially those that will keep his/her hands busy (e.g. drawing with crayons, doing jigsaw puzzles, playing with play-dough). Finally, by watching the child for a couple of days, all the situations and activities that are especially linked with the child's scratching are noted (e.g. getting dressed and undressed, sitting on the potty, watching TV). These are all listed in the handbook.

Treatment

The treatment programme is set out in the handbook. As for adults, it is important to optimize the use of topical treatment by reviewing its rationale, and giving clear instructions. For the first phase of habit reversal, a period of 4 days, planning is needed to involve enough people to ensure that the child has someone with him/her all of the time, night and day. A long weekend may prove ideal. During this period, as well as the use of optimized topical treatment with emollient and topical steroids, those involved take turns to ensure that the skin is left alone by the child for long enough, *without* ever saying "*Stop scratching!*" The emphasis needs rather to be on what *should* be done. Reference is made to the third list for ideas to use: habit reversal for a young child consists of distractions and diversions – with careful attention to those times and activities when scratching is known to be likely. With the young child, scratching while asleep is dealt with (e.g. by holding the hands, offering soothing encouragement and employing sufficient distraction until sleep continues without further scratching).

The night-time "sentry duty" is usually no longer necessary after the 4 days. Topical treatment needs to be continued with habit reversal measures during the day, as planned. The child is praised and given attention when seen to be playing *without* rubbing and scratching. There follows now a period of 4 weeks continuing treatment, even if during this time the skin appears to have healed completely. As with the programme for adults and older children above, it is important that younger children do not stop topical steroids too soon [5].

Follow-up

A review at 4 weeks often reveals that healing is sufficiently advanced to reduce the frequency of topical treatment. Attention and praise for not scratching is continued. After another 2 weeks of topical steroid treatment of chronic eczema, this should be discontinued, with emollient treatment continuing as required.

As with the programme for adults and older children, from now on progress is determined by treating all episodes of acute eczema promptly and thoroughly, with increased use of emollients and appropriate use of topical steroids. The factors listed initially that provoked acute eczema need remembering, and clear advice on recognition of the signs of acute eczema is given. If acute episodes are correctly treated, the chronic eczema can be prevented from returning, with the quality of everyone's lives improving as a result.

Finding out more about The Combined Approach

Copies of the patient handbooks for The Combined Approach to atopic eczema can be

Box 8.2 Eczema websites

- The Home of The Combined Approach (www.atopicskindisease.com)
- The National Eczema Society (UK) (www.eczema.org)
- National Eczema Association (USA) (www.nationaleczema.org)
- The Eczema Society of Canada (www.eczemahelp.ca)
- Eczema Association of Australasia (www.eczema.org.au)

obtained at the programme website (http://www.atopicskindisease.com), where details of The Combined Approach in The Manual for Practitioners can be referred to, and where there is available supporting information together with an opportunity to discuss approach with both practitioners and patients. General eczema information and support is widely available on the internet. Some of the websites are given in Box 8.2.

Habit reversal and other skin conditions

Habit reversal training can be helpful as part of the treatment of any skin condition complicated or caused by habitual scratching, rubbing and picking. This applies in particular to:
- acne excoriée – acne complicated by habitual skin picking (see Chapter 16);
- trichotillomania – hair pulling (see Chapter 10);
- onychophagia – nail biting;
- psychogenic excoriation – compulsive skin picking (see Chapter 16).

In all the above there is little or no itch. Habit reversal may be helpful too in some other conditions in which itch is usually very much part of the condition, e.g.:
- lichen simplex – itchy skin thickened by scratching;

- pruritus ani – troublesome itch around the anus;
- nodular prurigo – scattered very itchy nodules (see Chapter 22).

At assessment the variables that need to be taken into account include associated physical characteristics, especially associated itch, and any associated abnormality in the mental state or relevant personality characteristics. Depending on the condition, other treatments apart from habit reversal training may be equally important; just as for the successful management of chronic atopic eczema, The Combined Approach requires not only habit reversal but also optimal topical treatment.

PRACTICAL TIPS

- The Combined Approach to atopic eczema is a treatment programme.
- It is an educational approach that involves the patient learning how to treat themselves.
- As much attention is needed in optimizing topical treatment as in teaching habit reversal.
- The approach does not require specialist training in psychological therapy.
- Habit reversal is useful in treating other skin conditions caused by habitual behaviour.

References

1. Thomas K *et al*. Role of psychological interventions and patient education for atopic eczema. In: Williams HC *et al*. (eds) *Evidence-Based Dermatology*. Chichester: Wiley, 2008, pp. 152–155.
2. Norén P Habit reversal: a turning point in the treatment of atopic dermatitis. *Clin Exp Dermatol* 1995; 20(1): 1–5.
3. Bridgett C, *et al*. *Atopic Skin Disease: A Manual for Practitioners*. Bristol, PA: Wrightson Biomedical Publishing, Ltd, 1996.
4. Armstrong-Brown S. *The Eczema Solution*. London: Vermilion, 2002.
5. Bridgett C, Ogoo I. Habit reversal for habitual scratching in younger children with atopic eczema. *Dermatol Nurs* 2013;12(3): 28–30.

CHAPTER 9

Nursing interventions in psychodermatology

Fiona Cowdell and Steven Ersser

Faculty of Health and Social Care, University of Hull, Hull, UK

It is becoming increasingly recognized that skin conditions can have a major detrimental impact on psychological well-being and quality of life for patients as well as their partners, family and friends [1]. Most people manage the problem alone, but some seek advice from a primary care nurse or doctor, and only a small proportion is referred to a specialist. Given the prevalence of skin disease, it is likely that all nurses will care for patients with dermatological conditions. The focus of this chapter is therefore on nursing interventions to assess and address psychosocial issues for patients living with skin conditions, especially long-term skin conditions.

Psychosocial issues in skin conditions

Many patients with primary dermatological conditions will suffer secondary psychiatric co-morbidities and can benefit from psychosocial support (see Chapter 1). Nurses are in a prime position to work with the majority of patients to address their psychosocial issues. Patients with primary psychiatric disorders such as delusional infestation require more specialized care and are discussed in Chapter 14.

Suffering due to skin conditions may have both psychological and social elements. Psycho-logical distress refers to issues related to the mind and ways of thinking, and how the person copes with his/her surroundings and experiences. The social aspect is about how the person interacts with other people and how they function in the social milieu. The mind–body link is a well-established concept and was recognized in nursing long before more scientific investigation examined the nature of the relationship between the brain and skin.

People with skin conditions may experience many psychosocial issues (Box 9.1). Concerns about personal appearance are common and whilst it is easy to attribute these to "vanity", it should be acknowledged that caring for one's appearance is part of being human and integral to psychological well-being; its importance should not be underestimated. There is a reciprocal relationship between feelings and appearance; failing to address these can affect how we look, feel and function.

Effective consultations

Nurses will already have an extensive skill-set which will inform consultations. There are additional techniques that may be integrated into consultations to enhance communication and ensure that psychosocial issues are identified and addressed.

Practical Psychodermatology, First Edition. Anthony Bewley, Ruth E. Taylor, Jason S. Reichenberg and Michelle Magid.
© 2014 John Wiley & Sons, Ltd. Published 2014 by John Wiley & Sons, Ltd.

Box 9.1 Psychosocial conditions related to skin disease [1,2]

- Anger
- Anxiety
- Avoidance
- Bullying
- Depression
- Embarrassment
- Exhaustion
- Frustration
- Guilt
- Helplessness
- Increased alcohol intake
- Irritability
- Low confidence
- Low self-esteem
- Performance issues
- Poor body image
- Relationship issues
- Resentment
- Secretiveness
- Self-consciousness
- Sexual problems
- Sleep deprivation/sleeplessness
- Social isolation
- Stigmatization
- Stress
- Suicidal thoughts
- Suicide
- Teasing
- Unemployment
- Withdrawal

The overall objectives of the nursing consultation are two-fold:

- to provide support and education to patients with skin disease;
- to enhance their mental health and so enable them to manage their condition as effectively as possible.

A four-stage therapeutic consultation approach allows the person to be examined holistically [3]:

1. The clinical observation – global evaluation: How does the patient behave?; How are they talking?; What non-verbal language is noted?; How do they look?; How are they interacting with others?
2. The clinician's feeling – What is the atmosphere (what impression is there of the patient's mood and non-verbal communication)?; Are the atmosphere and what the patient is saying congruent?
3. Questions regarding sleep disturbance, appetite, weight change, quality of life, impact on work and social roles.
4. Questionnaires can help to more accurately assess problems and consequence of disease and serve as a basis for evaluating clinical outcomes of interventions (see below).

Communication is central in any consultation and there are three core conditions that need to be met [4]:

1. genuineness;
2. empathy;
3. unconditional positive regard (acceptance and support of a person regardless of what they say or do).

The patient must have the opportunity to express his/her thoughts and feelings. Any consultation should take place in a quiet, warm, comfortable environment in which there are no disturbances. Critical steps in the consultation include:

- Establishing rapport.
- Agenda setting (What does each person expect from the consultation?).
- Asking open-ended questions:
  ○ *"What are your feelings about your skin?"*
- Using reflective listening:
  ○ *"It sounds like you are feeling . . ."*
  ○ *"It sounds like you are having trouble with . . ."*
  ○ *"You're feeling that . . ."*
  ○ *"You're having a problem with . . ."*

Assessment of psychological health and quality of life

Quality of life can be defined as the differences between the person's hopes and expectations and his/her current experience. There are many validated tools to measure quality of life, ranging from holistic to disease specific. Measurement tools that are commonly used in dermatology are summarized in Chapter 5. They can be used as a guide for discussion and, when repeated serially, allow the patient and nurse to see change over time.

The Person Centred Dermatology Self-Care Index (PeDeSI) (Figure 9.1) is a behaviourally based tool to identify how the patient may best be helped to care for his/her skin condition. This simple, evidence-based questionnaire, which is completed collaboratively by the patient and

Name label: Condition: Topical treatment(s):

Please score each area of ability in discussion with the person using treatment(s) by ticking the relevant boxes.

PeDeSI number	Degree of independence				
Ability	**0 = No ability**	**1 = Some ability**	**2 = Sufficient ability**	**3 = Full ability**	**Agreed action plan**
1. Do you have an understanding of your skin condition?					
2. Do you know what things make your skin condition better and worse?					
3. What is this treatment(s) used for?					
4. Are you aware of how long initial treatment will take to be effective?					
5. Do you know what the common side effects of your treatment(s) are?					
6. Do you know how much cream/ointment/lotion should be applied each time and at what time(s)?					
7. Can you apply the treatment(s) to the affected areas? (demonstrate)					
8. Do you know how and when to adapt treatment/seek help if the condition gets worse?					
9. Do you know how to obtain a repeat prescription?					
10. Do you feel confident to use treatment(s) at home yourself?					

Total Score /30 (maximum total score)
Total scores in Range: 0–10 needs intensive education and support to develop knowledge, ability, and confidence
Total scores in Range: 11–20 needs some education and support to develop knowledge, ability, and confidence
Total scores in Range 21–29 needs limited education and support to develop knowledge, ability, and confidence
Total score of 30: has sufficient knowledge, ability and confidence to manage on their own

Signature   Date

Figure 9.1 The Person-Centred Dermatology Self-Care Index (© Ersser, Cowdell, Gradwell & Langford, December 2011).

nurse, identifies education and support needs that, if met, will enhance concordance and self-management. There is overwhelming evidence that changing people's health-related behaviour can have a major impact on physical and psychosocial well-being [5].

Psychological interventions

Following consultation, the nurse will have built up a picture of the patient, his/her support and education needs, and whether onward referral is necessary. If the patient's condition is amenable to nursing intervention, using elements from the following psychological techniques may be helpful. Such interventions are intended for use as an adjunct rather than a replacement for pharmacological therapies. The patient should be assured that behavioural therapies are complementary to dermatological treatment. One of the major advantages of having psychological support within a derma-

tology department is that such care may be "normalized" if provided in "normal" health-care settings. Reinforcement, perseverance and practice are essential.

Cognitive-behavioural therapy (see Chapter 5)

Cognitive-behavioural therapy (CBT) is based on the concept that the way we think about things affects how we feel and how we behave. The aim is to help patients focus on changing their unhelpful thinking patterns in order to change their behaviour and emotional state. It is categorized as a "talking therapy", but can be delivered face-to-face, electronically or via reading self-help materials. It concentrates on the present rather than trying to make links with the individual's past. Therapy requires a collaborative relationship between patient and nurse. The patient needs to be motivated to want to change, since this process takes significant effort on his/her part. One approach to CBT is summarized in Table 9.1.

Table 9.1 Six phases in the CBT process and allied activities [6]

Phase	Activity
1. Assessment	Conversation with patients and their families, assessing a series of self-reported measures to identify degree of psychosocial impairment and determine appropriate course of action The patient is helped to appraise the personal meaning and significance of events and consider his/her needs and reactions to specific situations
2. Reconceptualization	The nurse assists the patient to reframe his/her experiences; this may simply require the nurse to draw the negative response to the attention of the patient (e.g. *"I am a failure in life because I have bad skin"*)
3. Skills acquisition	Teach patients how to deal with day-to-day obstacles in their everyday life and how to avoid falling into a faulty thought pattern Patient needs to understand the direct connection between thoughts and feelings (having more positive thoughts is likely to lead to more positive feelings) and that physical/bodily feelings can be changed. Techniques may be used to support this (e.g. deep breathing)
4. Skills consolidation	Patients are given "homework" to help them reinforce newly acquired skills
5. Generalization and maintenance	Patient and nurse discuss and agree how the patient is going to maintain his/her skills
6. Post-treatment assessment follow-up	Nurse and patient monitor and evaluate how CBT skills have been incorporated into everyday life

Table 9.2 Habit reversal (HR) clinical intervention model for use in chronic scratching (data from Grillo *et al.* 2007 [7])

Stage of habit reversal	Actions
Habit concept education	Provide the patient with a straightforward explanation of what a habit is and why HR is useful
Itch–scratch cycle education	Patient's own itch–scratch cycle should be defined and details represented diagrammatically
Situation awareness training	Patient needs to become aware of his/her scratching behaviour by: • Asking the patient to keep a scratch diary for a fixed time period • Learning to recognize early moves to scratch
Behavioural assessment	Patients need to learn the difference between itch and scratch (as some use these terms interchangeably). Assessment should include: • How the patient actually scratches (with what, where, when, frequency, intensity, duration) • Scratching triggers/exacerbators identified (temperature, atmosphere, etc.) • Define thoughts after the itch • Consider the consequences • List the patient's goals (stop scratching, allow skin to heal, etc.)
Design brief	Plan for the competing response exercise can be developed, including: • Can be done in bed or in public • Incompatible with scratching • Lasts for a minimum of 1 minute • Allows normal activity to continue
Competing response practice	Should be used for at least 10 minutes per day and when scratch trigger is experienced
Symbolic rehearsal	Patient is asked to describe the itching and scratching in detail whilst performing the competing response

Habit reversal (see Chapter 8)

Habit reversal therapy (HRT) is a brief intervention based on the premise that an old habit can be broken by replacing it with a new more desirable habit. A habit is defined as a recurrent, often subconscious or automatic pattern of behaviour that is acquired through frequent repetition. HRT has been used successfully in dermatology primarily to manage the itch–scratch cycle in conditions such as eczema, but also for trichotillomania and skin picking. Table 9.2 outlines nursing-specific interventions.

Social cognitive theory

Social cognitive theory (SCT) underpins many behavioural interventions for long-term conditions, and focuses on the development of self-efficacy. Self-efficacy is the belief a person

has that they can successfully initiate and complete the actions required in specific situations to achieve particular outcomes. To achieve this, the individual must acquire sufficient knowledge, skills, and confidence to self-manage his/her skin condition as effectively as possible. Self-efficacy is measured in the PeDeSI. The elements of self-efficacy are summarized in Table 9.3.

Future research

Future research should include:
• Development of more sensitive measures of impact on well-being and quality of life.
• Robust testing of psychological interventions (anxiety management, mindfulness, CBT),

Table 9.3 Elements of self-efficacy and their application to dermatology practice

Element	Description	Application to practice
Mastery experience	Most effective way of creating a strong sense of self-efficacy Enables people to master tasks pitched at the right level for each individual. If too easy, people will expect instant success; if too difficult, they will be discouraged. Learning to overcome obstacles will lead to resilience	Break tasks down into component parts (e.g. if a person needs to learn to apply several creams to different areas of the body, he/she might first be taught how and when to use emollients) Person needs to practise this task repeatedly in different environments with the required support, encouragement and feedback. When they are confident in this element of the task, further actions may be added
Vicarious experience	Useful in people with little experience or confidence. Watching a similar someone successfully achieve a specific task can convince individuals that they can master the skills needed to be successful	In a group learning situation more experienced members may be able to demonstrate applying a topical treatment to a plaque whilst avoiding healthy skin
Social persuasion	Through effective communication and social persuasion, a patient may begin to accept how seemingly difficult treatments can be incorporated successfully into his/her life	Emphasize success as a personal gain. Patient goals, developed in partnership with nursing and documented, are most likely to be successful Encourage patients to consider carefully what they really want to achieve; goals may often be quite different from those anticipated by nurses
Emotional regulation	Teach patients how to interpret their physical and psychological states accurately. Patients must learn to avoid the conclusion that physiological and emotional reactions are signs of an inability to complete certain tasks. Positive mood enhances perceived self-efficacy; despondent mood diminishes it	Advise on stress management and relaxation techniques

integrated within nursing practice, to improve mental and physical well-being for people living with long-term skin conditions.

- Methods of educating nurses to deliver psychodermatological interventions and assessing the impact that such interventions have on patient health and well-being.

PRACTICAL TIPS

- Dermatology nurses can enhance patient care by integrating elements of psychological techniques into consultations.
- Use available measures, when possible, to assess the impact of a skin condition on a patient's quality of life (see Chapter 5).
- Dermatology nurses can assess individual education and support needs by using the Person-Centred Dermatology Self-Care Index. This useful tool can identify how the patient may best be helped to care for his/her skin condition, which can lead to better outcomes.

References

1. Schofield J, Grindlay D, Williams H. *Skin Conditions in the UK: A Health Care Needs Assessment.* University of Nottingham: Centre of Evidence Based Dermatology, 2009.
2. National Institute for Health and Care Excellence. *Management of atopic eczema in children from birth up to the age of 12 years.* 2007. Available at http://guidance.nice.org.uk/CG57 accessed 8.2.13.
3. Poot F, Sampogna F, Onnis L. Basic knowledge of psycho-dermatology. *J Eur Acad Dermatol Venereol* 2006; 21: 227–234.
4. Rogers C. *On Becoming a Person.* Boston: Houghton Mifflin, 1961, pp. 283–284.
5. National Institute for Health and Care Excellence. *Behaviour change at population, community and individual levels.* 2007. Available at http://www.nice.org.uk/nicemedia/live/11868/37987/37987.pdf accessed 8.2.13.
6. Gatchel R, Rollings K. Evidence informed management of chronic low back pain with cognitive behavioral therapy. *Spine J* 2008; 8: 40–44.
7. Grillo M, Long R, Long D. Habit reversal training for the itch-scratch cycle associated with pruritic skin conditions *Dermatol Nurs* 2007; 19: 243–248.

Skin diseases with secondary psychiatric disorders

CHAPTER 10

Psychological impact of hair loss

Paul Farrant[1] and Sue McHale[2]

[1] Brighton and Sussex University Hospitals (BSUH) Trust, Brighton, UK
[2] Department of Psychology, Sociology and Politics, Sheffield Hallam University, Sheffield, UK

Anybody who has spent time dealing with patients presenting with hair loss will be familiar with the psychological impact this can have. What is less well understood is how emotional and psychological stress can have an impact on hair growth and trigger hair loss. There are also psychiatric conditions that can present in the hair clinic as traumatic hair loss, such as trichotillomania (Table 10.1).

Whilst hair in mammals has an important role in temperature regulation and camouflage, the main role in humans is in appearance, sexual attraction and social interaction. Therefore, hair loss can have a significant negative impact on self-esteem, confidence and body image.

The hair cycle

Hair fibres are the result of a cycle of a growing phase (anagen), followed by a regression phase (catagen), a resting phase (telogen) and a shedding phase (exogen). The majority of scalp hairs (85–90%) are in the growing phase at any one time and this typically lasts 2–5 years (Figure 10.1). Hairs take around 3 months to pass through catagen, telogen and exogen.

Psychological stress as a cause of hair loss

There are times in life where hair follicles will synchronize and enter into catagen and telogen together. This can be a normal physiological phenomenon such as postpartum, where it is common for women to experience a marked increase in hair shedding 2–3 months after giving birth. Synchronization can also occur due to severe psychological and emotional stress. Separation, bereavement, financial worries or any major life event can lead to a disturbance in the hair cycle and a temporary increase in hair shedding or telogen effluvium (see below).

Patients often mention "stress" as a trigger for their hair loss. Patients will frequently question the relevance of a significant life event that occurred prior to the onset of the hair problem. Some of the scientific rationale for this is discussed below.

Assessing psychiatric impact of hair disease in the clinic

It should be noted that the majority of dermatology quality of life (QoL) tools are validated for psoriasis and eczema, and simply substituting the word "skin" with "scalp" or "hair" does not make the tool valid. There is a need to develop a specific hair QoL tool.

Clinical assessment of hair disease

The majority of patients with hair loss will have non-scarring hair loss, with either episodes of generalized hair shedding, thinning in a pattern

---

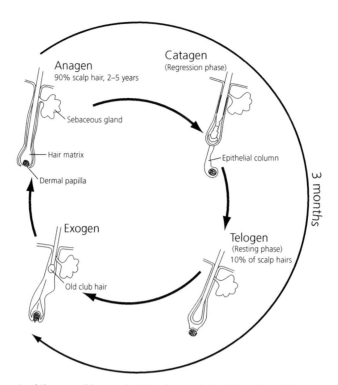

Figure 10.1 Schematic of the normal hair cycle. Disturbance of the hair cycle, which can result from physical and psychological stress, causes hairs to enter the resting phase (telogen) and ultimately to be lost in exogen after 2–3 months.

Table 10.1 Psychodermatology and hair disorders

Dermatological hair disease with psychosocial co-morbidities	Psychological and psychiatric disease that may affect the scalp and hair
• Alopecia areata • Telogen effluvium • Chemotherapy-induced hair loss • Male pattern balding • Female pattern hair loss • Scarring alopecia • Hirsutism	• Body dysmorphic disease (see Chapter 15) • Delusional infestation (see Chapter 14) • Trichotillomania • Post-traumatic stress disorder • Depression • Anxiety

Box 10.1 Clinical assessment

- Diffuse thinning over the vertex is a common presentation of genetic hair loss
- Generalized hair shedding in a diffuse pattern is more likely the result of a hair cycle disturbance and may point to an endocrine (e.g. thyroid) or nutritional abnormality, a side effect of medication, or psychological stress
- Patches of hair loss are the most common presentation of alopecia areata
- Loss of follicular openings, perifollicular erythema, pigment change, and scalp atrophy all point to a scarring cause of hair loss

or patches of hair loss (Box 10.1 and Figure 10.2).

Scarring hair loss is much less common and is characterized by loss of the follicular ostia, often leaving a shiny sclerotic or atrophic scalp.

Alopecia areata

Alopecia areata (AA) is considered an autoimmune disease that leads to hair loss. Typically AA starts with one or two circular patches of

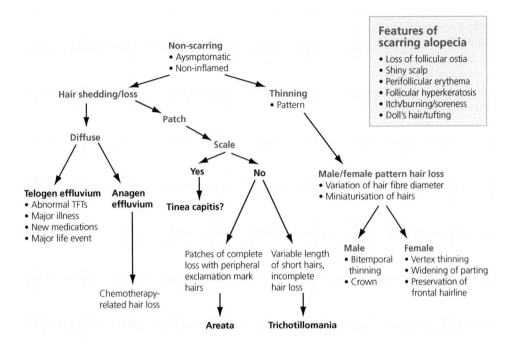

Figure 10.2 A clinical approach to non-scarring hair loss.

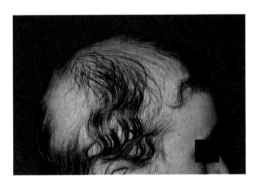

Figure 10.3 Alopecia areata typically presents with patches of hair loss that can spread to total scalp loss (totalis) or total scalp and body loss (universalis).

hair loss. Small broken hairs may be evident around the periphery of the patch and resemble an exclamation mark. Eyebrows, eyelashes and body hair can all be involved. It can spread to involve all the scalp hair (alopecia totalis) or result in loss of all scalp and body hair (alopecia universalis) (Figure 10.3).

It has long been postulated that psychological events may trigger attacks of AA in some individuals. It has been demonstrated in organ culture models of human scalp hair that the prototypic stress-associated neuropeptide, substance P, can induce collapse of the hair follicle immune privilege. Loss of immune privilege is a key first step in areata. Substance P is increased in early areata lesions, as are CD8 T cells that express neurokinin-1 receptor, which mediates substance P action.

There is however wide variation in case-controlled series of AA patients that have investigated the role of psychological stress. Some series have demonstrated a significant increase in stress (from bereavement, family dispute, etc.) in alopecia patients as compared to age- and sex-matched controls [1]. However, in larger series, stress has been identified as a potential trigger in less than 10% of patients [2].

There is no doubt that the hair loss associated with AA can have a profound effect on the psyche, and this may differ from other hair loss conditions for several reasons: AA may begin in childhood, leading to coping and bullying issues in schools; there is often an unpredictable remitting and relapsing pattern of hair loss; and medical treatments are limited and periods of positive response to treatment with hair growth can be swiftly followed by hair falling out once again. In a systematic review by Tucker, 17 of 19 studies demonstrated that AA had a negative impact on self-esteem, and increased levels of depression, anxiety, phobic reactions and paranoia. Some studies within this review demonstrated a greater impact in females, which has been attributed to the greater role that hair plays in female identity [3].

Age may have an effect on the type of psychological conditions found in AA, with a depressive disorder being more common in the young (less than 20 years old) and anxiety being more common in adulthood. This may relate to the effect of peer pressure in childhood and adolescence that has been linked with depression.

In addition to medical treatments, (e.g. topical, intralesional or oral corticosteroids) in AA patients with depression, there may be a beneficial response of hair regrowth with the use of antidepressants.

Telogen effluvium

Telogen effluvium (TE) refers to a disturbance of the hair cycle where hair follicles become synchronized and enter the regression (catagen) and resting phase (telogen) together. When hairs reach the end of the telogen phase (after 2–3 months), they enter into exogen and the old hair is lost before the follicle re-enters the anagen growth phase. Disturbances of the hair cycle are usually transient and there are few studies assessing the psychological impact. There is no doubt that a sudden increase in hair shedding, the hallmark of TE, is very distressing to the sufferer. However, for the majority of patients this is short lived and recovers.

What is more interesting from a psychological point of view is the role that psychological distress may play in triggering hair cycle problems. Mouse studies have shown that stress can inhibit hair growth and force hairs into catagen. It is likely that this is mediated by substance P and corticotrophin-releasing hormone. This finding extrapolated to humans could account for stress-induced TE. Stress-induced hair growth inhibition is promoted by nerve growth factor.

Male pattern balding

Male pattern balding (MPB) is a very common process that affects the majority of men with advancing age and is probably determined by genetic susceptibility. The frequency varies with race, with Caucasians being the most frequently affected. It is usually a gradual process that may begin in teenage years with bitemporal recession and thinning over the vertex. Studies have shown that bald men are seen as being older, less attractive and less confident than men with normal hair. Balding can preoccupy the sufferer and cause stress, lower body image satisfaction and lower self-esteem, and these effects are more marked in younger men, single men and those with an earlier hair loss onset. A negative impact on QoL is more pronounced in young men, although it is not restricted to this age group.

Medical treatments for MBP include topical minoxidil and oral finasteride. Surgical treatments and "weaves" are also available. Men who have successful treatment experience psychosocial benefits with improvements in self-esteem and perception of personal attractiveness.

Female pattern hair loss

Female pattern hair loss (FPHL) refers to the gradual thinning of hair over the central scalp, leading to decreased density and coverage

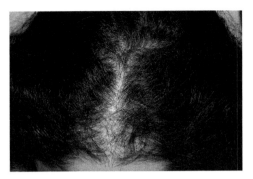

Figure 10.4 Female pattern hair loss presents with thinning over the vertex and widening of the parting.

(Figure 10.4). The miniaturization of hairs is akin to MPB but, unlike in men, it results in thinning rather than complete baldness. Whilst some women may have other symptoms associated with androgen excess such as hirsutisim and acne, most will not have any obvious abnormality of androgens. In addition to the possible role of androgens, it has been postulated that changes in oestrogen levels may play a role. The genetics of FPHL are still unclear, but it is common to have a first-degree relative with either MPB or FPHL.

FPHL affects around 50% of women over the age of 50 years. Whilst it is fashionable for men to have short hair cuts that may limit the impact of balding, in women it is far harder to mask the thinner areas with hair styling alone. FPHL has been shown to have a negative effect on daily life, lowering self-esteem and causing social co-morbidities. Studies comparing the impact of hair loss on men and women have shown that women suffer more emotional distress and make significantly more efforts to cope with hair loss [4]. This is likely to be explained by the fact that hair loss in women is not seen as a normal age-related process, as it is in men.

The impact of hair loss is not uniform and, in women as in men, can be affected by the severity, whether the hair loss is socially noticeable or not and by age (a younger age of onset has a greater psychological impact [4]). It is worth

mentioning that some women will have extreme reactions and this may entail a body dysmorphic disorder.

The treatment options for women are more limited. Topical minoxidil is the only licensed product. The role of antiandrogens is less clear than in men. However, it is more socially acceptable for women to use forms of camouflage such as keratin filaments or hairpieces to disguise their hair loss.

Chemotherapy-related hair loss

Chemotherapy works by stopping the division of rapidly dividing cells. Whilst this is beneficial in terms of killing the cancer cells, it also affects the rapidly dividing cells of the hair matrix, which produce the hair fibre. Hair loss usually begins within a couple of weeks of starting treatment and will start to regrow a few months after completing the course.

The impact of hair loss may be more profound than the surgical treatment of the cancer (e.g. mastectomy for breast cancer). The combination of alopecia and mastectomy may have a double impact on femininity, sexuality and attractiveness. For some patients the thought of hair loss can influence the type of chemotherapy or whether they have chemotherapy at all [5].

Chemotherapy-induced alopecia (CIA) has been shown to cause anxiety, depression, negative body image, lowered self-esteem and a reduced sense of well-being [5]. A woman's fear of rejection by her partner due to the hair loss has also been reported, even though this seldom occurs. The alopecia can also serve as a visible reminder of the actual cancer to both the patient and the public.

Some have a more positive outlook, viewing the alopecia as a sign that the treatment is working. As CIA is an inevitable consequence of treatment, patient's ideas, concerns and expectations should be explored before the onset of treatment. Strategies should be developed to deal with the anticipation of hair loss, the actual moment of hair loss and coping with hair loss and then regrowth [5].

Scarring hair loss

Hair loss can be separated into non-scarring and scarring. The latter is characterized by physical destruction of the hair follicle. This can be a primary process, where the stem cell compartment of the hair follicle is destroyed by inflammation at that site (e.g. lichen planopilaris or discoid lupus erythematosus; Figure 10.5), or secondary, where trauma to the scalp or other inflammatory processes destroy the follicle without the follicle being the primary target. Patients with scarring hair loss have no potential to regrow lost hair. The inflammatory conditions are often progressive and can be symptomatic, with itch and burning being the most common complaints. Effective medical treatments are limited.

As these are uncommon conditions, the psychological impact has been rarely studied, but in most clinician's experience, scarring hair loss is even more devastating than temporary hair loss as it is so final. For this reason it is very important to manage the expectations of the patient in terms of hair regrowth. It is also important to manage the inevitable psychosocial co-morbidities of hair loss.

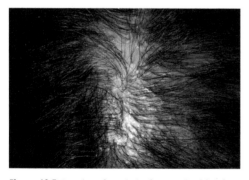

Figure 10.5 Scarring alopecia is characterized by the loss of the follicular ostia. Hair loss is irreversible.

Hirsutism

Hirsutism refers to excess coarse pigmented hair in a male pattern in women. This can be limited to the moustache and beard areas or more widespread, involving the chest, back and abdomen. Hirsutism can be a manifestation of abnormal hormones and is a feature of polycystic ovarian syndrome. In the setting of normal menses, hirsutisim is frequently idiopathic.

Excess hair can be self-treated with bleaching, depilatory creams, plucking, threading, waxing and shaving. Laser therapies and electrolysis offer a semi-permanent solution and some patients may respond to antiandrogen therapy and weight loss.

Hirsutisim is associated with greater levels of anxiety, lower self-esteem and decreased QoL. The social and relationship domains of QoL are particularly impacted and hirsutisim can dominate a woman's life, with women reporting that they constantly check mirrors or touch their skin. In addition, hirsutisim is associated with depression, poor social adjustment and a higher prevalence of eating disorders. QoL has been shown to improve with laser treatment (Box 10.2).

Box 10.2 Treatment of the psychosocial co-morbidities of hair loss/hirsutes

- Treat the hair problem appropriately (medically/surgically/via trichologists/via salons)
- Manage expectations immediately
- Use QoL assessments with care as they are not currently hair specific (but use them anyway where appropriate)
- Offer cognitive-behavioural therapy where appropriate (see Chapter 5)
- Consider treatment of affective disorders if necessary (see Chapter 13)
- Refer to a psychodermatology clinic or psychiatrist if there is higher risk/body dysmorphic disorder or delusional infestation (see Chapter 15 and Chapter 14, respectively)

Specific psychopathology leading to hair loss or presenting in the hair clinic

Body dysmorphic disorder

Body dysmorphic disorder (see Chapter 15) may involve a fear or belief that hair loss is progressive and baldness inevitable. Explanations about normal shedding patterns and use of standardized clinical photography can be very useful.

Delusional infestation

Delusional infestation (see Chapter 14), the belief that the hair is infested with insects, may present in the hair clinic. Some patients are very convinced that they hear the mites at night and will have associated auditory hallucinations. Most will bring specimens or will have digital auditory computer files or visual images to convince doctors about the presence of the infestation.

Trichotillomania

Trichotillomania is a heterogeneous disorder, although the main feature is pulling out the hair, most commonly one by one, resulting in alopecia and excoriations. Hair is most often pulled from the scalp, but eyebrows, eyelashes and even pubic hair can be targets (Figure 10.6 and Figure 10.7). Physical impairments include skin irritations, infection and bleeding. Individuals with trichotillomania generally have impaired psychological and social functioning, especially when trying to avoid exposing hair loss.

Three subsets of hair pulling have been identified: early onset, automatic and focused (Box 10.3) [6]. *Early-onset* hair pulling generally starts in children younger than 8 years old and generally stops without intervention. *Automatic* hair pulling frequently occurs during "risk activities", such as reading and watching TV. Individuals with *focused* pulling are aware of their hair pulling and this type is characterized by urges and tension around the hair-pulling

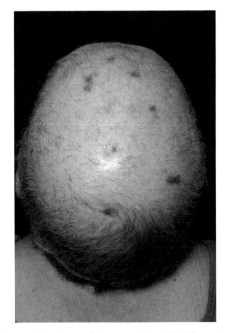

Figure 10.6 Advanced long-standing trichotillomania with extensive hair loss and excoriations.

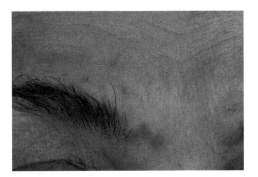

Figure 10.7 Eyebrow trichotillomania. Note the short and broken hairs and hairs of variable length (courtesy of Dr A. Bewley).

Box 10.3 Classification of trichotillomania

- Earlier onset (with limited progression)
- Automatic hair pulling
- Recalcitrant obsessive and focused hair pulling (patient may deny hair pulling)

act. The majority of patients report multiple attempts to resist hair pulling. The typical age of onset has been shown to be in late childhood (around the age of 13 years), although hair pulling can begin at any age. It is not clear how long hair pulling continues in those who start pulling at an early age, but many adult patients report starting the behaviour in childhood.

Trichotillomania is classified as an obsessive-compulsive and related disorder in DSM-5, and this reflects the compulsive nature of the hair pulling. The diagnostic criteria include significant pulling of the hair, increasing tension prior to, or in resisting hair pulling, followed by relief and gratification when pulling out hair. There is a suggestion that these last two criteria should be excluded from DSM-5. Currently, there is no universally accepted assessment for trichotillomania and a variety of measures have been developed [6].

The prevalence of clinically significant hair pulling remains unknown, although estimates vary between 4% and 10% in the general population. This is because patients often feel shame and stigma from the act of hair pulling and rarely present for treatment, and sufferers also go to great lengths to hide their habit from friends and family. Sex ratios of childhood trichotillomania are fairly even, although as age increases it is more prevalent in women [6].

Little is known about the onset of hair pulling, but it is thought to be the result of biological, psychological and social factors. Trichotillomania has also been reported to be associated with sudden loss or bereavement, or with life changing events. Hair pulling associated with childhood sexual abuse has also been reported. As such, a good psychosocial history focusing on stressful events precipitating the hair pulling behaviours should be taken, especially in children. Trichotillomania has been found in some cases to be co-morbid with mood, anxiety, eating and substance misuse disorders.

The majority of studies into treatment for trichotillomania are small scale, uncontrolled

Box 10.4 Management of trichotillomania

- Try to understand *why* this pattern has developed early in the course of the condition
- Offer cognitive-behavioural therapy early (see Chapter 5 and Chapter 16)
- Habit reversal has proved beneficial (see Chapter 16 and Chapter 8)
- Consider SSRIs where experienced/appropriate (see Chapter 13)
- Other psychotropic treatment via expert advice
- Treat the hair loss with physical measures where appropriate (weaves/appliances, etc.)

case reports. The most rigorously investigated treatments are behaviour therapies and pharmacotherapies (see Chapter 16) [6].

Behavioural therapies for trichotillomania are based on the premise that it is a learned behaviour and is maintained through classical and operant conditioning (Box 10.4) [6]. Flessner *et al.* found that the most widely used behavioural treatment for trichotillomania was cognitive-behavioural therapy (CBT) [7], although Bloch *et al.* have suggested that habit reversal training is the most effective intervention for trichotillomania [8]. Pharmacological treatments for trichotillomania vary widely and many drugs have significant side effects. Selective serotonin reuptake inhibitors (SSRIs) (e.g. fluoxetine) have proven ineffective in treating trichotillomania in a variety of studies. The dopamine-blocker pimozide and the carbohydrate inositol have been suggested for the augmentation of SSRIs in the treatment of trichotillomania. A double-blind placebo-controlled study into the use of the opioid antagonist naltrexone showed weak evidence of improvement of trichotillomania symptoms. The atypical antipsychotic olanzapine, known to be effective for the improvement of motor tics, has also shown promising results in treating trichotillomania. There are recent reports that N-acetylcysteine can be effective, with minimal side effects.

Psychological impact of appliances/wigs, camouflage and support groups (see Chapter 12)

Wigs are commonly used to camouflage hair loss. Wig use has been shown to improve quality of life and self-esteem in AA and androgenetic alopecia. They also have been shown to reduce the "sick aspect" in CIA. The psychological benefits of other camouflage methods such as keratin filaments and medical tattoos have not been widely studied.

There is no doubt that patient support groups can help patients deal with practical and psychological issues related to their condition, but published evidence of the effectiveness of these groups is lacking.

Support groups include:

- National Alopecia Areata Foundation (http://www.naaf.org)
- Alopecia UK (http://www.alopeciaonline.org.uk)
- Cicatricial Alopecia Research Foundation (http://www.carfintl.org)

PRACTICAL TIPS

- Hair loss frequently results in psychological morbidity.
- Anxiety, depression, lack of self-esteem and a negative impact on body image are common findings in patients with hair loss.
- The effect in women is often more profound than in men, and a younger age of onset is associated with more psychological sequelae.
- Assessing and managing anxiety and depression should be a routine part of clinical practice when dealing with patients with hair loss.

References

1. Manolaches L *et al*. Stress in patients with alopecia areata and vitiligo. *J Eur Acad Dermatol Venereol* 2007; 21: 921–928.
2. Van der Steen P *et al*. Can alopecia areata be triggered by emotional stress? An uncontrolled evaluation of 178 patients with extensive hair loss. *Acta Derm Venereol* 1992: 279–280.
3. Tucker P. Bald is beautiful? The psychosocial impact of alopecia areata. *J Health Psychol* 2009; 14: 142–151.
4. Cash T *et al*. Psychological effects of androgentic alopecia on women: comparisons with balding men and with female controls. *J Am Acad Dermatol* 1993; 29: 568–575.
5. Hesketh P *et al*. Chemotherapy Induced Alopecia: psychological impact and therapeutic approaches. *Support Cancer Care* 2004; 12: 543–549.
6. Duke D *et al*. Trichotillomania: A current review. *Clin Psychol Rev* 2010; 30: 181–193.
7. Flessner C *et al*. Current treatment practices for children and adults with trichotillomania: Consensus among experts. *Cog Beh Pract* 2010; 17: 290–300.
8. Bloch M *et al*. Systematic review: Pharmacological and behavioral treatment for trichotillomania. *Biol Psychiatry* 2007; 62: 839–846.

CHAPTER 11

Psoriasis and psychodermatology

Christine Bundy, Lis Cordingley and Chris Griffiths

Centre for Dermatology Research, Institute of Inflammation and Repair, University of Manchester, and Manchester Academic Health Sciences Centre, Manchester, UK

Epidemiology and defining features of psychological functioning

There is growing recognition that psoriasis is associated with a significant risk of both psychological and physical co-morbidities, such as cardiovascular disease (CVD) and the metabolic syndrome [1] (Figure 11.1).

There is a relative lack of research into the pathophysiological processes that link distress and psoriasis, but many individuals with psoriasis identify that stress or stressful life events can trigger both the onset and exacerbation of the condition. Anxiety in people with psoriasis is often high, with rates of pathological worrying reported to be around 25–30% [2]. Fear of negative evaluation by others and anticipatory avoidance of rejection may explain why some people with psoriasis have lower levels of social engagement and educational performance, and are restricted in their choices of and advancement in careers [3]. Even when psoriasis severity is reduced by effective treatment, patients may continue to report very low levels of emotional and social functioning.

Prevalence of low mood, depression and thoughts of suicide are higher in people with psoriasis than in those with other dermatological conditions such as acne, or indeed other non-dermatological long-term conditions [4]. Depressive symptomology has been identified in up to 62% of psoriasis patients, with rates of active suicidal ideation ranging between 5.6% and 7.2% [4]. Depression is more common in younger men with psoriasis. This group often has the highest alcohol use, which may imply a degree of self-medication for low mood. There is considerable anecdotal reporting of drug misuse amongst younger men with psoriasis, although to date this has not been subject to systematic examination.

Health professionals outside dermatology are often surprised at the levels of psychological distress and morbidity associated with psoriasis. The visible nature of the condition is a particular source of distress, although this goes largely unrecognized in general healthcare settings and rarely leads to appropriate management [5]. This in turn can lead to disengagement from formal healthcare by many individuals who may be either reluctant or unable to ask for help.

People with psoriasis are likely to engage in unhealthy lifestyle behaviours, such as low levels of physical activity, alcohol use, smoking, and be overweight. Poor motivation is associated with low mood, but feelings of embarrassment, stigma and shame, and direct experiences of rejection in public arenas such as parks, swimming pools or gyms contribute to reluctance to use public services. Another indicator of poor self-care may be lack of adherence to prescribed treatments. Adherence to topical treatments, the first line for most people with psoriasis, is very low [6]. Many report topical

Practical Psychodermatology, First Edition. Anthony Bewley, Ruth E. Taylor, Jason S. Reichenberg and Michelle Magid.
© 2014 John Wiley & Sons, Ltd. Published 2014 by John Wiley & Sons, Ltd.

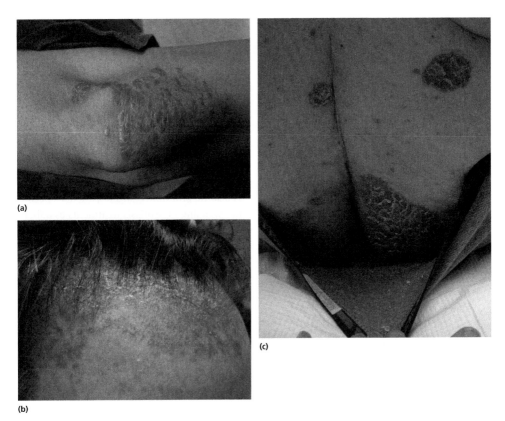

Figure 11.1 Classic signs of psoriasis on the (a) elbows and (b) scalp line. Though often overlooked, psoriasis on the buttocks (c) can greatly impact self-image and should be evaluated and treated along with the more visible areas (courtesy of Dr J. Reichenberg).

regimens as onerous and unpleasant, adding to the overall sense of disease burden.

Pathogenesis

There is little doubt that psychology – a person's thoughts, feelings and actions – plays an important role in the activity and management of psoriasis. Correlations between mood and behaviours with psoriasis flares are common, but more research is needed to establish causal relationships. However, there is a biologically plausible stress pathway linking beliefs and emotional arousal to skin activity, and this relationship may be moderated by health behaviours.

The biological route

Once an individual interprets the signs of a flare or the diagnosis of psoriasis as a threat to health, he/she formulates a cognitive and an emotional response to it. The cognitive response presents as five core beliefs (see below). These beliefs in turn drive an emotional response, including anxiety, anger or depression.

Physiologically, a real or imagined threat will result in activation of the hypothalamic–pituitary–adrenal axis. This complex neurohormonal cascade cannot be fully described here, but suffice to say that stress hormones, such as cortisol, are permissive of cutaneous immune responses in susceptible individuals. Cytokines and T cells are released to manage this increased local activity. This neuroendocrine and immune response sets up a vicious cycle of inflammation.

The behavioural route

As indicated above, unhealthy behaviours are common in people with psoriasis. These are known risk factors for CVD, which is associated with psoriasis [1], although whether psoriasis is an independent risk factor for CVD has not been clearly established.

Assessment

Assessing beliefs

A comprehensive psychological overview involving assessment of beliefs, mood and behaviour is important to guide the choice of appropriate interventions. Beliefs about illness are associated with worse health outcomes in long-term conditions, including worse functioning and greater utilization of healthcare. Understanding patients' beliefs about psoriasis and its treatment is key to the good management of psoriasis. Various tools based upon the Common-Sense-Self-Regulatory Model (CS-SRM) can be used for this (see also Chapter 5):
- Revised Illness Perception Questionnaire (IPQ-R);
- Brief Illness Perception Questionnaire (B-IPQ);
- Beliefs about Medicines Questionnaire (BMQ).
  The CS-SRM [7] is a useful framework to identify key illness and treatment beliefs. The five core beliefs are:
- what *caused* the initial onset or subsequent flare;
- *consequences* – personal, financial and social;
- main *symptoms* experienced;
- degree to which an individual believes they have personal *control* over flares and whether the treatment given will control flares;
- *timeline* or perceived trajectory of the condition over time.

The IPQ-R, which is based on the CS-SRM, is a well-established, valid and easy to use self-report instrument that is able to identify core beliefs about illness and help guide a suitable intervention. There is also a brief version (B-IPQ) that asks nine questions and may be more suitable in a busy clinical setting. The value of these tools is that they identify the *patient's perspective* of their condition, including gaps in understanding of psoriasis and the mechanisms that may trigger or maintain flares. It is also helpful to investigate patients' specific understanding of psoriasis treatments as adherence has been identified as a significant problem in psoriasis [6].

Beliefs do not act independently of each other; rather they cluster to convey an implicit logic, termed illness coherence. Many individuals hold adaptive and useful beliefs associated with positive coping. However, for some, their interpretation of the symptoms of their illness is closely associated with low mood and poor outcomes. Hence, assessment of illness beliefs should play a key role in psychological assessment.

Worries or concerns about medicines are associated with non-adherence across a range of long-term conditions and can be captured with the BMQ, a simple self-report measure that assesses four salient dimensions of beliefs about medicines.

Assessing mood

Mood can be a significant barrier to self-management behaviours, such as active maintenance of a healthy weight and medication adherence.

Both anxiety and depression are common emotional responses to psoriasis. The Hospital Anxiety and Depression Scale (HADS) is a well-established screening tool (see Chapter 5). In a busy clinic setting it may be more realistic to use the Patient Health Questionnaire (PHQ-2), which asks two screening questions for depression – *"Over the last 2 weeks, how often have you been bothered by (1) Having little interest or pleasure in doing things? and (2) Feeling down, depressed or hopeless?"* If the response to either question is affirmative, then further assessment using the HADS or the PHQ-9 is warranted. The nine-item PHQ-9 also probes experiences associated with depression, with one item that specifically asks about suicide or self-harm. Individuals attending either primary or secondary care report that the emotional aspect of living with psoriasis is the area they most wish they could discuss, yet distress is seldom raised by either them or the dermatology team. Contrary to common belief, low mood is not easy to detect unless it is actively assessed.

Assessing behaviour

If alcohol use is suspected to be a problem, then measuring actual alcohol consumption with the CAGE questionnaire for alcohol use or the Alcohol Use Disorders Identification Test (AUDIT) tool, both well validated and well used measures, is warranted (see Chapter 27).

The Dermatology Life Quality Index (DLQI) is used in the management and assessment of psoriasis and can provide a useful snapshot of how the disease impacts a patient's quality of life (QoL) (see Chapter 5).

Treatment

The six principles of a psychological-based intervention are (Box 11.1):

Box 11.1 Principles of treatment

- Use patient-centred communication
- Assess psychological functioning using validated measures
- Identify the "Think–Feel–Do cycle"
- Work with the patient to identify their goals and action plans for change
- Encourage "change talk" during the consultation
- Review progress with the patient

- *The first principle of any effective intervention is patient-centred communication* and this is especially true of psychological interventions. This implies more than just effective information gathering, and rather a structured attempt to understand and use the patient's perspective to guide later goal setting and action planning for change. There is good evidence that this approach is likely to lead to better outcomes than just demonstrating good communication skills alone. Allowing the patient to give an account of his/her views of the problem in his/her own words and in his/her own time will help to identify key illness and treatment beliefs. This provides an opportunity for the clinician to modify these beliefs if they are either incorrect or incomplete.

- *The second principle is to assess psychological functioning using validated measures.* An assessment combined with the patient's own account allows a more comprehensive problem formulation and enables the clinician to identify possible solutions. The National Institute for Health and Care Excellence (NICE) has produced recommendations for managing low mood and depression in patients with long-term conditions [8]. It recommends adopting a stepped approach, escalating treatment options as appropriate. The first step is to support self-management by encouraging the patient to become more active (behavioural activation), and to signpost to available specialist services, such as smoking cessation, weight loss or alcohol reduction.

- *The third principle is to identify the "Think–Feel–Do cycle",* identifying unhelpful behaviour patterns that can occur in response to beliefs and feelings about having psoriasis. For example, in an attempt to manage the distress of a psoriasis flare, patients may smoke more and drink more alcohol, which in turn disrupt sleep and perpetuate the flare. Patients may be unaware of these patterns, but when they are able to identify them they can often intervene early to stop them.

- *The fourth principle is to work with the patient to identify his/her goals and action plans for change,* preferably using specific, measurable, attainable, realistic and timely (SMART) techniques. Goals are more likely to be attained if they are realistic and the patient has identified potential solutions to overcome barriers. Suggestions need to come from the patients themselves rather than the clinician. Initially, aim to set easily achievable goals to boost motivation and intention to change. Follow this by addressing the (possibly) more important but more difficult goals. The experience of success increases motivation and the likelihood of other changes being made. Using techniques to increase motivation, such as simple verbal reinforcement comments (e.g. *"Well done for making a start"* and *"This is a significant step forward"*) from credible sources such as healthcare staff, can make a difference to a person's intention to persevere with change. Encouraging the patient to ask for help and share his/her plans with someone he/she trusts to be able to help also helps him/her to continue with the desired change (Figure 11.2).
- *The fifth principle is to encourage "change talk" during the consultation.* This means asking the patient to identify what he/she has been able to achieve in the past and gently discouraging any focus on failure. This simple task of attending to successes builds a patient's confidence or self-efficacy and helps him/her to refocus his/her attention on what he/she can achieve.
- *The sixth principle is reviewing.* Planning a session to review progress with the patient helps him/her believe he/she is being supported in the process. The information gathered from the assessment phase can help the clinician to guide the patient to make specific and detailed enough action plans to be successful. Action plans that are little more than wish lists are less likely to succeed than ones that have considered all the factors that could derail an otherwise helpful change plan and encourage the patient to have some options available for managing those factors. This relapse prevention strategy helps patients to think around potential problems in advance of the situation, rather than simply reacting to circumstances when the unexpected occurs.

Through the process of careful listening and planning for change, the patient is encouraged to believe that change is a deliberate and organized intervention rather than it being left to chance. There is evidence that this deliberate, structured support intervention will be more likely to result in actual change than a less structured conversation. If this step in the care pathway is not successful, then within the NICE guidance, moving onto an even more structured, brief intervention is indicated. This is likely to be the time to refer to specialist mental health service.

If the clinician is to incorporate this additional activity into the consultation, he/she will require training to successfully implement the intervention. Training does not need to be lengthy or onerous, but it does need to be systematic and accessible to non-mental health specialist staff with follow-up support.

Future research

Recent developments in new technology platforms for delivering psychological intervention, such as the electronic Targeted Intervention for Psoriasis (eTIPS) study [9], show promise. They may allow wider access to psychological therapy for people with psoriasis, but these alternative methods require more testing before they can substitute for face to face contact.

Mindfulness approaches in psoriasis also show promise [10] and further research in the form of fully powered randomized controlled studies are needed to demonstrate the extent of their promise.

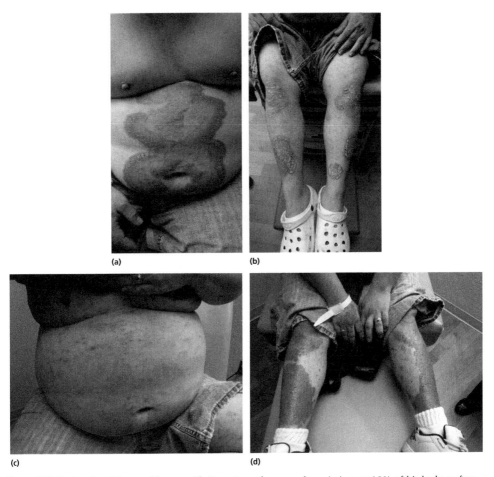

Figure 11.2 Patient is a 35-year-old man with Down's syndrome and psoriasis over 10% of his body surface area (a,b). The goals of his treatment were improvement of symptoms of itching and scaling. He was started on acetretin 25 mg daily, and over the next few months he showed dramatic improvement in symptoms, though some signs of his disease persisted (c,d) (courtesy Dr J. Reichenberg).

As with medical therapies, some of these approaches are more suitable for some groups of patients than others, and there is now a pressing need to determine which patients are likely to benefit from what kind of psychological interventions. Decisions should be based on careful and systematic assessment of beliefs, mood and behaviour, and consistent with a personalized or stratified approach to patient management.

PRACTICAL TIPS

- Assessment is key to formulating plans to support patients. Use validated assessment tools where possible and start to collect and record information routinely so that you can identify patterns or changes.

- Acknowledging your patient's distress or low mood in a consultation can be therapeutic. Check whether they believe it is directly associated with their psoriasis. Build good relationships with psychology or psychiatry services and refer where necessary.

- Use the *Think–Feel–Do* cycle. Ask your patients about their *beliefs* about psoriasis, how it makes them *feel* and how they *cope* or *behave*. It may help the patients to see links between these by writing their answers under each of these headings.

- If you *"feel stuck"* it is likely that this is how the patient is feeling. Ask the patient to list three things that he/she would like to change about the current situation and then to rank them in order of priority. Use this as the basis of treatment planning or referral.

References

1. Langan SM *et al.* Prevalence of metabolic syndrome in patients with psoriasis: A population-based study in the United Kingdom. *J Invest Dermatol* 2012; 132: 556–562.

2. Fortune DG *et al.* Pathological worrying, illness perceptions and disease severity in patients with psoriasis. *Br J Health Psychol* 2000; 5: 71–82.

3. Kimball AB *et al.* Psoriasis: is the impairment to a patient's life cumulative? *J Eur Acad Dermatol Venereol* 2010; 24: 989–1004.

4. Gupta M, Gupta A. Depression and suicidal ideation in dermatology patients with acne, alopecia areata, atopic dermatitis and psoriasis. *Br J Dermatol* 1998; 139(5): 846–850.

5. Nelson PA *et al.*, on behalf of the IT. Recognition of need in health care consultations: a qualitative study of people with psoriasis. *Br J Dermatol* 2013; 168: 354–361.

6. Thorneloe RJ *et al.* Adherence to medication in patients with psoriasis: a systematic literature review. *Br J Dermatol* 2013; 168: 20–31.

7. Leventhal H, Nerenz D, Steele D. Illness representations and coping with health threats. In: Baum A, Taylor S, Singer J (eds). *Handbook of Psychology and Health*. Hillsdale, NJ: Erlbaum, 1984, pp. 219–252.

8. NICE Clinical Guidelines for Depression in Adults. 2009 Available at http://www.nice.org.uk/CG90.

9. Bundy C *et al.*. A novel, web-based, psychological intervention for people with psoriasis: The Electronic Targeted Intervention for Psoriasis (eTIPs) Study. *Br J Dermatol* 2013; 169(2): 329–336.

10. Fordham B, Griffiths CEM, Bundy C. Can stress reduction interventions improve psoriasis? A review. *Psychol Health Med* 2013; 18(5): 501–514.

CHAPTER 12

Living well with a skin condition: what it takes

Henrietta Spalding, Wendy Eastwood, Krysia Saul and Susan Bradbrooke

Changing Faces, The Squire Centre, London, UK

"I was cripplingly shy as a child and things only got harder to deal with as a teenager. I felt very angry most of the time. It was a painful emotion to live with, and I began to isolate myself. It was only at university that I developed the social skills to cope and not let other people's attitudes dominate my life."

(woman in her 20s with a port-wine stain)

The aesthetic impact of a birthmark, a skin disease or the treatment of skin cancer can cause patients a range of psychosocial as well as functional difficulties, pain or discomfort [1,2]. The psychosocial impact of living with a skin condition can affect every aspect of a patient's life, including education, seeking and retaining employment, using public transport, making friends, forming relationships, social life, healthcare, shopping, swimming, intimacy and hygiene. This means that patients (and their families) often have to learn how to live with the visual effects of their medical condition in a society that attaches great importance to appearance.

This chapter uses the term "disfigurement" as a useful collective word to describe the visual impact of these conditions, but *not* to describe an individual's condition. So a "disfigurement" is the aesthetic effect of a mark, rash, scar or skin graft, or an asymmetry or paralysis to a person's face or body.

Living with a disfigurement

Living with a face or body that looks unusual, whatever the cause, is not always easy. Many people find it challenging to feel good about themselves, experiencing psychological distress when they encounter staring, comments, and awkward questions [3]. In turn, psychological distress can potentially exacerbate some skin conditions.

One study [4] found that participants with port-wine stains felt their skin lesions exerted negative effects on self-esteem (64%), social (36%) and sexual (53%) relationships, education (33%) and their ability to get a job (17%).

Changing Faces (www.changingfaces.org.uk) is a UK charity that supports and represents people with any condition that affects their appearance. It summarizes the psychosocial difficulties that these people experience as follows:

- *Intrapersonal* – in our appearance-focused society, any unusual appearance is a challenge to a person's self-esteem and sense of identity. Feelings of sadness, grief, guilt, anger and depression are frequent.
- *Interpersonal* – disfigurement poses many everyday challenges in social encounters, especially being stared at, avoided, asked curious questions, patronized, called names and worse – ridiculed or rejected. It has been

Practical Psychodermatology, First Edition. Anthony Bewley, Ruth E. Taylor, Jason S. Reichenberg and Michelle Magid.
© 2014 John Wiley & Sons, Ltd. Published 2014 by John Wiley & Sons, Ltd.

described as "attitudinal violence" [5]. If encounters go badly, a person can become socially anxious, withdrawn and isolated, leading to depression and occasionally even suicide. Making friends and intimate relationships is complicated, while getting work or promotion can be very challenging despite the fact that "severe disfigurement" is covered by the UK's Equality Act 2010.

The cultural background

Ninety per cent of the general public unwittingly judge people with disfiguring conditions unfavourably such that they and their families are often unfairly treated simply because of their looks. The assumptions – and the subsequent behaviours – mitigate against an equal relationship.

There are three big cultural assumptions – stereotypes or misconceptions – about people with disfigurements, which tend to be reinforced by the media, film, and advertising:
1. "Good looks" are the key to success and happiness, so people with disfigurements can expect to live only second-rate lives.
2. People with scars and disfigurements are "different", not "normal" – hence they are justifiably caricatured in film and literature as villainous or nasty.
3. Reconstructive (and cosmetic) surgery can transform people's faces, make them perfect and make them happy, so everyone with a disfigurement should get it "fixed" by medical or surgical treatments.

Ironically, people with an unusual appearance and their parents/families can often apply these same cultural assumptions to themselves – feeling pessimistic about their prospects, disliking their "less-than-good looks" and associating them with inferiority, even immorality.

Historically, beauty has been held in high regard and advertising images endorse this. The recent Government Inquiry into Body Confidence [6] found that the success of the booming beauty, cosmetic surgery, diet and fashion industries demonstrates how much people are prepared to invest in their appearance.

Television and film portrayals, computer games and children's stories perpetuate the myth that heroes and heroines are handsome and beautiful. Bad people are portrayed as ugly – with scars, warts or distortions. Cinderella [and her ugly (i.e. nasty) sisters] and the orcs in *The Lord of the Rings* illustrate this well, whilst the Bond and Batman movies frequently equate scarring with evil. There are also sad images, with the Phantom of the Opera living tragically in the sewers of society. Only a few antiarchetypes are portrayed sympathetically – Shrek and Harry Potter being the shining examples.

What does this mean for patients?

"I wish that during my hospital appointments I'd been asked about how I was actually coping. Whether my hair grew or not was often overshadowed by my deep sense of loss, sadness and depression caused by my significantly altered appearance."

(woman in her 50s)

It is important to state that many patients adjust well to their skin condition and even report positive consequences from living with a visible difference, such as personal growth and increased empathy with others [7]. The literature also indicates that most people do eventually adjust reasonably well to a disfiguring condition, though time is by no means an automatic healer. Most people, however, experience some psychosocial difficulties for some time (Box 12.1), as do their parents, partners and families. Research attests that failing to recognize or respond to these difficulties early on may lead to long-term damage.

The extent or severity of a skin condition does *not* correlate with the degree of emotional and social distress caused. This means that treating it medically or surgically (even virtually removing it) is no guarantee that the patient will adjust psychologically. Evidence highlights the importance of "perceived severity" or noticeability of disfigurement rather than objective severity as the critical indicator of good or poor outcome [8].

Box 12.1 Examples of patients' concerns

- How can I look good with my skin like this?
- What will make me "better"?
- What will other people think of me?
- Starting school, work, going out will be tough.
- How will I ever find a partner?

Several non-physical "protective" factors have been found to facilitate coping and adjustment:

- having or acquiring positive beliefs about future prospects;
- having – or learning – good communication skills to manage others' reactions;
- possessing, or obtaining, quality social support from parents, friends and professionals.

Any patient struggling to come to terms with his/her appearance needs to have ready access to services that can help him/her develop the coping strategies necessary to living confidently. These include:

- quality information;
- social skills training;
- advice and emotional support;
- self-help booklets;
- workshops to build self-confidence and self-esteem;
- skin camouflage (Box 12.2).

Box 12.2 Skin camouflage in action

"Amazing, amazing! . . . now that I have the covering of the make-up I just feel that my face is back, I can get back to life, and I don't really have to worry so much, and yeah you can maybe still see the slight sort of lumps and whatever, but I feel like no one's going to see it as much as before."

Skin camouflage – the application of specialist camouflage products in thin layers to the surface of the skin – is a non-invasive coping strategy that reduces the appearance of many skin conditions and can benefit patients in dermatology, as well as in other specialties. Such products are ideal for dermatology patients as sunscreen, topical medicines and emollients can still be used alongside the camouflage treatment [9]. There is an extensive range of shades, benefiting patients from all ethnic groups. When properly applied and set with powder, camouflage creams may remain on the body for up to 4 days, and on the face for up to 12 hours; they are also waterproof, allowing the wearer to swim or take a shower without removing the product.

Case study: a woman living with lichen planus on her legs for over 15 years had been absolutely

devastated by the condition. She had felt horrendous and her quality of life had been significantly impeded. After a session with a skin camouflage practitioner, she was totally overwhelmed, "It was absolutely wonderful . . . I could have cried." The transformation allowed her to go out, feel good about herself, enjoy her social life, go on holiday.

During an individual consultation, trained skin camouflage practitioners inform the client about the camouflage creams used and set realistic expectations for what they can achieve. A colour matching process follows and then a demonstration on how to apply the products, enabling the patient to reproduce the effect themselves. He/she is given an information sheet and a prescription form to present to his/her GP. Products are available on prescription at the GP's discretion, although they can also be purchased independently.

Having access to a trained practitioner, who is familiar with a variety of different conditions, recognizes appearance-related distress and is informed about the range of camouflage creams

(Continued)

and application techniques available, is extremely valuable. Moreover, for a patient whose skin may have been exposed to a range of treatments, painful surgeries and attitudinal violence (stares, comments), an hour with a dedicated practitioner can be very therapeutic.

Skin camouflage works better for some skin conditions than others, and so may not be suitable for everyone. Whilst wearing a product can help an individual feel more confident and less vulnerable in social situations, skin camouflage does not address the more deep-seated psychological issues that the wearer may experience [10].

Case study: a perspective from a user who had been injured in an accident during childhood in the 1960s. After considerable clinical intervention, the surgeon suggested that she might consider using cosmetics to help disguise the highly visible scar.

"I recall no concerns about my patchwork appearance whilst at school though some adults told my mother I should not be allowed out in public. Real awareness of my facial difference and the accompanying self-consciousness developed when I left the security of school to work in a large London bank which required travelling by public transport. I came to loathe such journeys, always trying to obtain a window seat so that my 'good' cheek was visible to the passenger sitting near me. I felt particularly uncomfortable by the close proximity of fellow train travellers. I learnt to avoid eye contact, bury myself in a book: I hid behind strands of hair intentionally grown long – anything to deflect the curious, persistent and sometimes hostile public gaze."

"The use of a camouflage product to disguise or alter one's appearance can be transformative – up to a point – although its efficacy will vary from one person to another. It may initially restore some measure of confidence and self-assurance for those struggling to adjust to an altered appearance, as it did for me. However, camouflage alone is unlikely to equip disfigured people with the coping strategies that enable them to deal with visible difference and society's reaction to them."

How to promote successful adjustment (see also Chapter 4 and Chapter 11)

Skin conditions can present serious and lifelong psychological and social challenges for many patients; health and social care professionals need to act on these to improve patient outcomes. Changing Faces indicates that the best long-term, psychosocial adjustments are achieved if patients have access to an effective package of help and support designed to promote living with confidence. The package is usually delivered by a trained professional but can also be in a self-help format. It is essentially a cognitive-behavioural approach combining a mix of psychoeducational direction and psychotherapeutic support, known as FACES:

- *F – Finding out:* to gain realistic information about their condition and its treatment
- *A – Attitude:* to develop a positive outlook and beliefs about the future
- *C – Coping* with feelings: to manage them better with help from a trained professional
- *E – Exchanging:* to share experiences with others in similar situations
- *S – Social skills:* to learn the skills to handle the reactions of strangers, friends, etc.

What does each element of FACES mean in practice?

A brief overview of FACES is given and how it works illustrated with the example of Amy, a young person who made contact with Changing Faces for support with the impact of her acne:

F – Finding out

Patients/families receiving treatment should have the opportunity to read about and discuss their condition. Medical staff have a major role to play in empowering patients to make the right decisions. Gaining realistic information also means that the patient:

- can explain things more easily to his/her family, friends, employers and others;
- is informed about and referred to other agencies (e.g. to a skin camouflage clinic, if appropriate);
- feels more in control of his/her condition.

Case study: Amy and her mother were provided with information from their GP and she tried a number of treatments, including creams, homeopathic remedies and mineral foundation to cover the acne. She was also referred to see a dermatologist.

A – Attitude

In our looks-focused culture, it is important for patients and their families to develop positive beliefs about their future and to debunk negative thinking about appearance issues. This can be done by attending workshops, looking at websites and reading self-help literature and/or people's personal accounts so the patient can:

- start thinking positively about his/her future;
- be encouraged to think about his/her strengths and interests, not just his/her appearance.

Case study: Amy was supported to explore what made "a good day". What is "a good day" like and what are the barriers to "a good day"? Relationships with her peers, the meaning of peer groups to Amy, and the risks/benefits of making new friends were explored. She started to see that her prospects in life need not be controlled by her looks.

C – Coping

Patients should have access to excellent psychotherapeutic support to help them manage their feelings. Health professionals can help by:

- acknowledging the problem – *"It will take time to get used to your skin"* rather than *"you are lucky not to need hospitalization"*;
- legitimizing – *"It's OK to feel upset when your skin is causing you discomfort"*;
- normalizing – *"Many people feel distressed following hair loss"*.

Case study: Amy was given space to talk freely and without judgement about her experiences on the phone. Her concerns were normalized and she was

provided with positive encouragement. A trusting relationship was established and support and reassurance given to Amy's mother as part of the overall intervention.

E – Exchanging

Patients and families should be offered the chance to connect with others going through similar experiences (not all will want to) through workshops or a relevant support group. This enables patients to gain mutual support.

Case study: Amy was directed to the Changing Faces webpages and online resources developed by young people, as well as to the website of a teenager with severe acne who blogs about how she has managed to deal with her condition.

S – Social skills

Patients need to learn new skills for handling others' reactions to their looks and develop effective strategies to manage social situations (e.g. through self-help guides and workshops covering topics such as assertiveness or intimacy). One of the factors clearly identified as predictive of good outcome is the number and variety of positive non-avoidant coping strategies employed by the individual [11].

Changing Faces has developed two models that can help. First, the Reach Out model consists of a toolkit of communication strategies that can prepare individuals for social situations, so as not to be caught off guard, and enable them to take the initiative:

- R – Reassurance: putting someone at their ease
- E – Energy: creating interest in what they are saying
- A – Assertiveness: taking the initiative
- C – Courage: being strong and taking control
- H – Humour: introducing fun or a joke
- O – Over there!: distracting away from the skin condition
- U – Understanding: being aware that seeing a skin condition can be difficult
- T – Tenacity: try again – use a different strategy if the first does not work

Second, 3-2-1 Go! prepares a patient with a visible difference with the following coping strategies:

- Three things to do if someone stares at you:
  - Look back and smile
  - Look back, smile and say, *"I'm sorry, do we know one another?"*
  - Ask them not to stare
- Two things to say if someone asks you what happened:
  - *"I have a skin condition but I'd rather not talk about it"*
  - *"I've had psoriasis for a few years but it's not contagious"*
- One thing to think if someone appears to turn away:
  - *"It's OK, they didn't mean any harm"*

Case study: Amy was encouraged to develop a number of strategies to try out with peers to start a conversation or deal with comments or questions about her acne:

- *Introducing a subject, use of a distraction technique "over there" – "What did you do last night?" or "What lesson have you got now?" These questions allow Amy to take control of the conversation.*
- *Assertive/confident responses – "Can we talk about something else?" or "I can think of more interesting things to talk about". These responses help to redirect the conversation.*
- *Having something to say – "I have acne. Sometimes it's brought on by stress."*

Application of FACES in the healthcare setting

The FACES model can be adapted to a hospital or community setting, and a graded approach is recommended with the setting of goals for those living with skin conditions. This helps them prepare and develop the number and variety of coping strategies with which they feel comfortable.

> "Just sitting and talking to somebody about this 'thing' that I felt had affected my life and that I have always kept hidden . . . that you are not alone . . . there are other people in the same situation . . . It doesn't have to have such a negative impact on your life."

The psychosocial aspects of skin disease are frequently a priority for patients and this needs to be recognized. Every member of the clinical team, its leadership and management have a role to play in promoting access to psychosocial care and interventions, overseen by a trained psychologist or similar (Table 12.1 and Box 12.3).

It is important that professionals consider how information can be sensitively conveyed to each patient and how they respond. For example, consider the detrimental impact on a patient recently diagnosed with vitiligo of being told *"What will happen is you will get patching on your face, it'll get worse, and you'll end up looking like a panda."*

Table 12.1 Roles of healthcare professionals

Tier	People and professionals	Role
1	Whole team (clinical and non-clinical staff)	Recognition of psychological needs (including privacy and boundaries)
2	Professionals with additional expertise, such as nurses, physiotherapists, occupational therapists, social workers	Identifying and basic screening for psychological distress in all patients, flagging up issues to Tier 3 specialists
3	Trained and accredited psychosocial professionals, e.g. counsellors, assistant psychologists, community psychiatric nurses	Assessment and diagnosis of all patients/families for psychological distress; management of basic psychopathology
4	Mental health specialists, such as clinical psychologists, psychotherapists and psychiatrists	Diagnosis and treatments of psychopathology; supervision of Tier 2 and 3 staff
5	Psychosocial care coordinators, such as consultant clinical psychologists or psychotherapists	Management of psychosocial rehabilitation for the whole team

Box 12.3 How can healthcare professionals support patients learning to live with their skin condition?

Assess a patient's psychosocial needs:

- Social support
- Coping mechanisms
- Self-esteem
- Anxieties
- Attitude
- Your own attitudes and terminology

Give:

- Full information and advice – especially when there are a variety of treatment options

- Hints and tips for dealing with comments, stares, unwanted attention

Refer:

- To other professionals for emotional support/ counselling as appropriate
- To patient/voluntary support networks or condition-specific support groups
- For social interaction skills training

PRACTICAL TIPS

- A patient can face psychosocial difficulties in every aspect of his/her life.
- The extent or severity of a skin condition does not correlate with the degree of emotional and social distress caused.
- To facilitate the best long-term, psychosocial adjustment, patients need access to effective help and support to promote living with confidence.
- All healthcare professionals play an integral role in facilitating good adjustment and best patient outcome.

References

1. Magin PJ. A cross-sectional study of psychological morbidity in patients with acne, psoriasis and atopic dermatitis in specialist dermatology and general practices. *J Eur Acad Dermatol Venereol* 2008; 22: 1435–1444.
2. Schofield JK. *Skin Conditions in the UK: A Health Care Needs Assessment*. Nottingham: Centre of Evidenced-based Dermatology, University of Nottingham, 2009.
3. Lansdown R. *Visibly Different: Coping with Disfigurement*. Oxford: Butterworth-Heinemann, 1997.
4. Troilius A. Treatment of hemangiomas and port-wine stains with emphasis on lasers. *Dermatol Ther* 2000; 13: 17–23.
5. Whittington-Walsh F. The broken mirror: Young women, beauty, and facial difference. *Women's Health Urban Life* 2006; 6(2): 7–24.
6. Reflections on Body Image. *All Party Parliamentary Group on Body Image*. Central YMCA, 2012. Available at ymca.co.uk.
7. Egan K. A qualitative study of the experiences of people who identify themselves as having adjusted positively to a visible difference. *J Health Psychol* 16: 739–749.
8. Kleve L. A survey of psychological need amongst adult burn-injured patients, *Burns* 1999; 25: 575–579.
9. McMichael L. (2012). Skin camouflage can play an important part in improving wellbeing for patients with permanent or chronic skin problems. *BMJ* 2012; 344: d7921.
10. Kent G. Testing a model of disfigurement: effects of a skin camouflage service on well-being and appearance anxiety. *Psychol Health* 2002; 17(3): 377–386.
11. Clarke A. (1999) 'Psychosocial aspects of facial disfigurement; problems, management and the role of a patient-led organisation' *Psychol Health Med* 4(2): 129–142.

CHAPTER 13

Chronic skin disease and anxiety, depression and other affective disorders

Steven Reid[1] and Wojtek Wojcik[2]

[1] Central and North West London (CNWL) NHS Foundation Trust, St Mary's Hospital, London, UK
[2] Royal Edinburgh Hospital, Edinburgh, UK

Common mental disorders such as anxiety disorders and depression, with a lifetime prevalence of up to 20%, are frequently co-morbid with chronic skin disease. However, the relationship between the two is complicated. In dermatology, the prevailing view is that skin disease causes distress, and likewise its treatment will reduce it. We witness, for example, increased suicidality in people with severe acne. However, it is also true that mental disorders such as depression can increase the subjective distress and disability caused by chronic skin disease, and can interfere with effective treatment adherence.

The classic cases described in psychodermatology are those where the psychopathology is inarguably causal to the presenting complaint, such as delusional infestation and dermatitis artefacta. However, the population health burden of co-morbid common mental disorder with chronic skin disease is much greater. A study of the UK General Practice Research Database involving more than 900 000 patients found that patients with psoriasis were 37% more likely to have a diagnosis of depression than matched controls, and that this increased with the severity of psoriasis [1]. A World Health Organization study involving 245 000 patients worldwide found that depression had a

larger impact on health scores than chronic physical disorders such as arthritis or asthma, and that depression co-morbid with a chronic physical illness (9–23%) had a greater health decrement than either alone [2]. Depression and anxiety commonly occur together.

Clinicians will commonly encounter distress and despair in the medical setting and determining at what point specific treatment is appropriate can be a challenge. In practice, two features are of particular importance: (i) the severity and duration of the symptoms and (ii) the impact on the patient's functioning and quality of life. Both anxiety and depressive states can be associated with increased perceptions of pain and distress that in turn accentuate the functional impairment of skin disease.

Defining features of key mood and anxiety disorders (see Table 13.1 for DSM-5 criteria)

The key disorders are:
- *Mood disorders:*
  - major depression;
  - bipolar disorder;
  - persistent depressive disorder (dysthymia).

Practical Psychodermatology, First Edition. Anthony Bewley, Ruth E. Taylor, Jason S. Reichenberg and Michelle Magid.
© 2014 John Wiley & Sons, Ltd. Published 2014 by John Wiley & Sons, Ltd.

- *Anxiety disorders:*
  - generalized anxiety disorder;
  - social anxiety disorder (social phobia);
  - specific phobia;
  - panic disorder.

Major depression

The core features of major depression are low mood, fatigue and anhedonia (inability to experience pleasure) lasting more than 2 weeks. Other symptoms (Table 13.1) include excessive guilt, poor concentration, suicidality, sleep disturbance and appetite or weight change. In severe illness, psychotic symptoms (e.g. delusions and/or hallucinations) can occur. Self-neglect may be a feature and this may include neglect of treatment regimens for skin disease.

Bipolar disorder

Bipolar disorder affects approximately 1–2% of the population and is defined by episodes of pathologically elevated mood as well as of depression (Table 13.1). Bipolar disorder is classed as Type I when manic episodes occur or Type II when milder hypomanic episodes feature. Elevated mood may also be an adverse effect of treatment with corticosteroids.

Persistent depressive disorder (dysthymia)

Dysthymia is a mood disorder characterized by symptoms that lack the severity necessary for a diagnosis of major depression, but which are chronic, persisting for at least 2 years (Table 13.1).

Table 13.1 DSM-5 classification of depression and anxiety disorders (source: Diagnostic and Statistical Manual of Mental Disorders, Fifth Edition. Reproduced with permission from American Psychiatric Association).

Major depression	Duration of 2 weeks or longer
	Either (i) depressed mood most of the day or (ii) loss of interest or pleasure
	Three or more of:
	• Weight loss >5% in a month or persistent increase/decrease in appetite
	• Insomnia or hypersomnia most days
	• Psychomotor agitation or retardation (restless or slowed down)
	• Fatigue, loss of energy
	• Worthlessness or excessive guilt
	• Reduced concentration or indecisiveness
	• Suicidal ideas
Mania	Duration of 1 week (or any if hospital admission required)
	Three (or four if mood only irritable) of:
	• Inflated self-esteem/grandiosity
	• Reduced need for sleep
	• More talkative
	• Subjective experience of racing thoughts or "flight of ideas"
	• Increased goal-directed activity or agitation
	• Increased distractibility
	• Increased risk taking in pursuit of pleasure:
Hypomania	Duration of 4 days or longer
	Three (or four if mood only irritable) of symptoms of mania (see above)
	Unequivocal change in behaviour uncharacteristic of the person when well
	Disturbance in mood is observable by others
	Episode is not severe enough to cause marked impairment in social/occupational function, hospitalization is not required, no psychotic features

Continued

Table 13.1 Continued

Persistent depressive disorder (dysthymia)	Duration of 2 years or longer Depressed mood for most of the day, for more days than not (1 year for children and adolescents) Two or more of: • Increased or decreased appetite • Increased or decreased need for sleep • Poor self-esteem • Poor executive functioning (i.e. decision making and concentration) • Hopelessness During the 2 year period the person has never been without the symptoms for >2 months at a time There has never been a manic episode, mixed episode, or hypomanic episode The criteria for cyclothymia have never been met The symptoms are not better explained by a psychotic disorder (e.g. schizophrenia, delusional disorder) Significant impairment in function
Panic attack	Four or more of the following (reaches a peak within minutes): • Heart racing • Increased sweating • Shortness of breath • Choking sensation • Gastrointestinal distress • Lightheadedness/dizziness • Feelings that things are not real (derealization/depresonalization) • Fear of "going crazy" • Fear that one is dying • Chills or hot flashes • Numbness or tingling
Agoraphobia	Anxiety about being in a place from which escape may be difficult (e.g. public transport, outside home alone, supermarket) The situations are avoided, endured with marked distress or require a companion Not better accounted for by another anxiety disorder.
Panic disorder	Recurrent panic attacks At least one attack followed by 1 month or more of: • Persistent concern about further attacks • Worry about implications of the attack ("having a heart attack," "going crazy") • Significant change in behaviour (May be with or without agoraphobia. If with agoraphobia, both diagnoses should be assigned)
Specific phobia	Marked, persistent, unreasonable fear cued by a specific object or situation Exposure to a stimulus provokes immediate anxiety response Recognized by the person as excessive or unreasonable Avoidance of phobic situation Significant impairment of function or marked distress May include phobias to: • Animals • Natural disasters • Blood/injection/injury • Situational (e.g. airplanes, elevators)

Table 13.1 Continued

Social anxiety disorder (social phobia)	Marked fear of social or performance situations featuring unfamiliar people or scrutiny by others. Fear of humiliation or embarrassment Exposure to the situation provokes anxiety, which may be a panic attack Recognized as excessive or unreasonable Avoidance Impaired function Not due directly to substance use, a medical condition or another mental disorder
Generalized anxiety disorder	6 months or more of excessive worry on most days about various events or activities Difficult to control the worry Three or more of: • Restlessness or feeling on edge • Easily fatigued • Poor concentration, mind going blank • Irritability • Muscle tension • Sleep disturbance The worry is not specific to the cues of another anxiety disorder or mental disorder (such as somatic symptom disorder or eating disorder) Significant distress or impaired function Not due to direct effect of substances, a medical condition (e.g. hyperthyroidism) and not occurring in the context of another mental disorder (e.g. depression)

Generalized anxiety disorder

The core feature of this disorder is constant irrational worry over which the person feels he/she has little control. Unlike with the phobias, there is no specific trigger for the onset of anxiety symptoms. Generalized anxiety disorder is usually associated with a range of somatic symptoms, including hyperventilation, tachycardia and sweating.

Social anxiety disorder (social phobia)

Social phobia is defined by crippling shyness and avoidance of social situations, often starting in adolescence (Table 13.1). It may feature particularly in presentations of skin disease with visible lesions.

Specific phobia

Specific phobias are characterized by persistent, excessive fears triggered by the presence or anticipation of a specific object or situation.

In healthcare settings, blood/injury/injection phobias, involving a fear of being injured, of seeing blood or of invasive medical procedures (e.g. blood tests or injections), are particularly significant given their propensity to compromise investigations and treatment.

Panic disorder

Panic disorder manifests with sudden, repeated attacks of fear (panic attacks) that last for several minutes. Sometimes the symptoms last longer. Panic attacks are characterized by a fear of disaster or of losing control, and are associated with marked somatic symptoms (Table 13.1). Panic attacks are often unpredictable and lead to constant fear of the possibility of another attack.

Agoraphobia

Agoraphobia may present as a fear of going outside and/or of being in crowded places, complicating attendance at clinic (Table 13.1).

Pathogenesis

Biological factors

Both anxiety disorders and depression have recognized heritability, although not to the same extent as bipolar disorder. Serotonergic pathways are implicated in both depression and anxiety states, with noradrenergic pathways diverging from the locus coreleus, particularly in anxiety. Increased sensitivity of the hypothalamo-pituitary (HPA) axis is involved in anxiety and some depression cases. Lower levels of brain-derived neurotrophic factor (BDNF) are reported in illness states and are linked to lower volume subcortical structures, such as the hippocampi in depression.

Psychological factors

Core beliefs about ourselves and the world impact on how we interpret, respond to and learn from events in life. A history of early neglect, abuse and relationship difficulties increase the likelihood that someone may not have optimal ways of coping with the world. A flare of a dermatological problem may activate self-critical beliefs and compound perceptions of disfigurement, which lead to social isolation and thus further risk of mental disorder. Avoidance secondary to anxiety or self-neglect in depression may delay presentation to dermatology. Public reaction to visible skin disease may potentiate feelings of shame and low self-worth.

Social factors

Significant life events are recognized precipitants for both depression and anxiety. They may also lead to exacerbations of chronic skin diseases. Life events include:
• breakdown of a relationship;
• family crises;
• bereavements;
• health problems;
• loss of employment;
• accommodation crises.

Clinical assessment

The assessment of mental disorders is by clinical interview, although screening questionnaires are commonly used to support this (see Chapter 2 and Appendix). Clinical assessment involves:
• use of screening tools in the waiting room;
• history and examination to establish the presence of criteria for diagnosis;
• further clarification of severity and risk of suicide;
• differential diagnosis;
• consideration of the interaction with cutaneous disease.

Screening questionnaires

Questionnaires can be filled in by patients before being seen in clinic. Commonly used scales include the Patient Health Questionnaire (PHQ), which is widely used in primary care in the UK, and the Hospital Anxiety and Depression Scale (HADS) [3,4]. In the US, the PHQ-9 and Beck Depression Inventory-II (BDI-II) are used frequently to screen for depression (see Chapter 2), and the Mood Disorder Questionnaire (MDQ) to screen for mania. These may serve as a guide to symptom severity, facilitate making a diagnosis and aid in monitoring response to treatment.

Useful screening questions for anxiety disorders include:
• Tell me how you are feeling at the moment?
• Is there anything that you worry about more than you think is reasonable?
• Do you often feel tense or find it difficult to relax?
• Is there anything you cannot do because of fear or worry?

History and examination

In addition to asking about the symptoms of anxiety and depression, enquire about how this is impacting the patient's daily life. Enquiry about suicidal thinking is always a standard part of assessment (see Chapter 6). The history taken will also consider what contributory or causal factors may be present (such as a flare of psoriasis, or recent marital break-up or unemployment). Where there is co-morbidity or a broad differential diagnosis, taking a careful history of how the symptoms started will usually clarify this, but a collateral history from a spouse or parent can be invaluable (see Chapter 2).

There should be specific consideration of treatments for skin disease that may have psychiatric adverse effects (e.g. isotretinoin and steroids) (see Chapter 3).

When enquiring about sensitive topics (e.g. suicidality), it is useful to remember that if the clinician is comfortable asking a question, the patient is more likely to feel comfortable answering it. Many clinicians working outside mental health initially find it awkward to ask about self-harm. For either depression or severe/generalized anxiety, this is essential (see Chapter 6). Mental health services should be contacted urgently if the following are elicited:

- *Suicidality* – ongoing suicidal thoughts, particularly if these involve planning of how to do it.
- *Psychotic symptoms* – such as persecutory delusions or the patient is distracted by hallucinations.
- *Clinician disquiet* – if the clinician finds him/herself feeling that there is something seriously wrong or unsafe, even if he/she cannot articulate it.

Differential diagnosis
Depression
- *Adjustment disorder* – "sub-threshold" psychological reaction to a life event, not meeting full criteria for depression, but significant depressive symptoms are present.
- *Dysthymia* – longstanding chronic depressive symptoms of over 2 years' duration.
- *Bipolar affective disorder* – elicited by taking a history of past episodes of elevated mood (mania). Bipolar depression requires a different treatment plan and psychiatric referral.

Anxiety
- *Adjustment disorder* – symptoms are milder, less chronic, and in response to a life event.
- *Substance use disorder* – history and examination will demonstrate use pattern and withdrawal symptoms (see Chapter 27).
- *Depression* – a full history should distinguish this, but psychomotor agitation in depression may present similarly to generalized anxiety. Depression and anxiety commonly occur together.
- *Obsessive-compulsive disorder* – presence of obsessions and ritualized compulsions which reduce anxiety when carried out (see Chapter 16).

Interaction with skin disease
Both mood and anxiety disorders may impact on skin disease through:
- self-neglect and decreased adherence to daily treatment;
- lower tolerance of side effects;
- increased perception of pain, itch or disfigurement;
- catastrophization of disfigurement.

Share these concerns with the patient, taking care to sound collaborative and not punitive. Involving the spouse or parent of a patient can be helpful.

Management

The treatment of anxiety and depression (Box 13.1 and Box 13.2) includes:
- education, self-help, and active monitoring (see Chapter 7);
- referral for psychological therapy (see Chapter 5);
- antidepressant medication – for anxiety disorders or depression (see Chapter 3);
- if not responding to treatment, expressing suicidal thoughts or severely functionally impaired, referral to specialist mental health services (see Chapter 6).

Box 13.1 Treatments for depression

- Education, self-help, active monitoring, support groups in primary care
- CBT (individual, computerized or group)
- SSRI antidepressant for moderate or severe depression
- If SSRI unsuccessful, consider venlafaxine or a second SSRI
- Contact mental health services if suicidality elicited, or not responding to treatment

Box 13.2 Treatments for anxiety disorders

- Education, self-help, active monitoring, support groups in primary care
- CBT (individual only for social phobia)
- SSRI antidepressant if psychological therapy unsuccessful or if patient preference. Consider pregabalin or gabapentin
- Consider co-morbidity, such as depression or substance misuse, if refractory to treatment

The first step is to discuss the anxiety or depression with the patient and explain your concern. It is important to put this in the context of the patient's situation, as often patients may find the suggestion of mental disorder alarming or unacceptable.

What is the clinician's role?

Referral by the hospital doctor or nurse to the general practitioner (GP) or psychodermatology service, if one is available locally, is appropriate. If the patient describes ongoing suicidal ideas or planning, seek urgent help.

A GP can establish initial treatment (see below) and coordinate onward referral to psychological services. Severe, complex or refractory cases are referred to mental health services.

Treatment approaches: self-help and community support, psychological therapy and medication

There are three evidence-based approaches to treatment. In the UK, these are usually tiered in a stepped-care model (see Chapter 7), where education and self-help is followed by psychological therapy or medication. Specialist services offer more intensive treatment for severe or refractory cases, including more intensive psychotherapy and third-line medication approaches.

Self-help and education with active monitoring

In cases of mild and moderate illness, initial education about the condition and self-help may initiate gradual resolution of symptoms, as the patient draws upon his/her resources and receives support from others. For example, the anxious patient who believes his/her gastrointestinal distress, headaches, poor concentration and dizziness herald a progressive physical illness may require a lot of education to accept he/she has a generalized anxiety disorder, but once there is acceptance, he/she may be far better able to self-manage symptoms and improve. Attending a community group can be helpful, as hearing the experiences of others can normalize a person's distress, and approaches for recovery can be shared. The GP can maintain active follow-up and progress to the treatments described below if needed.

Psychological therapies

The majority of good quality evidence for psychological therapy is specific to cognitive-behavioural therapy (CBT), with different tailored approaches for each diagnosis. The essence of this approach is to establish a collaborative partnership with the patient, which involves education and scrutiny of beliefs, thoughts and actions in daily life. Unhelpful thoughts are elicited through diary keeping and reflection, and modified by testing hypotheses with experiments. Behavioural experiments help modify learned fear responses and avoidance.

Medication

Antidepressant medication has good evidence of benefit in systematic reviews of randomized controlled trials in depression. Antidepressants are effective not just for depression, but also anxiety disorders and the treatment of chronic pain [5].

SSRI antidepressants

This class of antidepressant medication works on serotonin and is considered first line for pharmacotherapy of depression and anxiety disorders. It is noteworthy for its relative safety in overdose, in contrast with older antidepressants, such as tricyclics (e.g. amitriptyline). However, selective serotonin reuptake inhibitors (SSRIs) can induce significant "activation" symptoms in the first weeks of treatment before any clinical benefit is felt. If uninformed of these, the patient may discontinue the medication, particularly if he/she is anxious. Also, SSRIs are associated with a slightly increased bleeding risk, hyponatraemia and risk of an idiosyncratic reaction called serotonin syndrome (Box 13.3). For further reading, consult the Maudsley Prescribing Guidelines (UK) or the Physicians Desk Reference (US).

Failure to respond

Specialist referral is appropriate for patients who do not respond to standard therapy, including medication and CBT. The standard approach is to reassess the diagnosis, consider untreated co-morbidities and check which treatments have been trialled and whether these have been trialled fully. For example, a patient may have disengaged from SSRI treatment because side effects were inadequately explained, or the psychological therapy may

Box 13.3 Common side effects of SSRI antidepressants

- Nausea
- Loss of libido or erectile dysfunction
- Diarrhoea or constipation
- Restlessness and tremor
- Insomnia or hypersomnia
- Excessive sweating

have been discontinued prematurely. Ongoing stressors at home or work may complicate treatment (e.g. marital strain, debts, legal difficulties).

Treatment of specific disorders

Depression

Evidence-based treatment options are recommended by the National Institute for Health and Care Excellence (NICE) in the UK, which publishes guidance based on systematic reviews and health economic analyses of treatments (Box 10.1) [6]. It recommends stepped care as follows:

- *Initial self-help*, including bibliotherapy, exercise, social activities. Many patients with mild symptoms will improve with simple interventions like this, with active monitoring to confirm improvement.
- *Psychological therapy* – group or computerized CBT, or individual CBT. Some patients may prefer computerized CBT (e.g. if they have difficulty leaving home or co-morbid social phobia).
- *Pharmacotherapy* – trial an SSRI, then consider venlafaxine or duloxetine, or another SSRI if there is no response. Venlafaxine and duloxetine are antidepressants that work on norepinephrine and serotonin (SNRIs), and may be more potent antidepressants at higher doses than the SSRIs, but may have less tolerability.
- *If no response* – consider referring to mental health services for an opinion. Consider the diagnosis also; is there a co-morbidity such as alcohol, or a personality disorder, or is the diagnosis wrong (e.g. bipolar depression)? Note that response does not mean full resolution and that many patients may feel better on treatment but experience residual symptoms, particularly if perpetuating factors (such as financial and domestic stressors, poor coping skills) are present.

Anxiety

Treatment (Box 13.2) approaches for anxiety are similar to those for depression, and often both are treated in the same patient. Self-help can be beneficial (e.g. if a patient can restructure his/her perception of the danger of the aversive cues or somatic symptoms he/she experiences when anxious). Psychological treatment models have evolved for each disorder. Drug treatment (with SSRIs) often takes longer and may require a higher dose than for depression.

Agoraphobia

Psychological therapy involves evaluating thoughts and beliefs about the aversive situations, practising relaxation techniques and exposure to incrementally more aversive environments (from doorstep to supermarket).

Sertraline, escitalopram, citalopram, and paroxetine are licensed for agoraphobia with panic.

Generalized anxiety disorder

Self-education and bibliotherapy are often the first-line treatment. Psychological therapies or pharmacotherapy are second line. Psychological therapy includes education and experiments to test the benefit of worrying (worrying can become a coping skill in chronic patients), as well as relaxation techniques.

First-line pharmacotherapy is sertraline or escitalopram. Pregabalin is a second-line option in the UK. Pregabalin is an anticonvulsant with evidence and licence for treatment of generalized anxiety disorder, and is less addictive than benzodiazepines (which are not recommended for chronic anxiety symptoms).

If there is no response, consider co-morbidities and referral to specialist services. If harmful or a substance use disorder is identified, this should be treated first, as anxiety may then resolve.

Social anxiety disorder (social phobia)

Following self-help and education, individual CBT is recommended. Patients often have a history of social anxiety disorder dating back to adolescence, and deeply ingrained negative cognitions about how they are perceived and how others respond to them.

Pharmacotherapy is second-line treatment; escitalopram or sertraline are recommended.

Bipolar disorder

The treatment of bipolar disorder is initiated by psychiatric services and not covered here. However, first-line mood stabilizers are all associated with potential dermatological complications:
- *Lithium* – associated with exacerbation of, for example, psoriasis, but the prescribing psychiatrist may not note this co-morbidity.
- *Anticonvulsants* – valproate is a first-line mood stabilizer. Lamotrigine and carbamazepine are also being used as first- or second-line treatment. These and other drugs in this class are known to cause Stevens–Johnson syndrome, toxic epidermal necrolysis (TEN) and drug reaction with eosinophilia and systemic symptoms (DRESS).

Future research

There is much scope for further research on biological factors, psychological treatments and the shared social impact of cutaneous disease and mental disorders. Possibilities include:
- Evidence of an association between inflammatory factors and cytokines in depression may present hypotheses for future research into any biological factors mediating an association with dermatological disorders such as psoriasis or atopic eczema.
- Further research on the impact of perceived disgust and shame in acute skin disease on the risk of depression. Previous social psychiatry research indicated that "shaming" life events may be a particular risk for depressive illness.
- Improved collaborative models of psychological care may improve outcomes in patients with depression or anxiety co-morbid with skin disease. More tailored and collaborative approaches may be more effective.

PRACTICAL TIPS

- Depression and anxiety commonly occur together.
- A pervasive loss of interest or pleasure in doing things is a core feature of depression.
- Enquiry about suicidal thinking is an essential part of an assessment of mood.
- Antidepressants may be effective not just for depression but also for anxiety disorders and chronic pain.

References

1. Kurd SK *et al.* The risk of depression, anxiety, and suicidality in patients with psoriasis: a population-based cohort study. *Arch Dermatol* 2010; 146: 891–895.
2. Moussavi S *et al.* Depression, chronic diseases, and decrements in health: results from the World Health Surveys. *Lancet* 2007; 370: 851–858.
3. Kroenke K, Spitzer RL, Williams JB. The PHQ-9: validity of a brief depression severity measure. *J Gen Intern Med* 2001; 16: 606–613.
4. Zigmond AS, Snaith RP. The hospital anxiety and depression scale. *Acta Psychiatr Scand* 1983; 67: 361–370.
5. Taylor D, Paton C, Kerwin R. *The Maudsley Prescribing Guidelines in Psychiatry*. Oxford: Wiley Blackwell, 2012
6. National Institute for Health and Care Excellence. The Depression Pathway. Created May 2011. Last updated Sept. 2013 http://pathways.nice.org.uk/pathways/depression (accessed 10 December 2013).

Psychiatric disorders with secondary skin manifestations

CHAPTER 14

Delusional infestation

Peter Lepping,[1] Roland Freudenmann[2] and Markus Huber[3]

[1] School of Social Sciences and Centre for Mental Health and Society, Bangor University, and BCULHB, North Wales, UK
[2] Department of Psychiatry, University of Ulm, Ulm, Germany
[3] Department of Psychiatry, General Hospital Bruneck, South Tyrol, Italy

Delusional infestation describes a fixed, false belief by a person that he/she is infested with living or inanimate pathogens (Box 14.1). This belief is held despite a lack of medical evidence for such an infestation [1]. Patients often believe that the pathogens are living underneath or on their skin, which is the reason they commonly present to dermatologists. Less commonly, patients believe that the infestation is inside their body or in their immediate environment (e.g. house or garden). The descriptions of the alleged pathogens have changed over time, from scabies and worms, to bacteria, to insects, then to viruses. The 21st century has seen an emergence of inanimate objects such as fibrous strands, although insects are still the most commonly alleged source of infestation [2]. As is well known in psychiatry, delusional themes often change with cultural shifts.

Delusional infestation is estimated to have annual incidence rates of 2.37 and a prevalence of 17 per million inhabitants per year [1,3]. Most studies report a female-to-male ratio of 2.5:1 [1]. The median age is towards older patients, with very few cases having been reported in the under 30s. About half of all patients with delusional infestation present with what they believe is proof of their infestation, either in a container or as photography, the so-called "specimen sign" [4]. There is no particular association with socioeconomic status, education or childhood problems. Studies have also failed to identify any particular personality traits [1]. Risk factors include social isolation and visual impairment. About 90% of patients with delusional infestation seek help from a dermatologist (not a psychiatrist).

Defining features

Delusional infestation can occur as a primary or a secondary disorder. About half of all cases in large case studies are a primary delusional disorder described as a persistent delusional disorder (F22.0) in ICD-10 or a delusional disorder, somatic type (297.1) in DSM-5 [1]. The delusions are present for at least 1 month, and cognitive and social functioning is otherwise preserved. Secondary delusional infestation can arise in the context of medical disease, psychiatric disorders or substance misuse (Box 14.2).

Patients may use aggressive chemicals on their skin, such as bleach, which causes additional secondary skin problems and can in turn reinforce the belief of infestation. Sometimes patients believe they are contagious and avoid social contact, which can lead to significant social isolation. Delusions by proxy (the patient believes someone else to be infested) are not uncommon; particular care should be taken when children are presented with alleged

Practical Psychodermatology, First Edition. Anthony Bewley, Ruth E. Taylor, Jason S. Reichenberg and Michelle Magid.
© 2014 John Wiley & Sons, Ltd. Published 2014 by John Wiley & Sons, Ltd.

Box 14.1 Synonyms of delusional infestation (reason why they are misnomers)

- Ekbom's syndrome (eponymous)
- Delusional parasitosis (but other alleged pathogens now more common)
- Monosymptomatic delusional hypochondriasis (not explicit enough and not a neurotic disorder)
- Parasitophobia (not a phobia)
- Dermatozoenwahn – mixes the Greek words for animal and skin with the German word for delusion (less well-known internationally, and non-living pathogens are becoming more common)

infestation as child protection issues need to be considered (see below).

Pathogenesis

Most patients describe an event (e.g. the sighting of an insect) at the beginning of their illness. This can be a real sighting, a misinterpretation of a real perception (called "illusion" in psychiatry) or a true hallucination. Rather than dismissing the possibility of an infestation, errors of probabilistic reasoning occur, which may have a neurological basis, and reinforce the belief that there is a true infestation.

Magnetic resonance imaging (MRI) in patients with delusional infestation indicates a disruption in brain areas associated with the *interpretation* of perceptions rather than the perception itself. Disturbed functioning of the putamen and the associated dorsal striato–thalamo–cortical loop is thought to cause somatic delusions and tactile misperceptions, while frontal dysfunction is hypothesized to be responsible for disturbed reality testing. The involvement of the dopaminergic putamen and the therapeutic efficacy of D_2-dopamine antagonists (antipsychotics) in delusional infestation indicate dopaminergic dysfunction in delusional infestation. Patients with intoxication from

Box 14.2 Aetiology of delusional infestation (DI)

Primary DI
Persistent delusional disorder (ICD-10 F22) = delusional disorder somatic type (DSM-5 297.1)

Secondary DI
- Toxic – substance-induced psychotic disorder:
  - Illegal drugs: mostly amphetamines, cocaine, tetrahydrocannabinol (THC) (ICD-10 F1x.5)
  - Prescribed medications: usually dopaminergic agents, rarely antibiotics such as ciprofloxacin, clarithromycin or steroids (ICD-10 06.0/2)
- General medication conditions or those affecting brain function and/or inducing pruritus and paraesthesia:
  - Systemic infections, e.g. tuberculosis
  - Endocrine disorders, e.g. hypothyroidism
  - Solid tumours or haematological diseases
  - Chronic or acute liver or renal failure
  - Malnutrition and hypovitaminosis, e.g. vitamin B_{12} deficiency
  - Autoimmune disorders, e.g. systemic lupus erythematosus
  - Leprosy
- Brain disorders, e.g. tumour, cerebrovascular disease, stroke, traumatic brain injury, infections, etc.
- Dementia
- Delirium
- Psychiatric:
  - As part of a schizophrenic illness
  - As major depression with psychotic symptoms
  - As rarities: learning disabilities, borderline personality disorder, anxiety disorder

Special forms
- DI as a *shared psychotic disorder* (folie à deux, etc.) – as the inducer or as the receiver
- DI as *DI by proxy* – often presented in a child or a pet

substances influencing the dopamine transporter (e.g. cocaine, amphetamines, bupropion) may experience delusional infestation as well, further supporting this observation [5] (Figure 14.1).

Secondary delusional infestation is most frequently reported in elderly patients with

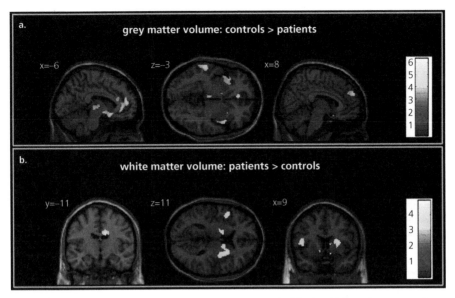

Figure 14.1 Grey and white matter volume changes in patients with delusional infestation compared to controls.

generalized brain atrophy or subcortical vascular encephalopathy, often in Type 2 diabetes and cerebrovascular disease. In stroke patients, delusional infestation often occurs following lesions of the right temporoparietal cortex, thalamus, and putamen [1].

Assessment (Box 14.3)

Patients with delusional infestation will frequently say that they will do anything to get rid of their infestation. However, they are often reluctant to see a psychiatrist. Clinics in Austria, Germany, the UK and the US have utilized the Psychodermatology Multidisciplinary Team model with varying success. In these clinics, psychiatrists have jointly assessed patients suspected of having delusional infestation with a colleague from dermatology or tropical medicine.

The general approach to a patient with psychocutaneous disease has been described in Chapter 2. There are more specific techniques

Box 14.3 Assessment of patients with delusional infestation

- Risk and suicidal ideation
- Risk to others – folie à deux, delusional infestation by proxy (children!), and factitious or induced illnesses
- Material patient brings
- Underlying disorders (organic and psychiatric)
- Substance abuse
- Real (genuine) infestations

for patients with delusional infestation (Box 14.4).

The first step in the assessment is to evaluate whether the onset has been acute or insidious. An acute onset would suggest an acute intoxication with cocaine or other illicit substances, the possibility of a delirium, or the new onset of neurological deficits or a cardiovascular accident. For a list of tests to be considered in a patient with delirium or mental status changes see Chapter 2. A careful history of prescribed

Box 14.4 Tips for the initial approach to patients suspected to have delusional infestation

- The first appointment will probably take longer than a normal new patient assessment. Prepare ahead of time if possible
- Take the patient's story seriously. Acknowledge the patient's suffering. Show empathy and offer to help to reduce distress!
- Take time for a careful history, including possible exposure to parasites on trips to tropical resorts
- Perform the diagnostic investigations needed (even if you are sure that the patient has no infection) and examine all specimens carefully
- Do *not* use words like "delusion(al)," "psychotic", "psychological" or "psychiatric", etc. Instead, paraphrase the symptoms ("your itch", "the sensations", "the crawling")
- Explore the patient's reasoning for his/her belief that he/she is infested
- Do *not* try to "calm down" the patient (e.g. "be happy it's not infectious", "it is only psychogenic"); this will upset them
- Do *not* overlook frank aggression against other healthcare professionals
- Do *not* forget to ask patients with despair and signs of manifest depression about suicidal ideation and to evaluate any risk to others

Box 14.5 Medications that can cause delusional infestation (known publications)

- *Illicit psychotropic drugs:*
  - Cocaine
  - Crack cocaine
  - Amphetamines
  - Amphetamines plus tetrahydrocannabinol (THC)
  - THC
  - Alcohol
- *Stimulant drugs:*
  - Pemoline
  - Methylphenidate
  - Amphetamine diet pills
- *Anti-parkinsonian drugs:*
  - L-DOPA
  - Peribedil
  - Ropinirole
- *Antibiotics:*
  - Clarithromycin
  - Ciprofloxacin
  - Erythromycin
- *Antiepileptics:*
  - Topiramate
- *Others:*
  - Corticosteroids
  - Interferon alpha 2b plus ribavirin
  - Phenelzine
  - Bromide intoxication

medication should also be taken as macrolide antibiotics, such as erythromycin, as well as corticosteroids, anti-parkinsonian drugs and antituberculosis treatment are associated with a sudden onset of delusional infestation. See Box 14.5 for a list of medications that have been associated with DI.

In the majority of cases the onset will be more insidious, in which case it is first necessary to exclude the possibility of a real infestation. This will always include a clinical examination (Figure 14.2), a careful history, including travel abroad, and routine lab investigations, including inflammatory markers (Box 14.6). It is important to investigate any specimens (Figure 14.3) presented by the patient microscopically and microbiologically. Bacterial super-infections

are common and may confuse the picture [1,6], as may bed bugs or scabies.

The examination of the patient and the specimens will help to form a trusting relationship, which will serve as the foundation for later treatment. This is paramount given that most patients with delusional infestation have been told in the past by others that their symptoms are "all in their mind". Many are therefore highly suspicious of any additional specialist opinion. It is important to make clear from the beginning that the patient's symptoms will be taken seriously and the possibility of an infestation will be seriously considered. However, if no clinical signs of infestation are found, this has to be clearly communicated, as there is never any therapeutic advantage in colluding with a patient's delusion.

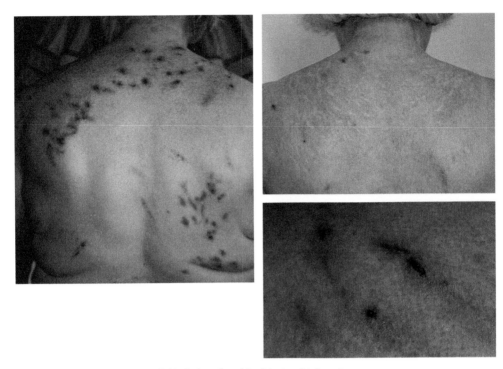

Figure 14.2 Typical distribution of skin lesions found in delusional infestation..

Box 14.6 Investigation of delusional infestation

Suggested:

- Full blood cell count
- Erythrocyte sedimentation rate
- C-reactive protein
- Serum creatinine and electrolytes
- Liver function
- Thyroid stimulating hormone
- Urine analysis (obligatory for illicit drug use testing) in particular testing for cocaine, amphetamines and cannabinoids
- Microscopical/microbiological examination of any specimens provided by the patient

Optional:

- Pregnancy testing – where appropriate
- B vitamins and folate

- Fasting glucose and lipids, ECG (especially if antipsychotics are considered)

To be considered in specific clinical constellations:

- Borrelia, treponema, hepatitis and human immunodeficiency virus (HIV) serologies
- Vasculitis screening
- Allergy testing
- Skin biopsy
- Skin scrapings
- Carbohydrate-deficient transferrin
- A chest X-ray and an electrocardiogram (ECG) can be necessary
- Electroencephalography (EEG)
- Cranial MRI to rule out brain pathology

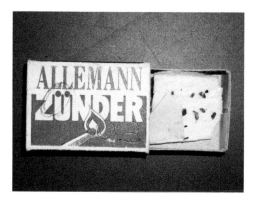

Figure 14.3 Example of the specimen sign.

In recent years some patients have started to advocate a new disease entity they call Morgellons disease. The possibility of an undiscovered pathogen, in this case fibres, was attractive to many sufferers and with the internet, the idea spread quickly. A recent study by the United States Center for Disease Control and Prevention, funded after pressure from self-declared Morgellon's sufferers, showed no evidence of real infestation or infection [7]. See Chapter 26 for a more extensive discussion of this phenomenon and the literature surrounding it.

Dermatologically, it is important to examine the patient's skin very carefully because there may well be a need for the treatment of secondary skin lesions or super infections. You should look for pruritis senilis (the elderly can have idiopathic pruritis), acne excoriée and dermatitis artefacta. Immunobullous diseases and contact dermatitis may be diagnosed with skin biopsy.

If these evaluations are negative, delusional infestation can be diagnosed. It is important to look for secondary causes of delusional infestation as well (see Box 14.6). Drug screens are helpful.

It is important to consider the possibility of delusional infestation by proxy when an inducer presents with his/her child, other relative, or pet with an alleged infestation. Conversely, you should ask whether the patient feels that other people might be infested as well, particularly when the patient has younger children who may be subjected to treatment against the alleged pathogens. Clinicians should be alert to child protection issues in this situation. It is vital to question patients about what treatments they are using or considering using on their children. If patients are acting on delusional beliefs in this way, they may be posing a risk to the wellbeing of any children in their care, and this concern must be raised with the appropriate child protection authorities for a full risk assessment.

Treatment

In the case of sudden-onset delusion, the treatment is to address the underlying illness or the cessation of the triggering substance. In cases of cocaine- or antibiotic-related delusional infestation particularly, the intensity of the symptoms can be so severe that it might be necessary to give emergency haloperidol for immediate relief.

With secondary delusional infestation, success depends on the successful treatment of the underlying illness (Figure 14.4). In cases of acute intoxication, it is usually sufficient to stop the substance that triggered the delusional symptoms.

Treatment of the skin must be concurrent with psychological and psychiatric treatments (Table 14.1).

If the delusion is shared by one or more other people, it is important to find the so-called inducer and treat him/her. Those sharing the delusions in a secondary capacity will usually improve with treatment of the skin only. In cases of delusional infestation by proxy where children are involved, it is highly likely that child protection procedures are necessary as discussed above.

For patients with insidious onset of DI, you should not attempt to treat the patient with psychiatric medication at the first visit. The follow-up visit should be used to continue to

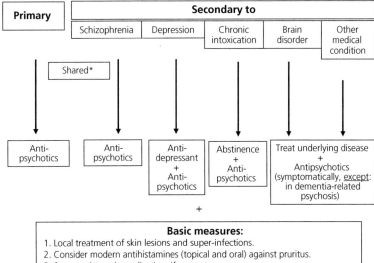

Figure 14.4 Treatment pathway (Source: Lepping and Freudenmann, 2008 [6]. Reproduced with permission of Wiley.).

Table 14.1 Concurrent treatment of delusional infestation [6]

Skin	Psychiatric disorder	Risk and underlying disorder
Emollients	Antipsychotics are first line (choose according to the lifestyle of the patient):	Suicidal risk
Antibiotics (topical and systemic).		Substance abuse (see Chapter 27)
Antihistamines		Of associated affective or cognitive disease:
Phototherapy	• Risperidone (0.5–4 mg)	
Try to avoid using antiparasite treatment such as ivermectin unless there is a genuine infestation	• Olanzapine (2.5–10 mg)	• Antidepressants
	• Amisulpride (200–400 mg)	• Acetylcholinesterase inhibitors for dementia
	Others	• Treatment of stroke
	• Haloperidol (2–5 mg)	Other underlying causes:
	• Pimozide (ECG and other monitoring essential)	• Antibiotics and prescribed medication
	• Antidepressants to treat secondary depression	

ECG, electrocardiography

establish rapport and discuss the results of any laboratory testing performed during the initial consult. Do not try to convince the patient that he/she does not have a real infestation as, by definition, he/she will have a fixed, false belief.

Psychiatric referral, albeit in theory the logical way forward, may lead to disengagement by the patient, particularly if tried early. For other tips for the approach to the treatment of delusional infestation, see Box 14.7.

Box 14.7 Tips for continued management of patients with delusional infestation

- At follow-up, explain the results of the specimens, biopsies or laboratory tests. If they are negative, tell the patient that you have not found any pathogens or infections so far, and indicate that there is currently no evidence for a known infestation
- Do *not* attempt *immediate* psychiatric referral or try to establish psychopharmacological therapy too soon
- Indicate that you are familiar with the problem and that you were able to help other patients, not instantly but after a while
- Use the terms "unexplained dermopathy" or "Ekbom's syndrome" if the patients asks for the diagnosis
- Indicate that this may be due to overactivity of the nervous system and normal neurone-adaptive processes in the brain. It can be useful to use analogies of other situations where sensations arise centrally from the brain in the absence of a peripheral stimulus (e.g. phantom limb or the sensation of a watch still being on the wrist after it has been removed). Some (but not all) patients can accept the suggestion that perhaps an infestation that was present

has now been eradicated, but because of overactivity in the sensation signalling systems they can still feel sensations on the skin. Medication can then be presented as a way of dampening down this overactivity and reducing the skin sensations
- Psychopharmacological treatment depends on the form of delusional infestation. Most, but not all, patients need antipsychotics
- If indicated, introduce antipsychotics to reduce the distress that people experience and the unpleasant skin sensations, indicating that such medication has helped many of your other patients with similar problems
- Antipsychotics can be helpful against the patient's distress and itching (antihistaminic component of many antipsychotics)
- Try and persuade the patient to be adherent with antipsychotic medication. It may be necessary to tell the patient that he/she has nothing to lose and to give it a try as nothing else seems to have worked
- Do *not* prescribe antibiotics or any other anti-infective without evidence of a real infection (this will further reinforce the delusion)

At this time, there are no psychological (talk) therapies that have been shown to be effective in delusional infestation. Pharmacological therapy is the mainstay of treatment. Antipsychotics appear to reduce distress and symptoms, but persuading the patient to take them is very difficult. Adherence depends on whether patients trust their treating doctor. Reported response rates to antipsychotic medication are 70–80% [8,9]. The average time to the onset of action is about 1–2 weeks [8]. The doses are by and large lower than those used in schizophrenia.

It has been virtually impossible to conduct any randomized controlled trials, as delusional patients are difficult to recruit. A randomized controlled trial of pimozide from the 1980s included 11 patients in a cross-over study. It showed good response to pimozide [10], which explains why pimozide was for such a long time

the treatment of choice. However, a Cochrane review found pimozide to have a higher likelihood of causing extrapyramidal side effects such as akathisia (restless legs) than other first-generation antipsychotics in the treatment of schizophrenia. Other problems with pimozide are QTc interval prolongation and drug interactions.

Most authors recommend the use of second-generation antipsychotics (risperidone, olanzapine, amisulpride) over first-generation antipsychotics (pimozide, haloperidol) due to their improved side effect profile [1]. Response rates for second-generation antipsychotics are in the region of 75% [8] compared with 60–100% for first-generation antipsychotics. First-generation antipsychotics were more likely to achieve full remission, while second-generation antipsychotics were move likely to result in partial remissions [9].

It can be a challenge to get a patient to agree to take medications as prescribed. Since most patients will read the information leaflet that comes with the medication, it is important to explain that antipsychotic medication is usually used for illnesses such as schizophrenia, but can also be used for other experiences or symptoms, such as distress or anxiety. Explain that anti-psychotic medication may ease the level of distress the patient experiences. Signs of depression or suicidal ideation should not be missed, given patients' level of distress over their impaired quality of life. You may consider using "SIGECAPS" or other depression screens (see Chapter 2 and Appendix).

It is possible to treat patients with delusional infestation outside of psychiatric settings. In a survey of British dermatologists, about 60% of patients accepted psychiatric medication. In an elderly sample, 89% adherence was achieved. We therefore very much recommend that treatment is initiated by the doctor who sees the patient first, rather than embarking on a patient journey of many referrals, which often ends with no effective treatment. If not already familiar with antipsychotic medication, it is worth familiarizing yourself with one (e.g. risperidone 2 mg nightly, amisulpride 200–400 mg/day, or olanzapine 10 mg nightly; see Chapter 3). Treatment goals need to be clear. Remission does not require full insight into delusional thinking (which rarely happens), but merely the cessation of symptoms.

Future research

Patients with delusional disorders are difficult to recruit into clinical research trials. Current research concentrates on imaging studies and significant progress has been made recently with matched cohort imaging studies. It would be desirable to replicate these and to extend the field to other mono-delusional disorders to see whether they have similar imaging findings to those for delusional infestation.

PRACTICAL TIPS (FOR TREATMENT WITH ANTIPSYCHOTICS)

- Evidence is limited but pimozide is *not* the agent of choice because of concerns about drug safety.
- Most experience is with risperidone and olanzapine. The dosage needed is usually lower than in schizophrenia (e.g. 0.5–4 mg risperidone or 2.5–10 mg olanzapine). Amisulpride is also a promising option (200–400 mg/day).
- Expect first effects after 1–2 weeks and maximum effects after 6 weeks on average (3 weeks in secondary delusional infestation, 10 weeks in primary delusional infestation).
- All second-generation antipsychotics are an off-label use in delusional infestation (they are only approved for treating schizophrenia or, sometimes, mania).
- Discontinuation of antipsychotic treatment within a year often leads to a relapse.
- Treat the skin appropriately at the same time as treating the delusional component.

References

1. Freudenmann RW, Lepping P. Delusional infestation. *Clin Microbiol Rev* 2009; 22(4): 690–732.
2. Bewley A *et al*. Delusional parasitosis: time to change the name of the condition to delusional infestation. *Br J Dermatol* 2010; 163(1): 1–2.
3. Trabert W. Delusional parasitosis. Studies on frequency, classification and prognosis [in German]. Dissertation. Homberg/Saar: Universität des Saarlandes, 1993.
4. Freudenmann RW *et al*. Delusional infestation and the specimen sign: a European multicentre study in 148 consecutive cases. *Br J Dermatol* 2012; 167(2): 247–251

5. Wolf RC, *et al*. Abnormal gray and white matter volume in delusional infestation. *Prog Neuropsychopharmacol Biol Psychiatry* 2013; 46: 19–24.

6. Lepping P, Freudenmann RW. Delusional parasitosis: a new pathway for diagnosis and treatment. *Clin Exp Dermatol* 2008; 33: 113–117.

7. Pearson ML *et al.*; Unexplained Dermopathy Study Team. Clinical, epidemiologic, histopathologic and molecular features of an unexplained dermopathy. *PLoS One* 2012; 7(1): e29908.

8. Freudenmann RW, Lepping P. Second-generation antipsychotics in primary and secondary delusional parasitosis: outcome and efficacy. *J Clin Psychopharmacol* 2008; 28(5): 500–508.

9. Lepping P, Russell I, Freudenmann RW. Antipsychotic treatment of delusional parasitosis: systematic review. *Br J Psychiatry* 2007; 191: 198–205.

10. Ungvari G, Vladar K. Pimozide therapy in dermatozoon delusion [in German]. *Dermatol Monatsschr* 1984; 170: 443–447.

CHAPTER 15

Body dysmorphic disorder

Emma Baldock and David Veale

Institute of Psychiatry, King's College London and the South London & Maudsley NHS Foundation Trust, London, UK

Diagnostic criteria

The fifth edition of the Diagnostic and Statistical Manual for Mental Disorders defines the criteria for a diagnosis of body dysmorphic disorder (BDD) (Box 15.1). The 11th edition of the International Classification of Diseases and Related Health Problems of the World Health Organization (ICD-11) will follow very similar diagnostic criteria.

Clinical features

The preoccupation with appearance in BDD is characterized by high levels of negative intrusive imagery and extreme appearance-related self-consciousness [1]. Appearance concerns may relate to any part of the body, but often include the skin (e.g. in 73% of more than 500 patients surveyed by Phillips [2]) (Figure 15.1). Insight may be poor and beliefs about appearance may be held with delusional conviction (sometimes termed body dysmorphic disorder without insight or delusional disorder, somatic type). Commonly reported appearance-related behaviours in BDD fall broadly into three categories:

- those that are aimed at restoring or enhancing a feature (e.g. cosmetic procedures);

- those that are aimed at avoiding, camouflaging or distracting attention away from a feature (e.g. the use of excessive make-up or distracting jewellery);
- those that are aimed at verifying how one looks (e.g. mirror-checking) [1].

Seeking dermatological, surgical or other medical treatment is one of the most common (up to 76%) appearance-related behaviours in BDD [2] (Box 15.2). Dermatological treatment in particular was the most commonly sought and received in this sample (in 55% and 45%, respectively), and antibiotics were the most commonly received intervention. In our own unpublished survey of 439 people with BDD attending a psychiatric setting in the UK, the most desired dermatological cosmetic procedures in order of popularity were laser resurfacing, laser hair removal, dermafiller, dermabrasion, scar treatments, botox injections and electrolysis.

BDD patients, particularly those seeking dermatological treatment, may also present with psychogenic excoriation or skin picking as a means of trying to "improve" their appearance.

BDD is associated with high rates of suicidal ideation and attempted suicide, and a high degree of functional impairment and distress (see Chapter 6).

Practical Psychodermatology, First Edition. Anthony Bewley, Ruth E. Taylor, Jason S. Reichenberg and Michelle Magid.
© 2014 John Wiley & Sons, Ltd. Published 2014 by John Wiley & Sons, Ltd.

Box 15.1 DSM-5 diagnostic criteria for body dysmorphic disorder

A. Preoccupation with one or more perceived defects or flaws in physical appearance that are not observable or appear slight to others
B. At some point during the course of the disorder, the person has performed repetitive behaviours (e.g. mirror checking, excessive grooming, skin picking, or reassurance seeking) or mental acts (e.g. comparing his/her appearance with others) in response to the appearance concerns
C. The preoccupation causes clinically significant distress or impairment in social, occupational or other important areas of functioning
D. The appearance preoccupation is not better explained by concerns with body fat or weight in an individual whose symptoms meet diagnostic criteria for an eating disorder

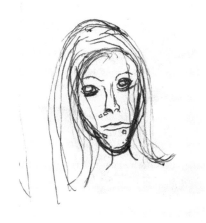

Figure 15.1 A self-portrait of a patient with BDD (courtesy of Dr D. Veale).

Box 15.2 Dermatological treatments sought by patients with body dysmorphic disorder

- Minoxidil (for perceived hair loss)
- Isotretinoin (for minimal acne)
- Antibiotics (for a variety of skin conditions)
- Surgical treatments (dermabrasion, fillers, botox, scar treatments)
- Other aesthetic treatments (lasers, others)

Epidemiology and presentation

The reported prevalence of BDD in community samples ranges from 0.7% to 2.4% [1]. The prevalence of BDD in dermatology clinics is substantially higher. For example, Conrado *et al.* [3] reported BDD prevalence rates of 7% in a general dermatology sample (n = 150) and 14% in a cosmetic dermatology sample (n = 150).

Bowe *et al.* [4] reported on a sample of 128 patients with acne aged 16–35 years and recruited from outpatient dermatology clinics. When more stringent criteria for acne were applied, 42 patients (32.8%) presented with minimal to non-existent acne, and 14.1% of this subgroup met diagnostic criteria for BDD. When less stringent criteria for acne were applied, 82 patients (64.1%) met criteria for mild acne and 21.1% of this sub-group met diagnostic criteria for BDD. There was a two-fold increased odds of BDD in patients requiring systemic isotretinoin therapy.

BDD patients present to mental health services an average of 10–15 years after onset of the condition, and before that are more likely to present to cosmetic surgeons, dermatologists and primary care physicians. This is likely to relate to poor insight, but also to a fear of being misunderstood and being seen as vain. Even in mental health settings, patients are more likely to present with depression or social anxiety unless they are specifically questioned about symptoms of BDD (Figure 15.2).

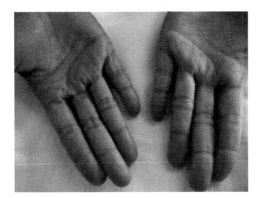

Figure 15.2 A 28-year-old Asian patient with (normal) hyperlinearity (increased skin markings) of the palms. This patient was severely depressed and responded eventually to SSRIs and CBT, together with attempts to improve the palmar appearance (courtesy of Dr A. Bewley).

Aetiology

There is very little evidence for specific risk factors in the development of BDD. In terms of a genetic contribution, rates of BDD are elevated in first-degree family members of BDD patients, as are rates of OCD, suggesting shared genetic vulnerability factors. Temperamental traits of an avoidant personality, anxiety, perfectionism and self-consciousness may be risk factors for BDD, but there are currently no prospective data to establish any causal link. Social anxiety typically precedes BDD in patients co-morbid for both disorders, suggesting a common pathway. Cross-sectional and retrospective research provides evidence for elevated rates of childhood adversity (including sexual, emotional and physical abuse), and childhood bullying (especially appearance-related) in patients with BDD. In our clinical experience there may be a link between the onset of BDD and dermatological or other stigmata in adolescence, but this is yet to be examined empirically. Another putative risk factor specific to BDD is heightened aesthetic sensitivity. BDD patients are more

likely than other psychiatric patients, and twice as likely as the general population, to have an educational or occupational history in art or design and to be more aesthetically sensitive. For a referenced review of aetiology, see Veale and Neziroglu [1].

Detection and assessment

Veale and Neziroglu [1] provide a detailed guide to the assessment of BDD in a specialist mental health setting. Here we provide guidelines on the detection and diagnosis of BDD in dermatological settings.

- In a dermatological setting, the observation of marked distress in a patient who has a feature that is hardly noticeable or not that abnormal should always trigger screening for BDD.
- The Cosmetic Procedure Screening Questionnaire (COPS; see Appendix A10) [5] can be used to screen for BDD in the cosmetic or dermatological setting.
- The Body Dysmorphic Disorder Questionnaire (BDDQ; see Appendix A11) is an alternative screening questionnaire that has been validated for use in dermatological as well as psychiatric settings [6].
- The COPS [5] can also be used to measure symptom severity and to track changes in symptoms over time.
- Always be mindful of potential suicidal ideation (see Chapter 6).

A list of key diagnostic screening questions is provided below (Box 15.3).

In the UK, evidence-based guidelines for the assessment and treatment of BDD recommend that people with suspected or diagnosed BDD seeking cosmetic surgery or dermatological treatment should be assessed by a mental health professional with specific expertise in the management of BDD [7]. In an ideal world, a clinical psychologist or cognitive-behavioural therapist would be attached to a dermatological clinic.

Box 15.3 Diagnostic screening questions

- Do you currently think a lot about your skin?
- On an average day, how many hours do you spend thinking about your skin? Please add up all the time that your feature is on your mind and make your best estimate.
- Do you feel your skin is ugly or very unattractive?
- How noticeable do you think your skin is?
- Does your skin currently cause you a lot of distress?
- How many times a day do you usually check your skin, either in a mirror or by feeling it with your fingers?
- How often do you feel anxious about your skin in social situations? Does it lead to you avoiding social situations?
- Has your skin had an effect on dating or an existing relationship?
- Has your skin interfered with your ability to work or study, or your role as a homemaker?

Box 15.4 Key principles of engagement

- Recognize stigma and correct any misunderstandings (e.g. BDD as vanity)
- Do not argue about the content of the patient's appearance concerns or the diagnosis of BDD
- Instead, focus on the impact of the patient's appearance concerns on their distress and functioning, and validate their experience in these terms

Engagement

Engagement skills are particularly important in assessing and treating people with BDD, whether in the dermatological, primary care, or mental health setting. This is because of the discrepancy that commonly exists between the patient's own view of the problem (their appearance) and its solution (e.g. corrective therapy or surgery) on the one hand, and other people's view of the problem (the patient's perception of their appearance) and its solution (e.g. psychological therapy) on the other hand. Some key principles of engagement are summarized in Box 15.4.

Psychological and psychiatric treatment

Evidence-based treatment options
The evidence-based UK guidelines for the treatment of BDD recommend a choice of individual

cognitive-behavioural therapy (CBT) or a selective serotonin reuptake inhibitor (SSRI) in the case of moderate functional impairment, and a combination of CBT and an SSRI where there is severe functional impairment [7]. Two randomized controlled trials with wait-list controls have demonstrated the superiority of CBT for BDD over no treatment, and a series of case-control studies and case series have also supported the effectiveness of CBT. Two randomized controlled trials of an SSRI have demonstrated superiority of SSRIs for BDD over placebo. There is thought to be a dose–response relationship, with higher doses tending to have a better response. However, there is a significant risk of relapse when an SSRI is discontinued. There is no evidence for the benefit of antipsychotic medication and this is not recommended even in delusional variants of BDD. There have been no randomized controlled trials comparing CBT to an SSRI or to a combination of the two. For a referenced review of evidence-based treatment options, see Veale and Neziroglu [1].

The main treatment approach used for skin picking in the context of BDD is the use of self-monitoring and habit reversal, although the effectiveness of this approach has not been systematically evaluated either for skin picking in the context of BDD or for skin picking in its own right. Chapter 16 provides further details on skin picking.

Box 15.5 Summary of key components of cognitive-behavioural therapy

- Engagement and formulation
- Imagery rescripting
- Modifying attentional biases
- Modifying cognitive processes
- Behavioural experiments with exposure and response prevention

Cognitive-behavioural therapy

The following brief overview is based on Veale and Neziroglu [1].

CBT is usually offered in 12–16 weekly outpatient sessions and involves the key components listed in Box 15.5.

A key method for engaging patients in CBT is to help them to develop and test an alternative understanding of their problem (the formulation). This is to see their problem in terms of *worry* about appearance or their body image, rather than appearance itself. The patient is encouraged to use therapy to test out this alternative theory, on the grounds that he/she can always return to treating it as an appearance problem at the end of therapy. In the formulation, key early experiences are identified (e.g. teasing about appearance), and how they have informed the patient's current body image is explored. The patient's current attentional, cognitive and behavioural responses to his/her appearance concerns are then identified, along with the consequences of these responses in maintaining appearance-related preoccupation and distress.

Following this formulation work, treatment usually begins with imagery re-scripting. This involves updating early experiences (e.g. of appearance-related bullying) and aims to de-couple the patient's current body image from such experiences.

A range of attention training techniques, including "detached mindfulness", is used to address cognitive processes such as rumination and worry, and also to shift the patient's attention away from him/herself and his/her body image and onto the external world (e.g. onto other people or the environment or an activity).

Behavioural experiments are used to generate new information and to test out the theory that the patient's problems may be better described in terms of *worry* about appearance, rather than appearance itself. Typically, the patient tests out the theory by entering situations he/she would normally avoid, dropping his/her usual responses such as camouflage and rumination, and applying his/her new techniques (e.g. an external focus of attention).

CBT is usually deferred in patients who are seeking a cosmetic procedure or other medical procedure, or the procedure is deferred until the end of CBT. Otherwise the procedure will interfere with the patient's ability to test out the theory that his/her problem is one of worry. A possible exception is where a patient has damaged his/her skin through skin picking. Phillips [2] suggests that in this case a combination of psychiatric and dermatological treatment may be indicated, but with a warning that the dermatological treatment is unlikely to bring any relief to BDD symptoms.

There are no prospective data available on the outcomes of dermatological treatments in patients with BDD, but retrospective data suggest that the symptoms of BDD do not tend to improve following such procedures, and that where patients are in fact satisfied with the outcome, their preoccupation tends to recur on the same or a different body part [8]. Phillips [4] surveyed 250 people with BDD who were receiving dermatological treatment, and found that BDD symptoms improved in 27 (9.8%), remained the same in 217 (81.9%) and worsened in 23 (8.3%). In the dermatology literature, BDD patients have been reported to respond poorly to dermatological treatment [9].

In a study comparing individuals without BDD who were satisfied with their rhinoplasty

Box 15.6 Guidelines on dermatological treatment and body dysmorphic disorder

1. Screen and assess for BDD
2. If you believe the patient has BDD following screening and assessment, share the diagnosis with them
3. Advise referral to a mental health practitioner for a full assessment and further advice
4. Explain the rationale for referral to a mental health practitioner in terms of the significant risk of dissatisfaction with the procedure, and the likelihood that preoccupation and distress will remain or move to another body area
5. Avoid arguing with the patient about whether his/her perceived "defect" is real or imagined
6. Express lots of empathy about his/her distress and preoccupation
7. Do not refer for a second opinion from another dermatologist; instead, discuss with a mental health practitioner and refer for a psychological or psychiatric assessment
8. Try and liaise with the patient and mental health professional to allow dermatological procedures to be completed prior to starting psychological therapy, or to postpone them until after psychological therapy or after a trial of SSRI medication
9. Consider co-working with a mental health professional, especially if there is damage from skin picking or if it helps to increase engagement

and BDD patients who craved rhinoplasty, the latter were more likely to believe that cosmetic surgery would significantly alter their life and more likely to be dissatisfied with other areas of their body [10]. Overall, patients are more likely to have a good psychological outcome if they can clearly describe the feature that concerns them, they are clear about the desired physical outcome, the outcome can be technically achieved and they have very modest psychosocial expectations from the procedure.

Summary guidelines for the management of BDD in dermatological practice are given in Box 15.6.

Future research

Two key priorities for future research are:
• prospective studies on outcome of dermatological treatments in patients with BDD;
• further trials on the effectiveness of the combination of CBT with SSRI medication.

PRACTICAL TIPS

• Seeking dermatological treatment is a common symptom of BDD.

• There is a significant risk of dissatisfaction with any dermatological treatment in patients with BDD, and appearance-related preoccupation and distress is likely to remain or to move to another body area.

• The COPS or BDDQ can be used to screen for BDD in the dermatology clinic.

• If BDD is suspected, the patient should be offered a referral to a mental health professional with specific expertise in BDD, for an assessment.

• The evidence-based treatment recommendation for BDD is CBT, combined with an SSRI where the functional impairment is severe.

• There should be liaison between physical and mental health professionals to avoid running dermatological procedures and psychological/psychiatric interventions in parallel, and to co-work where there is both BDD and genuine skin pathology.

References

1. Veale D, Neziroglu F. *Body Dysmorphic Disorder: A Treatment Manual*. Chichester: John Wiley & Sons Ltd, 2010.
2. Phillips KA. *The Broken Mirror: Understanding and Treating Body Dysmorphic Disorder*. Oxford: Oxford University Press, 2005.
3. Conrado LA *et al*. Body dysmorphic disorder among dermatologic patients: prevalence and clinical features. *J Am Acad Dermatol* 2010; 63(2): 235–243.
4. Bowe WP *et al*. Body dysmorphic symptoms among patients with acne vulgaris. *J Am Acad Dermatol* 2007; 57: 222–230.
5. Veale D *et al*. Development of a cosmetic procedure screening questionnaire (COPS) for body dysmorphic disorder. *J Plast Reconstruct Aesthetic Surg* 2012; 65(4): 530–532.
6. Dufresne Jr RG *et al*. A screening questionnaire for body dysmorphic disorder in a cosmetic dermatologic surgery practice. *Dermatol Surg* 2001; 27: 457–462.
7. National Institute for Health and Care Excellence (NICE). Obsessive-compulsive disorder: core interventions in the treatment of obsessive-compulsive disorder and body dysmorphic disorder. Clinical guideline no 31. London: NICE, 2005.
8. Veale D. Psychological aspects of a cosmetic procedure. *Psychiatry Med* 2006; 5(3): 93–95.
9. Cotterill JA. Review of body dysmorphic disorder. *Dermatol Clin* 1996; 14(3): 457–463.
10. Veale D *et al*. Cosmetic rhinoplasty in body dysmorphic disorder. *Br J Plast Surg* 2003; 56: 546–551.

CHAPTER 16

Pickers, pokers, and pullers: obsessive-compulsive and related disorders in dermatology

Jonathan S. Abramowitz and Ryan J. Jacoby

Department of Psychology, University of North Carolina at Chapel Hill, Chapel Hill, NC, USA

Obsessive-compulsive disorder (OCD) and a number of conditions thought to be associated with it [i.e. obsessive-compulsive related disorders (OCRDs)] are among the most impairing psychological conditions. The symptoms of these problems often interfere with work or school (e.g. missing deadlines), interpersonal relationships (e.g. repeatedly seeking reassurance), activities of daily living (e.g. using the bathroom), and – as we focus on in this chapter – can be associated with bodily injury (e.g. dermatitis). The psychopathology of OCRDs is also complex: affected individuals struggle against ubiquitous unwanted thoughts, doubts, and urges to perform senseless behaviors that are difficult to resist. This chapter will focus on the nature, assessment, and treatment of OCD and related symptoms, especially as they pertain to the field of dermatology.

Defining features

Obsessive-compulsive disorder

OCD is defined by the presence of *obsessions* and *compulsions* (Box 16.1) that produce significant distress and cause interference in role functioning [1]. Although washing/cleaning and checking rituals are most commonly observed,

rituals might involve ordering/arranging, counting, and reassurance seeking (Box 16.2).

The prevalence of OCD is about 2–3% in the adult population and its course is generally chronic, with waxing and waning of symptoms, often in relation to the degree of stress in the person's life.

Washing and cleaning rituals are among the most likely OCD symptom presentations to show effects on the skin. The most common dermatological effects of these behaviors include dermatitis, pruritis, and excoriation. However, a number of skin diseases have also been observed among individuals with OCD, including acne, eczema, lichen amyloidosis, drug sensitivity, effluvium, erythema, and nevus.

Body dysmorphic disorder

Body dysmorphic disorder (BDD) (see Chapter 15) involves excessive concern with an imagined or slight defect in appearance (e.g. a minor skin blemish). Although once categorized as a somatoform disorder, it is now classified as an OCRD in DSM-5 as it shares many features with OCD. Like OCD, thoughts of the defect lead to significant anxiety and subsequent compulsive behaviors [e.g. checking in mirrors, hiding perceived defect (camouflaging), and excessive grooming] to reduce anxiety.

Practical Psychodermatology, First Edition. Anthony Bewley, Ruth E. Taylor, Jason S. Reichenberg and Michelle Magid.
© 2014 John Wiley & Sons, Ltd. Published 2014 by John Wiley & Sons, Ltd.

Box 16.1 Obsessions and compulsions

Obsessions are intrusive thoughts, ideas, images, impulses, or doubts that the person experiences as senseless or disturbing and that lead to anxiety. Examples include unwanted thoughts of germs and contamination and unwanted doubts of violence or mistakes. Obsessional themes, however, vary widely from person to person and might also concern religion and morality, sex, order, harm, symmetry, and numbers.

Compulsions are urges to perform overt (e.g. checking, washing) or mental (e.g. praying) rituals according to certain rules that are designed to neutralize or prevent obsessional fears and reduce anxiety.

Box 16.2 Obsessive-compulsive disorders in dermatology

- Washing cleaning and checking rituals
- Hair pulling disorder (see Chapter 10)
- Skin picking disorder: acne excoriee, nodular prurigo (see Chapter 22), habit tic deformity of the nail

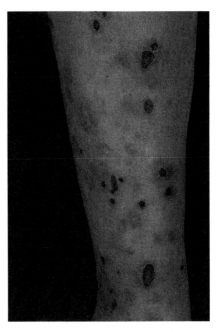

Figure 16.1 Skin picking disorder. Note the excoriated areas and areas at various stages of the healing process affecting the skin of this patient's legs (courtesy of Dr A. Bewley).

Trichotillomania (also known as hair pulling disorder; see Chapter 10)

Hair pulling disorder (HPD) is a behavioral problem in which the person pulls his/her hair to the extent that hair loss is noticeable. There is typically an increase in tension before pulling (or when attempting to resist), and gratification or relief afterwards [1]. Although the repetitive nature of the hair pulling might seem similar to compulsive rituals in OCD, there are no obsessions in HPD that drive the pulling. Rather, hair pulling might be precipitated by general tension, depression, anger, boredom, frustration, indecision, or fatigue [2], and may even occur outside of the person's awareness. Moreover, hair pulling leads to pleasurable feelings, a phenomenon not reported by OCD patients after completing rituals. HPD tends to affect females

more often than males. The prevalence rate is low (e.g. 0.6–1.5%).

Excoriation (skin picking) disorder (also known as pathological skin picking)

Skin picking disorder (SPD) is a problem in which the person engages in recurrent and repetitive picking of the skin, resulting in noticeable tissue damage, which causes significant social or occupational impairment or psychological distress (Figure 16.1). The major types of SPD in dermatology include nodular prurigo (see Chapter 22), acne excoriee, and habit tic deformity of the nail. In many, but not all individuals, the skin picking is triggered by specific situational cues, such as noticing a blemish or looking in the mirror. It might also have more general triggers, such as being alone, boredom, general distress, tension, or agitation. Similar to HPD, and unlike OCD, SPD is *not* characterized by persistent intrusive thoughts (obsessions). The picking behavior itself may be accompanied by feelings of gratification, relief, or pleasure in the short-term [3]. Although as many as one-fifth of the general population reports picking their skin to the point of causing tissue damage, clinically significant SPD has a prevalence rate in the range of 1.4–5.4%. The onset can be at any time, and tends to have a chronic yet fluctuating course. Moreover, it tends to affect women more frequently than men.

SPD can be associated with a number of dermatologic problems, including lesions, infections, and significant scarring. In extreme cases, SPD can have severe medical complications, such as exposure of muscles, vital arteries, and the need for amputation. Unfortunately, many individuals with this condition do not seek professional (mental or medical) help.

Acne excoriee (Figure 16.2), sometimes known as "picker's acne," is a form of SPD that occurs when someone with acne picks at the skin, resulting in a worsening of the blemishes and eventually a vicious cycle. The picking of acne blemishes might be motivated by appearance-related concerns or by the satisfying consequences (i.e. sensations) of picking. Such picking, however, often results in infection and further urges to pick that can be become very difficult to stop.

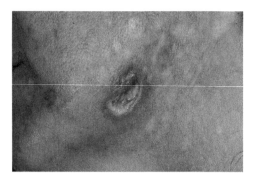

Figure 16.2 Acne excoriee. A patient with a very deep picked area on the cheek which she could not resist picking. Note the other adjacent scarred areas (courtesy of Dr A. Bewley).

Pathogenesis

The etiologies of OCD and the other conditions described in this chapter are largely unknown. One hypothesis is that biology plays a general role in creating vulnerabilities to these problems, whereas the individual's environment and learning history plays a more specific role in problem onset.

Contamination-related OCD

Although OCD is putatively associated with dysregulation in the serotonin and dopamine systems, neurotransmitter dysregulation has been implicated in many behavioral disorders and the results of studies have been inconsistent. Brain imaging studies suggest that the orbital cortex and the caudate nucleus might be associated with the expression of OCD symptoms [4], but findings are also equivocal. Behavioral models view contamination obsessions as arising from learning experiences in which once neutral stimuli (e.g. door knobs) are paired with fear and thus acquire the potential to trigger fear on their own (i.e. classical conditioning). Compulsive washing and cleaning behaviors, along with passive avoidance (e.g. refusing to touch "contaminated" objects), maintain the contamination fears by preventing their natural extinction. Cognitive-behavioral models emphasize the role of dysfunctional beliefs (e.g. "germs are lurking everywhere and I am vulnerable to illness") in the development and maintenance of contamination fears and washing behaviors.

Hair pulling and skin picking disorders

For both hair pulling and skin picking, a non-specific biological vulnerability might manifest in difficulty tolerating discomfort. Alterations in pain sensitivity (e.g. through up-regulation of the endogenous opioid system) might also influence the reinforcing quality of pulling behavior.

Behavioral models of HPD and SPD propose that these problems begin as normal responses to stress, but become associated with a variety of internal and external cues through conditioning mechanisms (e.g. [5]). Beliefs about the positive effects of pulling or picking (e.g. "hair pulling will make me feel better") or facilitative thoughts (e.g. "I'll just pick for a few minutes") may also cue episodes.

Assessment

There are no medical tests for OCRDs. The best way to determine whether OCD or a related condition is present in a dermatology patient is to conduct a careful clinical interview. In particular, it is important to understand behaviors that might be leading to skin problems, as well as the situations that trigger these behaviors and the consequences of the behaviors.

Contamination-related OCD

Washing and cleaning rituals, which can affect the skin, are usually triggered by obsessional fears of body secretions (e.g. urine, feces), dirt or germs, and environmental toxins (e.g., asbestos, household chemicals). Proximity to any stimulus that cues thoughts of feared contaminants, therefore, might provoke urges to wash or clean. Some patients fear becoming sick from the contaminants, and a subset worry that they will contaminate others. In other instances, a sense of disgust is more prominent than the fear of illness.

Rituals often involve excessive hand washing, showering/bathing, and use of handy wipes or disinfectant gels. Whereas some patients perform high frequencies of brief rituals (e.g. 50 brief hand rinses per day), others engage in fewer, yet more time consuming rituals (e.g. daily 90-minute rule-driven showers). Some patients establish sanctuaries (e.g. rooms) that they keep "uncontaminated." The use of barriers (e.g. paper towels, gloves) when touching surfaces or opening doors is common, yet patients may also take more exorbitant measures, including changing clothes and doing laundry excessively.

Accordingly, if contamination-related OCD is suspected, questions directed at identifying whether the above signs are present are appropriate:
- How many times do you wash your hands/shower each day?
- Do you have a special way that you wash?
- Are there other things you do to try to keep yourself clean?
- What concerns do you have about contamination or germs?
- What happens that makes you feel like you need to wash?
- What triggers the washing?
- What do you think would happen if you didn't wash your hands/shower in these situations?

In addition to these questions, the Dimensional Obsessive-Compulsive Scale (DOCS) [6] is a brief self-report instrument that assesses OCD-related contamination concerns (as well as other types of OCD symptoms) (see Appendix A9).

Trichotillomania

As with OCD, patients might be reluctant to disclose hair pulling, especially from certain parts of the body such as pubic area. Thus, if HPD is suspected, a straightforward and direct (asked in a matter-of-fact manner) and empathic approach to questioning is likely to yield more honest responses:
- How much time do you spend pulling each day and about how many hairs do you pull out each time?
- Where else on your body do you pull from? Some people pull from their pubic area – do you?

The MGH Hairpulling Scale (MGH-HPS) [7] is a seven-item self-report measure that assesses frequency, intensity, resistance, control, and distress related to hair pulling urges and behaviors (see Appendix A12).

Excoriation (skin picking) disorder

Patients with SPD typically pick at their skin in response to tension, which is reduced by the picking behavior. Patients might pick at healthy skin, or at scabs, acne, lesions, and other skin imperfections. The picking usually results in lesions at locations on the body that are easy to reach with the dominant hand (e.g. the face) and not in locations that are difficult to reach (e.g. the back). Patients might use their fingers or other objects (e.g. tweezers, scalpels, needles) to assist with skin picking. Depending on the method used, lesions or scars might be linear, round, or irregularly shaped. Moreover, whereas lesions from dermatologic diseases are usually symmetrical, those from HPD are often asymmetrical. Superficial erosions with underlying inflammation and erythema might be visible. Patients with SPD also often have long, ragged fingernails with staining and debris under the nails. The following questions might be helpful in identifying and understanding a patient's problems with SPD:

- How often do you pick at your skin?
- What parts of your body do you pick from?
- What else besides your fingers do you use to pick your skin?
- Tell me about the situations in which skin picking is likely to happen (Alone? In front of a mirror? Bored? Feeling stressed?)
- Do you usually plan to pick your skin or does it happen without your awareness?

In addition to these questions, the Skin Picking Scale (SPS) [8] is a six-item self-report measure assessing skin picking symptom severity (see Appendix A13).

Treatment (Box 16.3)

Obsessive-compulsive disorder

Meta-analyses of randomized controlled trials show that the most effective treatment for OCD is cognitive-behavioral therapy (CBT) using the techniques of exposure and response prevention (ERP). This treatment is associated with a

Box 16.3 Treatment strategies

Obsessive-compulsive disorder

- Cognitive-behavioral therapy:
  - Exposure
  - Response prevention
- Medication: serotonin reuptake inhibitors

Hair pulling and skin picking disorders

- Stimulus control:
  - Eliminate cues
  - Make picking/pulling more difficult
  - Eliminate positive reinforcements
- Habit reversal training:
  - Awareness training
  - Competing response training
  - Social support
- Cognitive therapy
- Medication:
  - Serotonin reuptake inhibitors
  - Olanzapine

60–70% reduction in symptoms on average. Exposure entails systematic, repeated, and prolonged confrontation with stimuli that provoke anxiety. In *situational* exposure, the patient encounters actual feared stimuli, such as toilets, door knobs, and floors. In *imaginal* exposure, the patient envisions anxiety-provoking obsessional thoughts, doubts, and images (e.g. of becoming ill or making a loved one ill). Response prevention means refraining from performing the compulsions. For example, a patient who fears contamination from chemicals such a pesticides would practice using such chemicals as directed in the house. They would also refrain from performing any rituals (e.g. washing, asking for assurance from "experts") to reduce anxiety or the chances of illness. The aim of ERP is to teach patients with OCD that they can manage obsessional anxiety (which will not persist indefinitely) and that avoidance and rituals are not necessary for averting harm.

Most medication trials for OCD show that serotonergic medications (e.g. clomipramine, sertraline) can be effective. Average symptom reduction rates, however, are only 20–40% and most treatment responders show residual symptoms after an adequate trial. Adverse effects and relapse after medication discontinuation are additional problems.

Hair pulling and skin picking disorders

Similar psychological (i.e. CBT) and pharmacological approaches are used in the treatment of HPD and SPD, and therefore we consider them together in this section. Most versions of CBT involve three components: stimulus control, habit reversal training, and cognitive therapy.

Stimulus control procedures involve three steps. First, situations (e.g. idle time alone) and stimuli (e.g. mirrors, tweezers) that are cues for pulling and picking behavior are identified and eliminated or attenuated from the patient's environment. Second, the pulling or picking response is made more difficult, such as by wearing a shorter hair style, putting bandages on fingers used to pull or pick, putting Vaseline on the eyelashes, or wearing gloves when in high-risk situations. Finally, reinforcing aspects of pulling or picking are identified and also attenuated. For example, patients who enjoy tickling their lips with hair after it is pulled might apply mild numbing agents on the lips in pulling prone situations.

Habit reversal training (HRT) [9] also includes three main components: awareness training, competing response training, and social support. Awareness training involves the patient describing in detail the act of pulling or picking, along with its antecedents (e.g. triggers and warning signs) and consequences. Antecedents might include physical settings (e.g. in the bathroom), early behaviors in the chain leading to pulling (e.g. stroking the hair, feeling the skin), and private sensations such as urges, tension, specific thoughts, or stress. After the antecedents and the subsequent act of picking/pulling are identified, the patient practices detecting the behavior until the clinician is confident the

patient is aware of them. Self-monitoring of pulling and picking is often assigned as homework to further enhance awareness. Next, the patient is taught to engage in a competing response – an inconspicuous behavior that is physically incompatible with the act of pulling or picking (e.g. fist clenching, using hands for something else) – for 1 minute or until the urge to pull or pick passes (whichever is longer) when they notice a warning sign, or when they begin to pull or pick. The social support component of HRT involves finding a significant other who can gently prompt the patient to use the competing response when they are seen pulling or picking, and praise the patient for correctly engaging in the competing response.

Cognitive interventions for HPD and SPD target dysfunctional beliefs that maintain the pulling or picking cycle, such as perfectionistic thoughts, beliefs about controllability of pulling or picking (e.g. "I can pull just one hair and then stop"), and rationalizations (e.g. "I need to get the bumps off my skin so I can be relaxed and study.").

Evidence for the efficacy of pharmacotherapy for HPD and SPD is limited. Open trials suggest that the atypical neuroleptic olanzapine and the selective serotonin reuptake inhibitors (SSRIs) fluoxetine, fluvoxamine, citalopram, and paroxetine might be effective for HPD. However, other more well-controlled trials using wait-list and placebo controls showed that fluoxetine was less effective than CBT, and only as effective as pill placebo. It is not clear if medications may be an effective adjunct to CBT.

Discussing treatment and providing referral information

When a dermatology patient appears to display the signs and symptoms of an OCRD, begin by presenting your impression that the skin complaints appear to be related to a psychological condition, and then describe the specific problem using the information presented earlier in this chapter. Provide a referral to a knowledgeable mental health professional who can further evaluate the patient to confirm the diagnosis. The organizations (and websites) listed in Box 16.4 are good places to turn when searching for a referral, as they provide lists of knowledgeable providers on their websites.

If the patient is concerned about having a mental health diagnosis, convey acceptance of patient's difficulties as legitimate, authentic, and treatable. When discussing treatment, if the patient reports that they have previously had psychological therapy, the adequacy of this treatment should be assessed and compared to the established CBT techniques discussed in this chapter.

Box 16.4 Organizations (websites) with searchable referral databases for OCRD treatment

- Association for Behavioral and Cognitive Therapies (www.abct.org)
- Anxiety and Depression Association of America (www.adaa.org)
- International Obsessive-Compulsive Disorder Foundation (www.ocfoundation.org)

The following steps can be followed during this conversation with the patient:

1. Define the OCRD and review the signs and symptoms as discussed in this chapter. Emphasize that this problem is typically chronic and unlikely to get better without effective treatment.

2. Tell the patient that the exact causes of the problem are unknown. Emphasize that biological and environmental factors probably contribute in tandem with one another.

3. Describe medications for the OCRD, including their advantages (e.g. they are quick and easy to take) and disadvantages (adverse effects, may not be beneficial).

4. Describe CBT for the OCRD, including the advantages (high probability of success, long-term benefit) and disadvantages (hard work, potentially anxiety provoking).

Future research

Given that treatment outcome research for HPD and SPD is still extremely limited, additional investigation of the efficacy of treatments for these conditions is warranted.

PRACTICAL TIPS

- If a patient displays the signs of an OCRD, present your impression that the skin complaints are related to a psychological condition, and then discuss the psychological problem with the patient.

- Asking the assessment questions in this chapter can help identify the extent to which a skin problem is associated with behavioral difficulties.

- Input from a relative or significant other can also help identify the extent to which psychological/behavioral problems are contributing to the dermatological problem.

- Consider psychological treatment (i.e. CBT) before or in addition to recommending medications as the former has a stronger long-term effect, while also producing no side effects.

References

1. American Psychiatric Association. *Diagnostic and Statistical Manual of Mental Disorders*, 5th edn. Washington, DC, 2013.

2. Mouton SG, Stanley MA. (1996). Habit reversal training for trichotillomania: A group approach. *Cogn Behav Pract* 1996; 3(1): 159–182.

3. Odlaug B, Grant J. Pathological skin picking. In: Grant JE *et al.* (eds.). *Trichotillomania, Skin*

Picking, and Other Body-Focused Repetitive Behaviors Washington DC: American Psychiatric Publishing, Inc., 2011, pp. 21–41.

4. Whiteside SP, Port JD, Abramowitz JS. A meta-analysis of functional neuroimaging in obsessive-compulsive disorder. *Psychiatry Res Neuroimaging* 2004; 132: 69–79.

5. Azrin NH, Nunn RG. Habit-reversal: a method of eliminating nervous habits and tics. *Beh Res Ther* 1973; 11: 619–628.

6. Abramowitz JS *et al.* Assessment of obsessive-compulsive symptoms: Development and validation of the Dimensional obsessive-Compulsive Scale. *Psychol Assess* 2010; 22: 180–198.

7. Keuthen NJ *et al.* The Massachusetts General Hospital (MGH) Hairpulling Scale: 1. Development and factor analyses. *Psychother Psychosom* 1995; 64: 141–145.

8. Keuthen NJ *et al.* The Skin Picking Scale: Scale construction and psychometric analyses. *J Psychosom Res* 2001; 50, 337–341.

9. Grant J, Donahue CB, Odlaug BL. *Treating Impulse Control Disorder: A Cognitive-Behavioral TherapyP.* New York: Oxford University Press, 2011

CHAPTER 17

Factitious skin disorder (dermatitis artefacta)

Jonathan Millard[1] and Leslie Millard[2]

[1] *South West Yorkshire Partnerships Foundation Trust, UK*

[2] *Hathersage, Derbyshire, UK*

Defining features

Dermatitis artefacta is a form of factitious disorder in which a fully aware patient creates his/her own skin disease and hides the responsibility for his/her actions from physicians (Box 17.1). The DSM-5 code used for this condition is 300.19, "Factitious disorder" under the larger category of "Somatic symptom and related disorders." This allows a distinction from other disorders in which there is also self-inflicted skin damage (Table 17.1). Patients with dermatitis artefacta intend to assume the sick role, but are doing so for their own internal motives, which are often psychological.

The epidemiology of factitious skin disorder is confounded by inclusion of these other syndromes in the assessment, with prevalence values ranging from 0.04% to 1.5% in dermatology clinics. There is a female predominance of up to 20:1, but for preadolescents and those over 50 years this ratio falls to 4:1 (likely due to confounding diagnoses). All racial groups can present with factitious disorder [1].

Pathogenesis and common co-morbid illnesses

Factitious skin disorder is invariably associated with a co-morbid psychological or psychiatric disorder. It is the identification and correct treatment of the co-morbid condition that helps towards resolution of the factitious disorder. Those conditions most frequently underlying a presentation of factitious skin disorder are described below.

Adjustment disorders

Adjustment disorders are psychological reactions to an identifiable stressor. The disorder must begin within 3 months of the stressor and terminate within 6 months of the stressor ending.

The pattern of an individual presenting with factitious skin disease associated with an adjustment disorder can thus be predicted from the five DSM-5 criteria that define the code for adjustment disorder. Factitious skin disorder in these circumstances would present within 3 months of a major life event (criterion A), along with marked distress and/or loss of social, occupational or other important areas of functioning (criterion B). There would be no other history suggestive of another psychiatric illness (criterion C) and the picture would not represent a normal bereavement reaction (criterion D). The factitious skin disorder would be expected to terminate within 6 months if the stressor were removed (criterion E) [2].

In practice, stressors sufficient to cause factitious skin disorder are often chronic in nature,

Practical Psychodermatology, First Edition. Anthony Bewley, Ruth E. Taylor, Jason S. Reichenberg and Michelle Magid.
© 2014 John Wiley & Sons, Ltd. Published 2014 by John Wiley & Sons, Ltd.

Box 17.1 DSM-5 diagnostic criteria for factitious disorder 300.19

> **A.** Falsification of physical or psychological signs or symptoms or induction of injury or disease associated with identified deception.
> **B.** The individual presents him/herself to others as ill, impaired or injured.
> **C.** The deceptive behaviour is evident even in the absence of obvious external rewards.
> **D.** The behaviour is not better explained by another mental disorder such as delusional disorder or another psychotic disorder.

Table 17.1 Differential diagnosis of dermatitis artefacta

	Distinguishing features for dermatitis artefacta
Self-harm	Intent is not to feign physical illness but to deliberately commit harm to the body, often with stated suicidal intent
Self-mutilation	May be unintentional, seen in some profoundly learning disabled, severely neurologically impaired, and dementia patients
Skin picking disorders	Damages skin for relief of tension
Skin damage secondary to psychosis	Damages skin in response to delusions or hallucinations
Skin damage secondary to body dysmorphic disorder	Damages skin in response to overvalued ideas of perceived imperfection
Malingering	External motive present

and neither client nor physician has the opportunity to observe whether symptoms, including those of the factitious skin disorder, persist in the absence of the stressor, as the stressor does not terminate.

Depressive disorders

Factitious skin disorder can be seen with the new onset of a major depressive episode, as part of a recurrent depressive disorder, or as part of a bipolar affective disorder. It is usually a complex interplay of genetic susceptibility (family history), vulnerable cognitive styles and adverse life events that trigger episodes of depression.

Key points from the history include a family or personal history of affective disorders, a tendency to think negatively in three key areas ("the self, the world, the future", often referred to as Beck's cognitive triad), and interpersonal problems that tend to be chronic and poorly resolved, such as relationship, employment, fiscal, and legal problems. The picture would be of a patient presenting with at least five depressive symptoms coinciding with the onset of the factitious skin disorder. If manic symptoms are present, this would indicate bipolar disorder, and management would be different. Depression and bipolar disorders are discussed in detail in Chapter 13.

Many medical conditions can produce depressive symptoms, and must be ruled out first. Similarly, substance misuse can closely mimic depression, especially alcohol misuse, and should be approached differently. Of note, drug misuse clients presenting with self-inflicted lesions are more likely to be frankly malingering to obtain pain medication.

Personality disorders

At least one-third of patients presenting with factitious skin disorder will have an underlying personality disorder [3]. Personality disorders are enduring patterns of behaviours that deviate from the expectations of the individual's culture. This pattern is inflexible, and affects interpersonal functioning, emotional response and impulsivity. They usually begin in adolescence or early adulthood, and have a significant impact on the individual's social and occupational functioning.

There are three main groups of personality disorders:

• *Cluster A* – paranoid, schizoid or schizotypal; patients present in an odd, aggressive or eccentric manner.

- *Cluster B* – antisocial, borderline, histrionic or narcissistic; patients are dramatic, emotional and unnecessarily theatrical.
- *Cluster C* – anxious, dependent or obsessive-compulsive; patients present as anxious, uneasy and restless.

All may present with factitious skin disorder, but the most recognized association is with borderline and histrionic personality disorder in females and personality disorder in males. Personality disorders are discussed in Chapter 2.

The presentation of a personality disorder with factitious skin disorder would be suggested by a long history of contact with healthcare services, especially psychiatry, copious or multiple volumes of notes and requests for numerous opinions. There may be long-standing civil, family or criminal legal problems. The management of these patients is for experts only and not for clinical dermatologists (see below).

Other psychiatric illnesses and factitious skin disorder

It is unlikely that patients with factitious skin disorder have a primary simple anxiety disorder such as social phobia or agoraphobia. Bipolar psychosis and schizophrenic psychosis are also not often seen with factitious skin disorder, so the presence of psychotic symptoms will lead away from this diagnosis. There may, however, be an association between factitious skin disorder of the penis and psychosis.

Clinical assessment

Taking the history is the "capture time" when the process of co-operative working with the patient is negotiated. The verbal shape and content of the clinical history is often as diagnostic as the physical signs of the skin artefact. Patients with factitious disease are anxious, secretive and guarded in their replies. There may have been some form of confrontation at a previous consultation elsewhere. The patient

and the accompanying relatives may also be aggressive. Patients will give a "hollow history". For example, the lesions appear fully formed, but there is no apparent prodromal or developmental state (i.e. the lesions appear overnight and exacerbations occur with no witness). Younger patients in particular develop lesions on the way back from school or reveal them at bathtime. Characteristically there are few significant symptoms of burning, itching or pain before the event. The lesions are monomorphic and appear in crops.

The common sites are the arms, hands and anterior thighs, and in women the breasts. Facial lesions are lateral rather than central, and are on the cheeks, neck and chin. The nose, lips and eyes are not commonly involved. Genital involvement in factitious disease is uncommon and is more likely associated with severe psychotic illness. There may be a preference for the lesions to be on the non-dominant side and an absence of involvement on inaccessible areas such as the centre of the back.

The shape of the skin lesion is determined by the mechanism of production. You should not dwell excessively on the exact method of production but use characteristic appearances of lesions to support the diagnostic premise of factitious disease. Friction and scarification with abrasives produce irregular, linear, superficial, oozy/crusty lesions of uniform appearance in a surprisingly regular distribution, the areas being roughly equidistant rather than randomly distributed (Figure 17.1).

Blunt trauma produces bruises, often in the shape of the offending object. The corner of a table, for example, will form a star-shaped area and metal tools the shape of the instrument head (Figure 17.2).

Corrosive liquids such as bleach or battery acid cause acute blistering with impressive erythema, crusting and an eschar, which can be very adherent if the tissue necrosis is very deep. Characteristically a "drip sign" may be present because application of liquids is difficult to

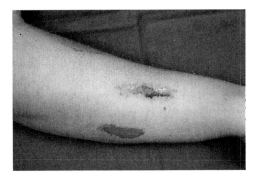

Figure 17.1 Scarification from friction instrumentation.

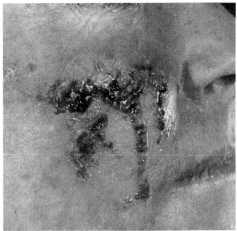

Figure 17.3 Drip sign from application of corrosive liquid.

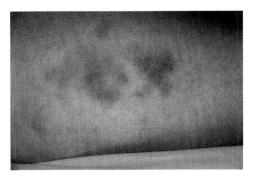

Figure 17.2 Bruising from external instruments.

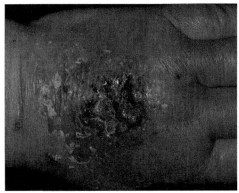

Figure 17.4 Injection of chemicals into the hand.

control when applied in these circumstances (Figure 17.3).

Chronic indolent lesions are more difficult and puzzling clinically. They resemble a panniculitis with boggy inflammation surrounded by a woody, hardened area that will eventually necrose and discharge. This clinical appearance can be the result of covert injections of milk, excreta, cosmetic oils, talc or, occasionally (in men), automotive lubricants. These are often on the anterior thighs, abdominal wall, breasts and non-dominant arm (Figure 17.4).

When simple surgical wounds such as biopsy sites, endoscopy incisions or wound closures fail to heal, one of the differential diagnoses should be factitious interference. This is important to consider when revisionary surgery has failed on many occasions. Factitious interference with a wound is far more common than genetic immune suppression or the growth of obscure bacteria, both of which can be ruled out by laboratory testing. Look for acute interference haemorrhages (from instrumentation, commonly needles or scissors) around the edges of the wound, or occasionally in the absolute centre of the wound (Figure 17.5).

Rubbing damage will show as a glazed polished area around the periphery where granulation tissue has been removed. Occasionally, colonization by odd bacteria such as faecal organisms will give a clue to contamination.

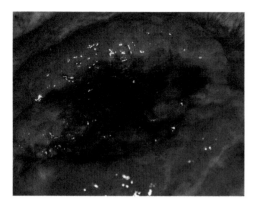

Figure 17.5 Central interference haemorrhage in a wound.

The clinical appearance of self-inflicted injuries often bears a passing resemblance to diseases the patient recognizes, so called "models to copy." In some cases patients covertly reproduce a disease they have suffered from, so-called dermatological pathomimicry (e.g. drug reactions by secretly taking the medicine they know they are allergic to; contact dermatitis from exposure to an allergen they have reacted to previously; or prolonging chronic leg ulceration by removing dressings). These patients may eventually induce a *real* clinical complication as a result of chronic interference (e.g. fistula formation in a wound). In dermatitis simulata, patients do not damage themselves but use their artistic talents to create camouflage that resembles disease, such as scaly skin (using glue), a birthmark (using paints) or a skin infection (using theatrical make-up).

Investigations

Most importantly, a primary skin disease should be ruled out. For patients with a likely diagnosis of dermatitis artefacta, any laboratory investigations will focus on promoting skin healing. A secondary benefit of these tests may be to give some clues as to the mechanism of damage and support a belief that the disease is factitious. Skin cultures can identify secondary infection and any curious organisms that may have been introduced (e.g. *Escherichia coli* from faeces). A biopsy of the lesions may help classify the type of damage, the depth, and the tissue reaction to such damage. Abrasions show as predominantly epidermal disruption with acute and some chronic inflammatory infiltrate. Acute necrosis may be evident and with chronicity, ulceration and signs of attempted epidermal repair.

Corrosive blisters show characteristic necrosis and acute cell death with an abrupt transition to normal skin. Suction and friction bullae, whilst clinically resembling a disease state, show the traumatic separation at the dermal–epidermal junction. Cryogenically-induced bullae (as from an asthma inhaler, or industrial or domestic aerosol) will show identifiable keratinocyte nuclear distortion. The haemorrhages from trauma are usually superficial and discrete, but sometimes extend into muscle. The deep panniculitis from foreign body injections may resemble a granuloma, but can be characterized with special techniques: lipids from milk or baby oil show as clumps of vacuoles with variable inflammatory response depending on the type of lipid and chronicity of the lesion, and talc granules show up on polarized light. Some complex substances such as toothpaste may provoke such an extensive reaction that histologically it resembles a T-cell lymphoma; in these cases, clinicopathological correlation is vital.

Treatment

The management and treatment of factitious disease is an almost unique experience for physicians, in that the patient is actively deceiving the healthcare team from whom he/she is seeking assistance. Direct confrontation has no place in the initial clinical management. The most important factor to remember is that this is *not* a criminal investigation that needs solving, but a psychological illness that requires identification and treatment.

The first objective is to offer an open, non-aggressive atmosphere that will allow a non-judgemental analysis of the problems. The patient's anxiety and suspicion can be allayed by permitting them to give an uninterrupted history (even when obvious anomalies exist) and an opportunity to discharge feelings of dissatisfaction at past treatment failures. Often relatives are outraged that previous consultations have suggested self-harm. Learning about the situation surrounding the initial onset of the disease may provide the physician with insight into the patient's initial psychological state. The aim is to gradually build up trust and a therapeutic rapport such that underlying psychosocial factors are uncovered and can then be addressed.

At the initial visit, it is important that the provider and patient agree on a forward strategy to consider all aspects of the illness, and that anger is displaced by positive optimism. The patient is given "homework" to think of any mechanisms that may be causing the disease, both physical (however unlikely) or psychological (even if it is painful to contemplate). This homework allows the patient to offer a positive contribution to the process of resolution rather than the negativism that comes with defence from suspicion.

Not uncommonly the patient may return with a "quasi-explanation" as a cause, and this should be taken as an invitation to discuss both the physical and psychological elements of the illness further. Dermatologists are extremely good at assessing visual and tactile clues, but perhaps lack the same verbal negotiating dexterity as psychiatrists and psychologists to convey these thoughts. A few useful phrases that are not antagonistic, but nevertheless powerful, may prove helpful (Box 17.2).

The physical repair of the skin should not be forgotten. Analgesics and antibiotics (both topically and systemically) can be helpful and where possible, occlusive dressings can be used.

Box 17.2 Approaching the patient with factitious disorder

- Defuse anger and suspicion. *"Can we start afresh from now to help you?"*
- Agree to a forward strategy. *"Can we consider all aspects of the illness including the stress that you must be under?"*
- Do not hurry. *"Sometimes this takes time to resolve. Can we work together to do this?"*
- Set a programme of mutual objectives, including *homework*. *"After we have talked, there may be other things that occur to you about possible causes for this reaction. Let's consider them, however unlikely they may seem."*

These clinic appointments to assess skin healing are valuable contact time to build rapport, but the effort invested in the skin care should not become the primary purpose of the consultation at the expense of the essential evaluation of the psychological state of the patient. At this stage, enquiries at an appropriate time during the consultation can elicit relevant predisposing, precipitating and perpetuating factors. Seeing the patient jointly with a psychiatrist in the skin clinic is the ideal setting for initial management. This joint management is better managed initially in the dermatology setting before a transfer to formal psychiatry care over many weeks. As the emphasis of the consultation shifts from repair of the skin to a focus on underlying psychopathology, a helpful analogy to provide the patient with is one of other illnesses that can be triggered by stress, such as migraine headaches or asthma.

Although confrontation is usually to be avoided, and certainly initially, there may be a point in the management where the potential benefits of direct discussion about the self-inflicted nature of the lesion outweigh the potential adverse consequences. This sometimes happens if a previous doctor has suggested that the lesions are self-inflicted, or perhaps a family member has done so. Confrontation should only be done by those very experienced in psychodermatology. The physician can suggest that sometimes people do things of which they are completely unaware (e.g. in their sleep or in a dissociated state such as sleepwalking) and when they are dealing with intolerable stressors or emotions. This is not to suggest that factitious patients have a dissociative disorder – rather it is a means for them to "give them an out" in a non-threatening environment. This line of approach may allow the patient to own the behaviour without fear they will be regarded as a malingerer or a liar. The acceptance of some form of quasi-explanation is only valid if it is followed by a discussion about vulnerability, perhaps provoked by elicited stressors.

Various other techniques have been described in the psychiatric literature, e.g. paradoxical intervention, but these should only be practised by an experienced psychiatric practitioner.

The treatment of adjustment disorders is primarily psychological. Techniques include guided self-help, computer-based therapy and in-person relaxation therapy. Medication can be helpful in the symptomatic relief of associated anxiety, but is not often recommended as monotherapy.

In depressive disorders, the use of antidepressants is well recognized (see Chapter 3 and Chapter 13). However, increasingly, there is a recognition that psychotherapy, especially cognitive-behavioural therapy (CBT), is as effective, if not more so, in some forms of the illness (see Chapter 5).

Treatment of personality disorders is complex and needs to be undertaken by appropriately trained practitioners in a setting with proper arrangements for supervision. These patients may be aggressive, disruptive and endlessly problematic. They may not only invade your professional space, but also the personal life of clinic staff. There are no recognized pharmacological therapies for personality disorders, and it is important not to commence inappropriate pharmacological treatment due to confusion over the diagnosis. Therapies for personality disorder have been developed in both individual and group modes, and many therapy modalities have been suggested, including CBT, schema-based therapy, transference-based therapy and skills-based therapies. Both single and group therapies have shown promise, especially small groups of patients treated in specialist settings. Often, treatment of personality disorders remains with those departments and psychotherapists with a special interest. Whilst effective in these settings, to make further impact in clinical situations such as factitious disorder, the development of strategic programmes to allow the treatment or referral of patients to appropriate settings (e.g. joint psychodermatological clinics) with appropriate supervision, is an important goal. For example, dialectical behaviour therapy (DBT) specifically for borderline personality disorder has been widely studied, and its beneficial effects repeatedly demonstrated. Given the prevalence of borderline personality disorder amongst patients with factitious disorder, the use of DBT techniques within these joint clinics is one of many potentials for the future. These cases are best managed by a team approach but in practice, one practitioner frequently assumes a major responsibility. There is a risk with many of these manipulative patients that the collaborative decisions reached by the group may be suborned if an individual allows a patient to cross professional boundaries into their personal spaces (e.g. accepting gifts or giving preferential treatment). Referral back to the team is advisable in these circumstances.

Future research

It will be helpful to assess the long-term cost–benefit analysis of psychodermatology multidisciplinary team clinics in the management of patients with suspected factitious disorder. Research is also needed to explore the relationship/boundaries between factitious disease and malingering.

PRACTICAL TIPS

- Factitious disorder is a specific entity in which patients cause harm to themselves in order to assume the sick role. In dermatology, it presents as self-inflicted skin damage, known as "dermatitis artefacta".
- Not all self-injury is a factitious disorder.
- There are dermatological clues that a factitious disorder may be present. However, confrontation is rarely helpful.
- Factitious disease is invariably associated with psychiatric/psychological disease (especially personality disorders) and treatment of the underlying psychological condition is vital to improvement.

References

1. Millard L, Millard J. Factitious skin disease. In: Burns T *et al.* (eds) *Rook's Textbook of Dermatology*, 8th edn. Oxford. Wiley Blackwell, 2010, pp. 64.34–64.55.

2. *Diagnostic and Statistical Manual of Mental Disorders*, 5th edn. Arlington: American Psychiatric Association, 2013.

3. Casey P, Kelly B. Personality disorders. In: *Fish's Clinical Psychopathology*, 3rd edn. London. Gaskell, 2007, pp. 106–120.

SECTION 5
Cutaneous sensory (pain) disorders

CHAPTER 18

Medically unexplained symptoms and health anxieties: somatic symptom and related disorders

Angharad Ruttley,[1,2] Audrey Ng[2] and Anna Burnside[2]
[1] Imperial College Healthcare NHS Trust, London, UK
[2] West London Mental Health NHS Trust, London, UK

"Medically unexplained" symptoms (MUS), also known as somatic symptom and related disorders in DSM-5, is a term used to describe physical symptoms where no clear pathology can be demonstrated or the symptoms cannot be fully explained by a known disease process. As such, the symptoms remain "medically unexplained". At least a third of somatic symptoms are medically unexplained, and of patients in this group, around 20–25% have recurrent or chronic complaints. The prevalence tends to be higher the more specialized the clinical setting [1]. In frequent attendees to outpatient clinics, the number of MUS is high, and the more symptoms the patient reports, the greater his/her functional disability. In patients presenting to outpatient clinics, the prevalence of somatic symptom disorder is around 12%, which is up to 100 times that in a comparable community sample [2].

Defining features

Attempts to categorize MUS can be challenging. However, somatic disorders may be characterized by repeated presentations with physical and pain symptoms and requests for medication and investigations, despite reassurance and negative investigation results (Box 18.1). There are various subtypes described in the two main diagnostic systems of DSM-5 and ICD-10.

DSM-5 has some minor differences from ICD-10, but in essence describes the same disorders. In the newly released DSM-5, the term hypochondriasis has been dropped due to its pejorative connotation that threatens an effective therapeutic relationship between the patient and doctor. The alternative "illness anxiety disorder" is preferred and dampens down the traditional mind versus body dualism that can be unhelpful in management.

Pathogenesis

Predisposing factors are female gender, childhood experience of parental illness, childhood abdominal pain, and poor care or adverse experiences in childhood. A consistent finding is that patients have fewer years of formal education than the general population [3].

There are high rates of "life events"' in the period leading up to the onset of symptoms, and MUS is commonly co-morbid with anxiety, depression and personality disorders.

Practical Psychodermatology, First Edition. Anthony Bewley, Ruth E. Taylor, Jason S. Reichenberg and Michelle Magid.
© 2014 John Wiley & Sons, Ltd. Published 2014 by John Wiley & Sons, Ltd.

Box 18.1 Medically unexplained symptoms in dermatology

- **MUS** – psychogenic pruritis, genital pruritis, dermatitis artefacta (see Chapter 17), psychogenic-elicited urticaria, anaesthetic skin areas, pseudoallergic reactions
- **Illness anxiety (hypochondriacal) disorders** – cancer (melanoma) phobia, candida phobia, venereophobia, AIDS phobia, syphilis phobia, borrelia phobia, delusional infestation (see Chapter 14), body dysmorphic disorder (see Chapter 15)
- **Delusional disorders** – somatic subtype – body dysmorphic disorder – psychotic subtype, primary delusional infestation
- **Somatic symptom disorders:**
  - *Ecosyndromes* such as multiple chemical sensitivity, sick-building syndrome, light allergy, amalgam phobia, food allergies
  - *Somatic pain disorders* – cutaneous dysaesthesia (see Chapter 19) such as glossodynia and vulvodynia (see Chapter 20)
  - *Somatic autonomic dysfunction* – hyperhidrosis, erythrophobia, goosebumps, undifferentiated somatoform idiopathic anaphylaxis

The cognitive-behavioural model of "health anxiety" has been further developed over the last two decades and is accepted as the most promising conceptualization of the disorder [4]. This can be applied broadly to MUS. The model includes four main interlinking domains; cognitive, perceptual, affective and behavioural. There is misattribution that occurs with regards to the somatic symptoms and the onset and maintenance involves the complex interaction of several factors [5].

Previous experience with ill health (e.g. death of a family member or friend from a disease; childhood experience of own/parental ill health) can be the start of the formation of dysfunctional assumptions. As a result, sufferers develop negative cognitions and overt illness behaviour.

Disproportionate amounts of time are spent checking for bodily changes (e.g. scrutinizing skin blemishes in minute detail) to the extent that benign changes and sensations are misinterpreted in a catastrophic manner.

Persistent thoughts and images of disease fuel the anxiety and accompanying physiological changes (e.g. palpitations or erythema) strengthen the patient's conviction. Reassurance seeking from physicians or significant others is common, as is the need for repeat medical investigations. Clinicians may feel uncertain as to how to respond to such anxiety and inadvertently reinforce it by ordering more investigations or dismissing the complaint.

Avoidance behaviour is common – sufferers avoid activity that they believe will exacerbate the condition, often to an excessive level. Conversely, some avoid medical consultation altogether as they fear confirmation of their beliefs. Typically, the illness beliefs tend to fluctuate in severity between periods of extreme anxiety and those of relative calm.

This cognitive-behavioural model can be used across most MUS syndromes, and has the advantage of being simple and understandable to patients. Specific explanatory models are given in Box 18.2 for hypochondriasis and for other MUS and conversion disorders in Box 18.3.

Assessment (Box 18.4)

Patients with MUS may develop additional physical pathology and the two may frequently co-occur; therefore, it is important not to lose sight of this. However, the most frequently missed diagnoses are psychiatric.

General advice from the literature on assessment recommends taking a careful history, including all symptoms. It is helpful to keep asking about other symptoms until the patient completely exhausts his/her symptom list. Allow enough time for the patient to tell the full story and acknowledge the patient's suffering. This will help the patient to feel understood,

Box 18.2 Pathogenesis of illness anxiety disorder (formerly known as hypochondriasis)

- **Cognitive** – e.g. recent death in family or friend with melanoma activates anxiety
- **Perceptual** – increased sensitivity to minor skin blemishes and awareness of bodily sensations exaggerated; benign changes are misinterpreted in a catastrophic way
- **Behavioural** – disproportionate amounts of time spent checking for bodily signs/symptoms, reading medical textbooks and websites that fuel anxiety; reassurance seeking and "physician shopping": short-lived relief but consolidates maladaptive behaviour
- **Affective** – recurrent images and thoughts of disease cause physiological change such as erythema, which serves to strengthen conviction of disease, and/or increasing distress causes more negative thinking and therefore more dysfunctional cognitions

Box 18.3 Theories of medically unexplained symptoms including conversion and dissociative disorders [6]

- **Psychoanalytical** – unconscious drives that "convert" unbearable and unresolved emotions into physical symptoms. Primary gain is the "psychic" relief conferred to the sufferer
- **Learning theory** – this looks at avoidance of responsibilities and assumption of the "sick role", i.e. seeking unconscious secondary gains
- **Sociocultural factors** – in western societies, dissociation may be the equivalent of "trance and possession" states, which are common in other cultures. Established gender roles in society may also play a part (e.g. it may not be acceptable for men to show emotional distress)
- **Neurobiological** – evidence suggesting that the frontal cortical and limbic activation associated with emotional stress may act via inhibitory basal ganglia–thalamocortical circuits to produce deficits in sensory and motor functioning

demonstrating that you believe him/her and take his/her problems seriously.

Asking a patient to take you through a typical day is a useful way to gauge the level of disability and focuses on the impact of the symptoms. Psychosocial stressors should be carefully sought and a thorough physical examination performed [7].

There is some evidence in patients with irritable bowel syndrome that a positive patient–doctor interaction reduces subsequent attendances. Factors that promote this are exploration of the psychosocial history, discussion of test results, and reassurance about the diagnosis [8].

The emphasis in the psychosocial history should be on predisposing, perpetuating and precipitating factors, using a biopsychosocial model (Table 18.1). You should establish a good chronology of life events and symptoms – drawing a timeline of these (*"to help me get your story clear in my head"*) can be a useful visual aid

Box 18.4 Assessment approach in medically unexplained symptoms

- Take a careful history including an exhaustive symptom list
- Seek out and explore psychosocial stressors
- A collateral history is valuable where obtainable
- Perform a thorough physical examination
- Perform investigations only where necessary, and discuss results with the patient – including what normal results mean
- Seek out a patient's fears about his/her symptoms and use this as a basis for reassuring him/her
- Do not invalidate the patient's symptoms; instead, work with him/her to find an explanation that is useful and acceptable

Table 18.1 Example biopsychosocial assessment grid

	Predisposing	Precipitating	Perpetuating
Biological	Genetic – family history of somatic disorders	Acute illness	Inactivity, physiological arousal
Psychological	Childhood adversity Childhood illness Parental illness	Recent bereavement/ illness in family/friends	Negative illness beliefs/ behaviours
Social	Low levels of formal education	Life events	Isolation Burden of care for others

to promote understanding of the links between the physical and psychological symptoms for both you and the patient.

A basic psychiatric evaluation should be carried out, including an assessment of risk and mood (see Chapter 2, Chapter 6, and Chapter 13).

Keep investigations to those clinically indicated and to a minimum. If investigations are required, discuss the possible outcomes and their meanings in advance. It is important to know that repeated investigations are unlikely to reassure patients, and may even make things worse (*"there must be something seriously wrong if I need more tests"*), so should only be carried out if there is a specific clinical indication [9].

Where there is suspicion of a somatic symptom and related disorder, questionnaires such as the Patient Health Questionnaire-15 (PHQ-15; see Appendix A8) (not to be confused with the PHQ-9, used in primary care in the UK for the diagnosis of depression) may be a useful adjunct to history taking, particularly where it is difficult to obtain a clear history.

Treatment

The main components of management are to find an explanation that is helpful to the patient, enable exploration of ways of managing morbidity and distress, and the avoidance or reduction of iatrogenic factors which are unhelpful and costly.

Reassurance is an important part of treatment for MUS; however, do not tell the patient that there is *"nothing wrong"*. Encourage the patient to talk about his/her fears and beliefs around his/her symptoms, and be open about uncertainty but reassuring that a serious cause is unlikely. Preparing patients for the possibility that investigations may not show a disease process can help with discussions around managing symptoms if a test is returned as normal. Help the patient to understand that MUS is common and that there is not always a disease explanation for symptoms.

When you have identified that a patient has MUS, a useful step is to book some time to discuss the patient with his/her primary care physician, who will have an important role in coordinating care. If the patient is being seen by other specialists across multiple systems, communication and collaboration is essential. For particularly complex patients, a case conference can be a useful way to ensure consistent care. Patients should be involved in all discussions around their care, including correspondence and care plans.

Reducing medical contact can minimize iatrogenic harm and wasted resources through inappropriate information, over investigation and over treatment, particularly the perpetuating cycle of assessment, discharge and rereferral to another specialty. In addition, while this continues, it may delay appropriate psychiatric treatment.

Box 18.5 Management strategies for somatic symptom disorder [11]

- Alcohol use disorders are commonly co-morbid with somatic disorders and should be sought for and treated. Patients with such problems can be referred to local substance misuse clinics or to voluntary sector organizations such as AA (see Chapter 27)
- Antidepressants are unlikely to be helpful unless there is co-morbid anxiety or depression
- CBT can be beneficial in reducing symptoms and attendances, as well as improving function
- Regular, scheduled appointments with the patient's GP can also be a useful management strategy to build a therapeutic alliance with a medical practitioner and reduce unscheduled contact

Box 18.6 Management strategies for illness anxiety disorder (hypochondriasis) [12,13]

- Avoid conflict around the cause of the symptoms
- Repeated reassurance is unhelpful as it may encourage further reassurance-seeking behaviour
- CBT is effective in reducing symptoms and improving function
- SSRIs have been shown to be helpful even in the absence of a co-morbid depressive disorder

Box 18.7 Management strategies for conversion disorders [14]

- Ensure that organic and other psychiatric disorders have been ruled out
- Medication is not recommended in the absence of a co-morbid depression or anxiety disorder
- Psychoeducation and CBT have been reported to be beneficial
- Hypnosis and analytical psychotherapy have also shown some benefit
- However, there is no robust evidence base for any treatment

Patients should be involved in the decision to bring investigations to a close and be reassured that in certain circumstances investigation may be warranted in the future (presentation of new or changing symptoms that are suggestive of a disease process).

It is important to prepare the patient adequately before referral to psychiatry or psychology services as patients may not readily perceive the need for, or usefulness of, this. Using the patient's own words and explanations can be helpful, as well as reassuring him/her that psychiatric and psychological treatments are in wide use for conditions such as diabetes, chronic pain and heart disease, where they have been found to improve symptoms and outcomes.

Co-morbid anxiety and depressive disorders should be treated with antidepressants or cognitive-behavioural therapy (CBT) where appropriate. Citalopram can be a good choice as it has few side effects, can be started in a therapeutic dose of 20 mg and interacts little with other medication. Escitalopram has even fewer side effects but is expensive. Choice of antidepressant is discussed in Chapter 3.

Management strategies for somatic symptom disorder, illness anxiety disorder and conversion disorders are covered in Box 18.5, Box 18.6 and Box 18.7, respectively.

Specific disorders that may present in dermatology clinics

Factitious disorders and malingering

Factitious disorder is the term used in ICD and DSM classifications to denote the creation or simulation of physical (or psychiatric) symptoms in oneself or others – as in Munchausen-by-proxy. This is thought of as being driven by unconscious processes resulting in deliberate

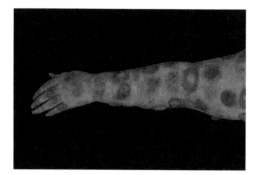

Figure 18.1 Patient with dermatitis artefacta blisters on the arms. The patient could not account for how these lesions appeared.

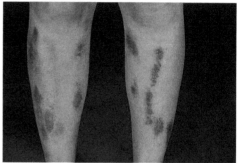

Figure 18.2 Patient who has self-induced superficial linear erosions on the leg, which appeared around the time of appointments with doctors. This patient was signed off sick from work as a healthcare practitioner as these lesions were thought to represent an infection risk. Between appointments, the lesions tended to resolve (courtesy of Dr A. Bewley).

illness or injury. The secondary gain is to "play the sick role".

This is a rare disorder, with prevalence estimated at 0.05–0.4%. It is usually observed in adolescent or young adult women. In the dermatology clinic, this is likely to present as dermatitis artefacta (Figure 18.1; see Chapter 17).

Patients with suspected factitious disorder should be referred to psychiatry when possible. This may be difficult as such patients often avoid psychiatric evaluation and may simply disengage from the healthcare setting, or seek care elsewhere. Should there be risk of serious iatrogenic harm, consideration should be given to circulating the details of the patient to local emergency departments and other dermatology clinics. This should always be done with the patient's consent following the principles of "Good Medical Practice". If consent is not possible and the risk is deemed serious, discussion with the appropriate legal authority should be sought (see Chapter 6). Child protection issues must be considered in situations of factitious disorder by proxy where a parent presents a child with factitious symptoms (see Chapter 6).

Malingering, by contrast, is defined as intentional and conscious creation or feigning of physical symptoms (Figure 18.2) in order to achieve a specific gain (e.g. compensation after injury or sickness benefit). The presence of secondary gain is often obvious enough to alert you to the possibility of malingering, and inconsistencies in the history may provide further evidence. Such patients are not motivated to participate in psychotherapy.

Persistent delusional disorders – somatic type

This group of disorders is defined by the presence of a persistent (>3 months according to ICD-10) delusion or set of related delusions. Other psychopathology is absent except for intermittent depression in some cases. However, the delusion or set of delusions must be the primary symptom and persist when there is no mood disturbance. Olfactory and tactile hallucinations may occur. There must be no other symptoms of schizophrenia, e.g. prominent auditory hallucinations or thought disorder, and no organic brain disease. Persistent delusional disorder can occur with different delusional themes, e.g. jealousy, but the somatic subtype involves delusions focused on the body, e.g. patients may have hypochondriacal delusions, believing some part of the body is diseased, or they may have delusional beliefs that a part of the body is deformed or abnormal in some way. Body dysmorphic disorder (see Chapter 15) may be psychotic, in which case it can often be classified as a persistent delusional disorder.

Disorders related to smell and body odour

Phantosmia and cacosmia

Phantosmia is the perception of an odour where no physical odour is present. Where the odour is unpleasant it is called cacosmia. Patients occasionally present in dermatology clinics with cacosmia. Cacosmia can be caused by a problem in the olfactory tract peripherally, e.g. malfunction of olfactory neurones, or a central pathology in the brain, e.g. epilepsy and neuroblastoma. Patients may retain or lack insight. It can also be associated with functional psychiatric disorders, e.g. schizophrenia or psychotic depression, and with dementias, e.g. Alzheimer's disease and Lewy body dementia.

Olfactory reference syndrome

Olfactory reference syndrome (ORS) is characterized by a person's persistent and distressing preoccupation with the belief that he/she *emits* an unpleasant body odour, in the absence of objective evidence of body odour. The syndrome has been consistently described across cultures and time (e.g. in Japanese culture it is called Jikoshu-kyofu). ORS is briefly mentioned in DSM-5 under "Other specified obssessive-compulsive and related disorders". It is not mentioned in ICD-10. It is unclear how it should be classified, but it is suggested that it is closely related to body dysmorphic disorder and social anxiety disorder [10].

Researchers have proposed the diagnostic criteria listed in Box 18.8. According to these criteria patients retain insight, but some patients will lack insight and present with delusions that they smell.

Box 18.8 Lochner and Stein proposed criteria for olfactory reference syndrome [15]

- A preoccupation with body odour or halitosis that persists despite reassurance that it is not perceived by others
- In someone who recognizes that the preoccupation is unreasonable or excessive
- Which causes significant distress or impairment in function
- And does not occur as secondary to another disorder (e.g. depression, anxiety disorders) or as a result of substances or other organic cause

Clinical assessment of presentations involving abnormal odours

When undertaking a clinical assessment, a sympathetic manner and a curious, interested approach using "what, when, where, why" type questions is a good way to engage with the patient. Questions perceived as querying the reality of the symptom could be met with hostility. This is understandable as patients may have been dismissed by doctors previously, or be anxious about not being believed or being labelled as having a mental illness. However, it is important not to miss a treatable physical or psychiatric disorder.

It is also important to remember that smells may vary with intensity or not actually be perceptible by the clinician, and therefore not detectable at consultation. This can be the case with trimethylaminuria (TMAU), a genetic disorder in which the body is unable to break down trimethylamine, which smells like rotting fish. As it builds up in the body, it causes affected people to give off this odour in their sweat, urine and breath. Asking the patient to explain the quality of the smell and carefully establishing the chronology of the problem can therefore be a helpful approach. In patients with TMAU careful history taking may reveal the problem as present from birth, or in females worsening around puberty, menstruation, when taking oral contraceptives or around menopause. Dietary supplements such as L-carnitine may exacerbate the problem and rarely liver or kidney disease can play a role.

Patients with cacosmia arising from a problem in the olfactory tract commonly have some pre-morbid loss of their sense of smell, often in the ipsilateral nostril [16].

Patients can develop an olfactory *hallucination* and may believe *"the smell is coming from me"*. Alternatively, they may develop a *delusional* belief that they smell, and that others can smell them, without actually having any olfactory hallucination. A description can help disentangle whether an odour is hallucinatory or delusional, and the strength of conviction with which the belief is held. For example, *"I smell burnt tyres all the time"* versus *"I smell terrible, I know, because at my office, I've started to notice that my boss won't get in the lift with me"*.

In psychosis, the key clinical finding is the unshakeability of the belief and the lack of insight the patient shows into his/her symptom. Cacosmia may occur as a mono-symptomatic delusional disorder or in other psychotic disorders such as schizophrenia. It can also sometimes be seen in severe depressive disorder with psychotic symptoms. The odours in this latter case are often described as of rotting flesh or earth and may be accompanied by the nihilistic delusion that the patient is actually dead or in the process of decomposition. This is typically found in the elderly, and symptoms can worsen with frightening rapidity.

In ORS the patient may be able to accept evidence against the belief that he/she has an unpleasant body odour, but still persists with obsessive worry about the smell. He/she may constantly monitor him/herself (e.g. for sweat or bad breath), engage in compensatory behaviour (avoiding others, seeking treatment for sweating), and monitor the response of those around him/her. Anything may become evidence to support the belief (e.g. a friend cancelling a meeting). As a consequence,

patients may become increasingly socially isolated.

Patients can also develop a secondary depression, so it is important to establish if the mood worsened before or after the onset. When asking about mood, you can normalize the question using phrases like: *"This sounds very difficult for you to live with, I wonder if it is affecting your mood?"*

For all patients, ask about suicidal ideation. Leopold [16] reports that around half of patients referred to an ENT clinic with phantosmia and seeking surgery have considered suicide due to the effects on their life. Should there be significant concerns, the patient can be referred on for specialist psychiatric evaluation.

Alzheimer's disease and other dementias (particularly Parkinson's or dementia with Lewy bodies) may also produce phantosmia/cacosmia, so in elderly patients or those with a strong family history, it is important to check cognition. Many quick screening tests are available, including the Mini Mental Status Exam (see Appendix A5). Be aware however that low scores on cognitive testing can also occur if a patient is significantly depressed.

Finally, ask about social functioning, as patients may increasingly isolate themselves due to embarrassment and distress associated with the smell.

For all patients, a head and neck examination should be carried out, with attention to the middle ear, nasal mucosa, airways and tongue. An ENT referral may be appropriate.

Investigations

A simple urine test can identify TMAU. Genetic testing can also be performed to look for the impaired *FMO3* gene (flavin-containing monooxygenase 3 gene).

If a patient has a possible dementia, blood testing should be carried out to search for reversible causes of impaired cognition, including thyroid function, vitamin B_{12} and folate deficiency, as well as HIV/syphilis testing. Referral to a memory service for more detailed neuropsychological testing is indicated.

Table 18.2 Differential diagnoses for disorders involving abnormal perception of smell [17]

Psychiatric	Central	Peripheral
• Delusional disorder, somatic type • Severe depression with psychotic symptoms • Olfactory reference syndrome • Schizophrenia/schizoaffective disorder/other functional psychoses • Dementias	• Seizure disorders • Brain tumour • Head trauma • Trimethylaminuria (fish odour syndrome)	• Chronic rhinosinusitis • Allergic rhinopathy • Upper respiratory tract infection

Imaging of the brain and nasal cavity should be performed to rule out tumours, infections and obstructions.

Differential diagnosis of disorders of smell

The literature contains an extensive list of causes of abnormal smell, including as sequelae to radiotherapy, surgery and medications, but the main causes of concern are listed in Table 18.2.

Management of disorders of smell

Management clearly depends on the underlying aetiology, and may involve more than one speciality, including primary care, otolaryngology (ENT), dermatology or psychiatry.

In patients who also have loss of sense of smell, it is important to counsel them regarding measures they can take to manage the associated risks (e.g. smoke detectors, using best before dates regarding spoiled foods, etc.).

If the cacosmia/phantosmia disappears on nasal occlusion, normal saline or oxymetazoline nasal drops can be used for temporary relief of symptoms.

For patients with TMAU, dietary restrictions form the mainstay of treatment and low-dose antibiotics to reduce the amount of gut bacteria can also be used. Genetic counselling can help sufferers better understand the condition. Be aware that depression can be associated with this distressing condition and should be treated if present.

If a psychiatric cause is found, and the symptoms are troublesome, referral to mental health services is indicated. You should take a careful history of suicidal thoughts and self-neglect, and ideally check with a relative or caregiver before you conclude that it is safe to send the patient home. If you are concerned, contact your liaison psychiatry service or on-call psychiatrist at your site for advice on where the patient can be seen for immediate psychiatric assessment. Organizing a joint psychodermatology outpatient clinic appointment or referral to a liaison psychiatry outpatient clinic situated in the acute hospital may be an acceptable approach for patients anxious about referral to a mental health professional.

In patients in whom no underlying disorder can be identified, the symptoms may disappear on their own over months or years, and it is important to explain this and offer the option of "watchful waiting". This should be done with assurance of follow-up from the GP and rereferral if needed. The patient should be sent a copy of the letter, with advice on what to do should the symptoms worsen or become distressing or disabling.

Dissociative form of pseudoangioedema or undifferentiated somatoform idiopathic anaphylaxis

Angioedema is a vascular reaction involving the deep dermis or submucosal tissues resulting in localized oedema, clinically characterized by swelling of the lips, tongue, larynx, genitals or peripheries. It can be caused by histamine- or bradykinin-mediated mechanisms. Histamine-dependent angioedema may occur with or without other features of anaphylaxis, such as urticaria, wheeze, diarrhoea and hypotension, and it is usually caused by mast cell degranulation. Angioedema caused by bradykinin is not accompanied by urticaria and it results from C1 inhibitor deficiency or as a side effect of angiotensin-converting enzyme (ACE) inhibitor drugs. There are idiopathic forms of both histamine- and bradykinin-mediated angioedema [18]. Swelling involving the larynx and/or upper airways may cause death from asphyxiation and hence represents a medical emergency. Angioedema of the viscera causes intractable abdominal pain akin to an acute abdomen. Between attacks, patients show no evidence of swelling. While laboratory investigations are useful in the diagnosis of some types of angioedema [e.g. allergic (IgE mediated) angioedema and C1 inhibitor deficiency), in others the diagnosis is made clinically and there are no available diagnostic tests (e.g. hereditary angioedema with normal C1 inhibitor function, idiopathic angioedema) [18]. Pseudoangioedema is the medical term that describes disease states that mimic angioedema. The differential diagnosis is wide and includes contact dermatitis, thyroid disease and connective tissue disease.

A small number of patients present to emergency and specialist services, sometimes repeatedly, with histories compatible with angioedema, but careful examination reveals that they have no objective evidence of swelling. Depending on the specialist setting in which the evaluation is undertaken, these patients may be diagnosed as having a dissociative form of pseudoangioedema or undifferentiated somatoform idiopathic anaphylaxis [19]. In a few cases the symptoms are factitious. These patients are challenging because they frequently present to emergency departments out of hours, complaining of severe abdominal pain or upper airway swelling. Due to the attending medical staff's perceived need for immediate treatment, these patients have often received epinephrine (adrenaline) and/or treatments for C1 inhibitor deficiency before imaging or expert assessment can be achieved. Diagnosis relies on a careful history and examination of the patient during and between attacks by physicians experienced in evaluating angioedema. In some cases, the symptoms resolve when the patient is reassured that there is no serious underlying disorder. Some patients may benefit from a psychiatric evaluation, while others are highly resistant to the diagnosis [19].

Acknowledgement

The authors are grateful to Dr Hilary Longhurst, Consultant Immunologist and Dr Ania Manson, SPR Clinical Immunology, Department of Immunology, Barts Health NHS Trust, Royal London Hospital, London, UK for the section on angioedema.

PRACTICAL TIPS

- Give patients time to explain all their symptoms fully.
- Reassure the patient that you take his/her symptoms seriously.
- Take time to understand the patient's beliefs about illness and his/her particular symptoms.
- Investigate only where clinically indicated.
- Do not say there is nothing wrong if tests cannot identify a disease process; there is something wrong, or the patient would not have come to you in the first place.
- Find an explanation that is helpful to the patient, and involve the patient in decision making and plans.
- Communicate with other professionals involved in the patient's care.

References

1. Kroenke K. Patients presenting with somatic complaints: epidemiology, psychiatric comorbidity and management. *Int J Methods Psychiatr Res* 2003; 12(1): 34–43.
2. Page LA, Wessely S. Medically unexplained symptoms: exacerbating factors in the doctor–patient encounter. *J R Soc Med* 2003; 96: 223.
3. Hatcher S, Arroll B. Assessment and management of medically unexplained symptoms. *BMJ* 2008 May 17; 336: 1124–1128.
4. Salkovskis PM, Warwick HMC. Morbid preoccupations, health anxiety & reassurance; a cognitive behavioural approach to hypochondriasis. *Behav Res Ther* 1986; 24: 597–602.
5. Warwick HMC, Salkovskis PM. Hypochondriasis. *Behav Res Ther* 1990; 28: 105–117.
6. Harvey SB *et al.* Conversion disorder: towards a neurobiological understanding. *Neuropsychiatr Dis Treat* 2006; 2(1): 13–20.
7. Sharpe M. Medically unexplained symptoms and syndromes. *Clin Med* 2002; 2: 501–504.
8. Owens D *et al.* The irritable bowel syndrome: longterm prognosis and the physician–patient interaction. *Ann Intern Med* 1995; 122: 107–112.
9. Howard L, Wessely S. Reappraising reassurance – the role of investigations. *J Psychosom Res* 1996; 41: 307–311.
10. Feusner JD *et al.* Olfactory reference syndrome: issues for DSM V. *Depress Anxiety* 2010 27(6): 592–599.
11. Oyama O *et al.* Somatoform disorders. *Am Fam Phys* 2007; 76(9): 1333–1338.
12. Barsky AJ, Ahern DK. Cognitive behaviour therapy for hypochondriasis: a randomised controlled trial. *JAMA* 2004; 291: 1464–1470.
13. Fallon BA *et al.* Fluoxetine for hypochondriacal patients without major depression. *J Clin Pharmacol* 1996; 13: 438–441.
14. Ruddy R, House A. Psychosocial interventions for conversion disorder. *Cochrane Database Syst Rev* 2005 ; 4: CD005331.
15. Lochner C, Stein DJ. Olfactory reference syndrome: diagnostic criteria and differential diagnosis. *J Postgrad Med* 2003; 49: 328–331.
16. Leopold D. Distortion of olfactory perception: Diagnosis and treatment. *Chem Senses* 2002; 27(7): 611–615.
17. Seiden A. *Taste and Smell Disorders*. Stuttgart: Thieme Medical Publishers, 1997, p. 4.
18. Grigoriadou S, Longhurst HJ. Clinical immunology review series: An approach to the patient with angio-oedema. *Clin Exp Immunol* 2009; 155(3): 367–377.
19. Choy AC *et al.* Undifferentiated somatoform idiopathic anaphylaxis: nonorganic symptoms mimicking idiopathic anaphylaxis. *J Allergy Clin Immunol* 1995; 96(6 Pt 1): 893–900.

CHAPTER 19

Dysesthetic syndromes

Sara A. Hylwa,[1] Mark D.P. Davis[2] and Mark R. Pittelkow[2]

[1] Department of Dermatology, University of Minnesota, Minneapolis, MN, USA
[2] Department of Dermatology, Mayo Clinic, Rochester, MN, USA

Dysesthetic syndromes comprise a wide variety of neurocutaneous disorders that cause unwanted or uncomfortable sensations within the skin, often with little to no attendant skin change. These sensations are often described by patients as burning, tingling, itching, prickling, pins-and-needles, or electrical jolts, and less often as frank pain. In this chapter, we will discuss several cutaneous dysesthesias, though many others exist (Box 19.1).

Treatment for dysesthetic syndromes should be guided by the underlying etiology. A simplified approach utilizes topical medicaments aimed at minimizing neuronal stimulation or signaling (e.g. lidocaine patches) in addition to systemic therapies to lessen spontaneous nerve impulses (e.g. gabapentin) (Table 19.1). There are no robust evidence-based approaches to the treatment of dysesthetic syndromes; all therapeutic regimens are the product of clinical observation and expert consensus.

Sensory mononeuropathies

Sensory mononeuropathies are defined by dysesthetic sensations experienced by a patient along the distribution of one nerve. The two most common sensory mononeuropathies encountered in dermatology are notalgia paresthetica and meralgia paresthetica.

Symptoms should fall along the course of a defined nerve; symptoms outside of that distribution would be abnormal. Failure to respond to the standard treatments discussed below would evoke the possibility of an underlying psychiatric diagnosis, such as a conversion disorder, hypochondriasis, somatic symptom disorder (see Chapter 18), factitious disorder (see Chapter 17) or a chronic idiopathic pain disorder (see Chapter 20).

Notalgia paresthetica
Defining features
Notalgia paresethetica is a unilateral sensory neuropathy characterized by tingling, burning, pruritus, or hypo- or hyper-esthesia of the subscapular and occasionally interscapular region of the back. The left subscapular area is more frequently involved than the right. Occasionally, patients may have a subtle hyperpigmented patch overlying the affected area. Females are affected more often than males; median age of presentation is 52–64 years [1].

Pathogenesis
The etiology of notalgia paresethetica is not well understood, but is generally believed to be due to impingement or trauma to the T2–T6 spinal nerves as they course through the muscles of the back precariously at right angles. Alternatively, primary spine (or vertebral column) pathology can be causative (e.g. degenerative disc disease, disc herniation, spinal stenosis, or scoliosis).

Practical Psychodermatology, First Edition. Anthony Bewley, Ruth E. Taylor, Jason S. Reichenberg and Michelle Magid.
© 2014 John Wiley & Sons, Ltd. Published 2014 by John Wiley & Sons, Ltd.

Box 19.1 Dysesthetic disorders

- Sensory mononeuropathies:
  - Head & neck – mental neuropathy, trigeminal neuropathy (trigeminal neuralgia, trigeminal trophic syndrome), greater auricular neuropathy, scalp dysesthesia
  - Extremities – meralgia paresthetica, gonyalgia paresthetica, brachioradial pruritus, cheiralgia paresthetica, digitalgia paresthetica
  - Trunk – notalgia paresthetica, thoracolumbar radiculopathy, incisura scapulae syndrome
- Erythromelalgia
- Chronic regional pain syndrome
- Palmoplantar erythrodysesthesia (hand–foot syndrome)
- Red ear syndrome
- Groin dysesthesia (red scrotum syndrome/ scotodynia)
- Infectious:
  - Herpes simplex, post-herpetic (zoster) neuralgia, Hansen's disease (leprosy), Lyme disease, HIV neuropathy
- Vascular:
  - Temporal arteritis/giant cell arteritis, peripheral arterial disease, venous stasis dermatitis
- Autonomic neuropathies:
  - Inherited – familial amyloid polyneuropathy, hereditary sensory autonomic neuropathy, Fabry disease
  - Acquired – idiopathic distal small fiber neuropathy, amyloid neuropathy, diabetes mellitus-associated neuropathy, uremic neuropathy, vitamin B_{12} deficiency, alcohol-related neuropathy

Notalgia paresthetica-associated skin hyperpigmentation is the result of chronic rubbing, which results in epidermal basal layer degeneration with pigment incontinence and deposition of keratin-derived amyloid within the papillary dermis [1].

Assessment

Notalgia paresethetica is a clinical diagnosis. The differential diagnosis includes contact dermatitis, fixed drug eruptions, lichen simplex chronicus, hyperpigmentation, and tinea versicolor. You should also consider the neuropsychiatric disorders listed earlier.

Treatment

Standard treatment for mild to moderate neuralgia paresethetica includes topical capsaicin cream. In one study, 70% of patients treated with capsaicin experienced symptom improvement compared to 30% with placebo. Unfortunately, discontinuing the cream led to symptom relapse within 1 month [2]. Alternative topical therapies include topical lidocaine or doxepin [3].

Patients with mild to moderate notalgia paresthetica may also benefit from exercises that support the muscles of the back. Case reports have shown that daily strengthening of the scapular muscles (rhomboid, trapezius, and latissimus dorsi) while stretching the pectorals (essentially encouraging proper posture), can improves or resolve symptoms within 1 week, most likely as a result of alterations in muscle alignment that ease the course of the nerves within the muscle [3].

For moderate to severe disease, gabapentin or pregabalin should be initiated. If these do not provide sufficient relief, oxycarbazepine can be substituted [1].

For refractory cases, transcutaneous electrical nerve stimulation (TENS) with five sessions per week for 2 weeks or acupuncture can be attempted. Narrowband UVB three times per week is an alternative. Regional intradermal botulinum toxin, type A has been reported to relieve symptoms as well [4]. Lastly, surgical procedures to repair degenerated discs can be considered, although there are few reports documenting response to this treatment.

Meralgia paresthetica
Defining features

Meralgia paresthetica is a cutaneous dysesthetic disorder characterized by unilateral numbness,

Table 19.1 Summary of features for common medications for dysesthesias

Medication	Common dose	Side effects	Contraindications/warnings
Capsaicin 0.025% cream	Apply to affected area five times per day	Burning, stinging, transient erythema with application	Wash hands after applying
Lidocaine 5% patch	Apply up to three patches on affected area once for up to 12 hours within a 24-hour period	Irritation, redness, swelling Serious hypersensitivity is rare	Contraindicated with other cardiac antiarrhythmics (especially Class I) Use with caution in hepatic disease Heat can cause increased drug release
Doxepin 5% cream	Apply to affected areas qid	Burning, stinging; drowsiness if applied to >10% BSA	Contraindicated if using selegiline Contraindicated in narrow-angle glaucoma and patients with urinary retention
Gabapentin	Start at 300 mg po daily, increase by 300 mg to a maximum of 300 mg tid Must adjust dose for renal impairment	Dizziness, fatigue, ataxia	Can potentiate other sedatives Do not discontinue abruptly
Pregabalin	50-100 mg tid	Dizziness, somnolence Drug dependency possible	Potential male-mediated teratogenicity Must gradually discontinue (taper) and monitor for withdrawal
Carbamazepine	400–800 mg/day in divided doses Should try to discontinue every 3 months during treatment period Maximum dose: 1200 mg/day	Ataxia, dizziness, drowsiness, nausea, vomiting	Black box warnings for TEN/SJS, especially in Han Chinese patients with HLA-B*1502 (this should be tested for before starting) Multiple contraindicated drug–drug interactions
Oxcarbazepine	Start 150–300 mg po daily and can uptitrate to 300 mg tid as tolerated	Dizziness, headache, nausea, vomiting, drowsiness, ataxia, vertigo, vision changes	Warn regarding risk of suicidal ideation Must be withdrawn gradually Many serious drug interactions Can render OCPs ineffective
Amitriptyline	25 mg nightly, increased by 25 mg every week to maximum of 100–200 mg/day	Dry mouth, drowsiness, anticholinergic effects	Black box warning as antidepressants can increase suicidal ideation Contraindicated with severe cardiovascular disease (including arrhythmias), narrow angle glaucoma, MAOIs; Possibly EPS and NMS

BSA, body surface area; MAOI, monoamine oxidase inhibitor; EPS, extrapyramidal symptoms, NMS, neuroleptic malignant syndrome; OCP, oral contraceptive pill; TEN/SJS, toxic epidermal necrolysis/Steven–Johnson syndrome burning, or stinging along the anterolateral thigh(s), possibly with associated alopecia secondary to rubbing. Patients often report exacerbation of symptoms with erect posture and prolonged standing, and these are relieved by sitting. Median age of presentation is 30–40 years; males are affected more commonly than females [5].

Pathogenesis

Meralgia paresthetica is due to compression or trauma of the lateral femoral cutaneous nerve, which provides sensory innervation of the anterolateral thigh. The most common etiologic factor is increased intra-abdominal pressure, as seen with obesity and pregnancy. For 25% of patients, anatomic variations in nerve course and location predispose the nerve to entrapment and injury and thus symptoms [5]. Surgery (especially gastrointestinal), internal tumors, or external pressure from tight-fitting clothes or equipment, have also been implicated as a cause.

Assessment

The diagnosis of meralgia paresthetica is clinical. Confirmatory measures include exacerbation of the symptoms upon tapping of the inguinal ligament or extending the thigh posteriorally, or resolution of pain with a local anesthetic block. Further confirmation can be made by sensory nerve conduction velocity studies if necessary [5].

If meralgia paresthetica is accompanied by a neurologic deficit, tenderness over the sciatic notch, or if a straight leg raise test is positive, alternative diagnoses such as spinal disease, pelvic neoplasm, or occult gastrointestinal infections must be considered [5]. You should also consider the neuropsychiatric disorders listed earlier.

Treatment

For most cases of meralgia paresthetica, lifestyle changes aimed at weight loss and avoidance of tight-fitting clothing paired with local nerve blocks should suffice. Blocks of bupivicaine 0.25% ± methylprednisolone are recommended. Topical capsaicin or lidocaine patches can also be considered. For resistant disease, oral gabapentin or a tricyclic antidepressant can be added [5]. Recently, treatment with intradermal botulinum toxin has shown benefit [6].

Surgery should be considered in patients with a known anatomic variant of the nerve, all pediatric cases, and cases refractory to medical treatment. Conservative medical management results in symptom improvement for 60–90% of individuals, with 40–50% of the refractory cases improving after nerve decompression [5].

Trigeminal syndromes

The trigeminal nerve supplies cutaneous sensation to the face and motor innervation to the muscles of mastication. Dysfunction of this nerve can cause two different dysesthetic disorders.

Trigeminal neuralgia
Defining features

Trigeminal neuralgia consists of brief paroxysms of unilateral severe pain in one or more distributions of the trigeminal nerve. It is one of the most painful conditions described in medicine. Symptoms often begin as an electrical-type shock – often described as like a lightning bolt going off in the face – that then progresses to an excruciating stabbing pain with resultant uncontrolled facial twitching [7,8], historically referred to as "tic douloureux." Attacks last roughly 20 seconds and are followed by a refractory period. The paroxysms of pain come in cycles, with the number of attacks and length of cycles varying widely. Attacks may number a few to hundreds per day; cycles may last several days to years. Remissions between cycles do occur and generally last weeks to months, with the length of remissions decreasing with time [9].

Pain is most commonly experienced along the maxillary nerve, and can be provoked by trigger points or everyday activities such as talking. Trigeminal neuralgia is most common after the age of 40 years and is almost twice as common in females.

Pathogenesis

Abnormalities within the trigeminal nerve, nerve root, or ganglion are responsible for trigeminal neuralgia. Frequently, a vascular structure compresses the nerve causing damage; disordered remyelination results in an excitation of the nerve that lasts beyond the duration of the external stimulus [7].

Assessment

The diagnosis of trigeminal neuralgia is made clinically. Criteria for diagnosis include paroxysms of intense, sharp, superficial or stabbing pain that lasts from a fraction of a second to minutes and affects one or more divisions of the trigeminal nerve. Attacks may have specific triggers and/or may be stereotyped in the individual patient [10]. If sensory or motor deficits, autonomic dysregulation, or stigmata of infection are observed, an alternate diagnosis should be pursued. Once a diagnosis of trigeminal neuralgia is made, magnetic resonance imaging (MRI) of the head should be performed to identify any nerve-impinging vascular structures that would be amenable to surgical decompression. As discussed for sensory mononeuropathies, if the pattern of distribution or response is atypical, alternative psychiatric diagnosis may need to be considered.

Treatment

Carbamazepine is the gold standard for medical treatment of trigeminal neuralgia and can provide complete pain relief within a few days, but is commonly associated with side effects. Oxcarbazepine, lamotrigine, phenytoin, and pregabalin are second-line agents [9].

If this medical management fails, cutaneous nerve blocks with lidocaine, alcohol, phenol, or streptomycin can be attempted, although the duration of response is typically only a few months [8].

Surgical management should be attempted in patients who have failed medical management; it may also be considered earlier in patients with evidence of vascular nerve compression on MRI. Alternative therapies include percutaneous ablation of the trigeminal ganglion or stereotactic radiation. All surgical options carry the risk of nerve damage or anesthesia dolorsa – intractable facial pain frequently perceived as worse than the original symptoms [8].

Having one episode of trigeminal neuralgia does not condemn an individual to future recurrences, and subsequent attacks do not predict the likelihood of future attacks [7]. Mortality is not increased in this patient population, though there are profound psychosocial consequences to living with this disease. Fear of provoking an attack often limits daily activities, such as basic dental care or eating. Support groups such as the Facial Pain Association (fpa-support.org) and Living with Trigeminal Neuralgia (livingwithtn.org) can help.

Trigeminal trophic syndrome
Defining features

Trigeminal trophic syndrome (Figure 19.1) is a rare type of neuropathic itch that results after injury to a peripheral or central branch

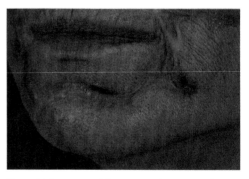

Figure 19.1 65-year-old patient with trigeminal trophic syndrome and depression (courtesy of Dr A. Bewley).

of the trigeminal nerve with resultant cutaneous anesthesia, intractable pruritus, and thus uncontrolled scratching. The painless scratching leads to self-induced ulceration of the skin – classically a non-inflamed crescent-shaped ulcer of the lateral nasal ala. Any area of the face may be affected, though the tip of the nose is often spared [11,12].

Trigeminal trophic syndrome is twice as common in females and mean age of presentation is 57 years (range 14 months–97 years) [13]. Median time to ulcer formation after nerve injury is 1 year [11].

The differential diagnosis for an ulcer on the face is broad, and it is important to rule out infections, neoplasms, inflammatory conditions, and psychiatric disease.

Pathogenesis

Injury to the trigeminal nerve is required for the development of trigeminal trophic syndrome. Why some patients develop trigeminal trophic syndrome while others do not is unclear.

The two most common etiologies of nerve injury are iatrogenic ablation for trigeminal neuralgia (one-third of cases) and stroke (one-third of cases) [12]. The last third of trigeminal trophic syndrome patients may have any one of a number of underlying etiologies (Figure 19.2), a summary of which is provided in Table 19.2.

Table 19.2 Factors underlying trigeminal trophic syndrome [12]

Peripheral nerve	Central nerve
• Post-herpetic itch • Leprosy • Syphilis • Amyloid • Trauma	• Multiple sclerosis • Neoplasm • Abscesses • Syphilis • Post-encephalitis • Parkinsonism • Amyloid • Vascular insufficiency (e.g. stroke) • Post-surgical (e.g. ablation) • Trauma

Assessment

The diagnosis of trigeminal trophic syndrome is made clinically after a thorough history and physical examination, with skin biopsies performed as indicated. Neurologic referral for detailed nerve testing can be considered. As discussed above, you should also consider psychiatric diagnoses when assessing these patients. Trigeminal trophic syndromes are the most difficult to differentiate from factitious disorders. You should also consider the neuropsychiatric disorders listed earlier – a history of trigeminal ablation or imaging studies consistent with stroke should lean you toward a diagnosis of trigeminal trophic syndrome.

Treatment

The treatment of trigeminal trophic syndrome requires a multidisciplinary approach involving dermatology, neurology, psychiatry, and surgery. Treating physicians frequently meet resistance from the patient to the concept of self-induced ulceration as patients are often unaware of scratching. Patient education regarding disease etiology and cessation of scratching are vital to change the course of the disease. Hand mitts may even be necessary to prevent unconscious picking [13].

Medications may reduce pruritus and curtail scratching. Options include carbamazepine or

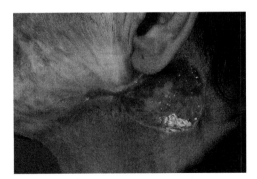

Figure 19.2 Patient with atypical trigeminal trophic syndrome (with no underlying cause) that extends beyond the usual borders of the trigeminal nerve (courtesy of Dr A. Bewley).

oxcarbazepine, gabapentin, pregabalin, amitriptyline, or pimozide [13]. Surgical grafts or flaps can be used to cover the ulcerated area, but are futile if the patient continues to pick.

The prognosis of trigeminal trophic syndrome is dependent upon patient responsiveness to treatment and the original extent of tissue destruction.

Erythromelalgia

Defining features

Erythromelalgia is defined by episodes of erythema accompanied by paroxysms of an intense burning sensation in the extremities. Feet (Figure 19.3), legs, and hands are most commonly affected, but cases involving the ears, neck, and face have also been described [14]. Attacks typically occur one to two times per week, although symptoms may be more frequent or even constant in some patients.

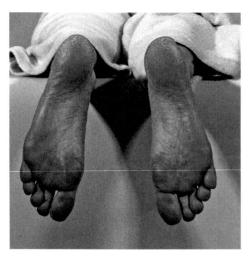

Figure 19.3 Erythromelalgia in a 65-year-old patient. Note the dusky erythema of the extremities (courtesy of Dr A. Bewley).

Provoking and exacerbating factors include heat and exercise; relief often comes with cooling the extremities. Between attacks, the extremities may feel normal or may be mildly cool, cyanotic, or uncomfortable [14].

Erythromelalgia is more common in females, and average age of presentation is 60 years, although diagnoses have been made in children. The incidence of erythromelalgia is 1.3 per 100 000 persons per year [15].

Pathogenesis

There are primary, secondary, and familial causes of erythromelalgia. Primary erythromelalgia is frequently idiopathic, and is the most common diagnosis in pediatric cases. More recently, however, many patients with primary erythromelalgia were found to have a distal cutaneous small fiber neuropathy that diminished sudomotor function (sweating). It has been postulated that this neuropathy also diminishes the sympathetic vasoconstrictive response, which results in a 10-fold increase in acral blood flow and an increase in cutaneous temperature by $7\,^{\circ}C$. As a result of this shunting, less oxygen and nutrients are delivered to the tissues, further provoking symptoms [16].

Secondary erythromelalgia is often due to an underlying leukemia, thrombocytosis, or polycythemia vera, with symptoms either proceeding or succeeding the diagnosis. In this subset of patients, increased microvascular viscosity is felt to be the cause [16]. Other secondary causes may include neuropathy (of many types), connective tissue diseases, medications and poisons, and pregnancy.

Familial cases of erythromelalgia rarely occur, and are thought to be due to an inherited neuron ion channelopathy. Onset of erythromelalgia is earlier in these patients [16].

Assessment

The diagnosis of erythromelalgia is established clinically. Work-up should include a complete blood count to assess for myeloproliferative disease. Differential diagnoses include complex regional pain syndrome, Raynaud's, cellulitis, palmoplantar erythrodysesthsia (chemotherapy-associated), and vasculitis [14].

Treatment

Treatment of erythromelalgia is difficult and must be tailored to the individual. Often combinations of therapies are needed. For patients with thrombocytosis or polycythemia vera, aspirin should be started [17].

When symptoms are mild, topical treatment may suffice, such as topical amitriptyline 1% with ketamine 0.5% gel, lidocaine patches, or capsaicin cream. For moderate cases, topicals should be combined with oral systemic therapy with gabapentin, sertraline, venlafaxine, amitriptyline, or nortriptyline [17]. When severe, erythromelalgia carries significant morbidity for the patient and merits collaboration with a pain specialist, systemic infusions with lidocaine, sodium nitroprusside, or prostaglandin can be considered. For patients not responsive to medical therapy, invasive procedures such as sympathetic blockade, sympathectomy, or dorsal cord stimulation may be considered [17].

Independent of severity, all patients should be educated to avoid provoking factors, such as warmth, dependent positioning, exercise, and alcohol. Cognitive-behavioral therapy and biofeedback techniques are also useful [17]. Relief from discomfort during episodes can be achieved through elevating the extremity and/or light cooling, such as with cold paper towels or limited immersion of the extremity in cool – but not ice cold – water. Education regarding cold injuries is especially important as many patients with erythromelalgia have evidence of cold injury from immersing their feet for prolonged periods in ice water. Cold injury causes maceration and edema that may progress to severe ischemia or sepsis, which may eventually require amputation [14].

An equal number of patients with erythromelalgia improve as remain *status quo* or worsen. There is an increased mortality in this patient population, with death often the result of an underlying myeloproliferative or connective tissue disease, sepsis, or patient suicide [14].

PRACTICAL TIPS

- Dysesthetic syndromes are varied in nature and level of morbidity to the patient.
- Sensory mononeuropathies are abnormal or unpleasant sensations within the skin experienced by a patient along the distribution of a nerve, with little or no attendant skin changes, and can often be managed conservatively.
- Primary erythromelalgia patients often have a distal cutaneous small fiber neuropathy resulting in massive blood shunting and symptomatology. Treatment is best achieved through education and therapy tailored to the individual.
- Trigeminal neuralgia and trigeminal trophic syndrome cause significant patient distress. Partnering with the patient and having a multidisciplinary approach may help achieve both patient- and physician-directed goals.
- For most dysesthesias, gabapentin, pregabalin, or amitriptyline are a reasonable first therapeutic approach.

References

1. Pérez-Pérez LC. General features and treatment of notalgia paresthetica. *Skinmed* 2011; 9(6x: 353–358.
2. Wallengren J, Klinker M. Successful treatment of notalgia paresthetica with topical capsaicin: vehicle-controlled, double-blind, crossover study. *J Am Acad Dermatol* 1995 32(2 Pt 1): 287–289.
3. Fleischer AB *et al*. Notalgia paresthetica: successful treatment with exercises. *Acta Derm Venereol* 2011; 91(3): 356–357.
4. Weinfeld PK. Successful treatment of notalgia paresthetica with botulinum toxin type A. *Arch Dermatol* 2007; 143(8): 980–982.
5. Harney D, Patijn J. Meralgia paresthetica: diagnosis and management strategies. *Pain Med* 2007; 8(8): 669–677.
6. Dhull P, Tewari AK. Botulinum toxin for meralgia paresthetica in type 2 diabetes. *Diabetes Metab Syndr* 2013; 7(1): 1–2.
7. Katusic S *et al*. Incidence and clinical features of trigeminal neuralgia, Rochester, Minnesota, 1945-1984. *Ann Neurol* 1990; 27(1): 89–95.
8. Zakrzewska JM, Linskey ME. Trigeminal neuralgia. *Clin Evid (Online)* 2009 ; 2009pii: 1207.
9. Zakrzewska JM, McMillan R. Trigeminal neuralgia: the diagnosis and management of this excruciating and poorly understood facial pain. *Postgrad Med J* 2011; 87(1028): 410–416.
10. The International Classification of Headache Disorders, 2nd edn. *Cephalagia* 2004; 24 (Suppl 1): 9–160.
11. Sadeghi P *et al*. Trigeminal trophic syndrome–report of four cases and review of the literature. *Dermatol Surg* 2004; 30(5): 807–812.
12. Curtis AR *et al*. Trigeminal trophic syndrome from stroke: an under-recognized central neuropathic itch syndrome. *Am J Clin Dermatol* 2012; 13(2): 125–128.
13. Rashid RM, Khachemoune A. Trigeminal trophic syndrome. *J Eur Acad Dermatol Venereol* 2007; 21(6): 725–731.
14. Davis MD *et al*. Natural history of erythromelalgia: presentation and outcome in 168 patients. *Arch Dermatol* 2000; 136(3): 330–336.
15. Reed KB, Davis MD. Incidence of erythromelalgia: a population-based study in Olmsted County, Minnesota. *J Eur Acad Dermatol Venereol* 2009; 23(1): 13–15.
16. Davis MD *et al*. Erythromelalgia: vasculopathy, neuropathy, or both? A prospective study of vascular and neurophysiologic studies in erythromelalgia. *Arch Dermatol* 2003; 139(10): 1337–1343.
17. Durosaro O *et al*. Intervention for erythromelalgia, a chronic pain syndrome: comprehensive pain rehabilitation center, Mayo Clinic. *Arch Dermatol* 2008; 144(12): 1578–1583.

Chronic idiopathic mucocutaneous pain syndromes: vulvodynia, penodynia, and scrotodynia

Peter J. Lynch[1] and Libby Edwards[2]

[1] UC Davis Medical Center, Sacramento, CA, USA

[2] Carolinas Medical Center, Charlotte, NC, USA

Chronic idiopathic pain disorders can involve any organ, including the skin and mucosa. Neologisms have been created with the site of pain as the prefix and the term "-odynia" (from the Greek for "pain") as the suffix. In this chapter, we use the terms "vulvodynia," "penodynia," and "scrotodynia". By definition, these disorders are idiopathic.

Regardless of the site involved, chronic idiopathic mucocutaneous pain disorders tend to share a number of common characteristics (Box 20.1). These shared characteristics suggest that all of these disorders have a common, as yet unknown, etiology and pathophysiology.

Chronic idiopathic genital pain is often accompanied by psychological, sexual, and social problems. The question, of course, is which causes which. Unfortunately, the answer to this "chicken and egg" problem is uncertain at this time.

Vulvodynia

The International Society for the Study of Vulvovaginal Disease (ISSVD) has defined vulvodynia as: "vulvar discomfort, most often described as burning pain, occurring in the absence of relevant visible findings or a specific, clinically identifiable, neurologic disorder" [1]. In that same publication, the ISSVD suggested that vulvodynia be classified as "generalized" or "localized" and, within each of these two categories, be identified as "provoked," "unprovoked," or "mixed" [1]. "Provoked" indicates that the pain is triggered by physical contact (sexual, non-sexual or both). "Unprovoked" means that the pain arises spontaneously without a specific physical trigger [1]. This definition and classification have become widely accepted, although many now think that the individual categories overlap to a greater degree than was believed originally.

Although studies vary somewhat, approximately 8% (range 3–14%) of women of all ethnicities and all ages from adolescence to late adult life have idiopathic, chronic vulvar pain at any one point in time [2]. The majority of these patients have provoked vestibular pain (provoked vestibulodynia) [2]. The annual incidence of vulvodynia is approximately 3% [3] and, over a lifetime, up to 25% of women will experience vulvodynia [2]. The mean and median age at onset is approximately 30 years [2]. For some women with vulvodynia, the pain starts with either first intercourse or first tampon use (primary vulvodynia), whereas for others, the pain arises later after having had satisfactory

Practical Psychodermatology, First Edition. Anthony Bewley, Ruth E. Taylor, Jason S. Reichenberg and Michelle Magid.

© 2014 John Wiley & Sons, Ltd. Published 2014 by John Wiley & Sons, Ltd.

Box 20.1 Characteristics commonly shared in patients with oral and genital chronic mucocutaneous pain disorders

- Pain is idiopathic; there is no recognizable underlying disease
- Pain is chronic and has been present for months or years
- Pain is unresponsive to conventional oral and topical anti-inflammatory analgesics such as aspirin, non-steroidal anti-inflammatory agents (NSAIDs) and topical steroids
- Pain interferes with falling asleep but does not cause awakening
- Patients with the pain often have painful co-morbidities such as chronic fatigue syndrome, fibromyalgia, irritable bowel syndrome or chronic pain at other sites
- Patients are preoccupied with the pain and find that it interferes with one or more aspects of their lives
- Patients deny the possibility of a psychological etiology

Table 20.1 Differential diagnosis for mucocutaneous genital pain in the absence of visible lesions

Diagnosis	Differentiating Features
Lichen planus	Visible lesions/ulcerations
Lichen sclerosus	Visible lesions/color changes
Pudendal neuropathy/ nerve entrapment	Pain occurs primarily in the distribution of the pudendal nerve Pain is often unilateral Pain is worsened when sitting and is relieved by standing or lying down Pain is relieved with anesthetic nerve blockage Diagnostic magnetic resonance neurography can be used in equivocal cases
Post-herpetic neuralgia	History of herpes zoster in the lumbo-sacral area 1–2 months previously Pain is unilateral Sensory changes may be present on neurologic examination Antibodies to varicella-zoster virus are elevated

intercourse and/or tampon use (secondary vulvodynia).

Defining features and assessment

A diagnosis of vulvodynia is one of exclusion, but can usually be established on the basis of history and examination. The usual history is that of pain of more than 3 months' duration. It is most commonly described as "burning," though the terms "rawness," "stinging," or "irritation" are sometimes used. Itching is not frequently present. The pain severity is remarkably high, with scores on a 0–10 visual analog scale clustering at the level of 9–10 [4]. Patients with vulvodynia are much more likely than those without vulvodynia to have other chronic pain conditions, such as interstitial cystitis, irritable bowel syndrome, chronic fatigue syndrome, and fibromyalgia; 25% have more than one of these conditions [5].

Examination generally occurs with the patient in stirrups and with lighting that is horizontally positioned. A number of dermatologic

and gynecologic disorders can cause vulvar pain (Table 20.1), most of which can be excluded based on visual examination [6]. If uncertainty exists, a wet mount preparation, potassium hydroxide (KOH) preparation, cultures or biopsy should be performed. Some authors consider that all patients with vulvar pain require a speculum examination and KOH preparation in order to rule out atrophic vaginitis, vaginal lichen planus, and desquamatory inflammatory vaginitis.

Evaluation of the pain is performed by asking the patient to touch the area(s) that is painful, followed by an examiner's gentle probing with a cotton-tipped applicator. The most common presentation is pain localized to the vestibule (vestibulodynia, clitorodynia), but more diffuse pain may be present over some, or all, of the vulva. Redness within the vestibule can be a

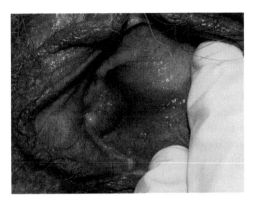

Figure 20.1 Deep red color in the vulvar vestibule – this is within the normal spectrum for vestibular color change. When present in a woman with vulvodynia, it is not indicative of pathologic inflammation and therefore cannot be considered as an explanation for the pain that is present (Reproduced with permission of Libby Edwards, 2013).

normal examination finding (Figure 20.1) and should not be seen as a sign of inflammation if found in isolation. Moreover, biopsies of the vestibule in women with and without vestibulodynia revealed similar numbers and types of inflammatory cells. Digital evaluation to evaluate the pelvic floor musculature is desirable in most instances of vulvodynia [7].

Pathogenesis

Currently, vulvodynia is considered to be an idiopathic disorder with a multifactorial pathophysiology [8]. Some of these factors include defective embryologic development, genetic abnormalities, hormonal abnormalities, infection, trauma, neuropathy, pelvic psychosexual dysfunction, and, most importantly, pelvic floor muscular abnormalities [6,7,9]. Other triggering factors include dyspareunia (not meeting the definition of vulvodynia), urinary tract infection, estrogen deficiency, and inflammatory disorders, especially that of vulvovaginal candidiasis [3,10].

Though vulvodynia was originally thought to be due to inflammatory damage to peripheral nerve receptors, the current concept is that the condition is due to damage to the neural pain fibers bringing a signal to the brain [8]. There is also evidence for "central sensitization," with changes in the way that the brain perceives the pain [8,11,12]. This would explain why these patients also report allodynia (the perception of pain to a normally non-painful stimulus), hyperalgesia, and chronic pain syndrome at non-vulvar sites.

Psychological, social, and sexual aspects

Most patients with vulvodynia have some degree of psychosocial or sexual impairment [13,14].

Patients with vulvodynia are more likely to report a history of depression than women with other vulvar disorders [10]. Antecedent depression and anxiety increase the subsequent risk of developing vulvodynia, and the presence of vulvodynia increases the risk of both new and recurrent onset of psychopathology [15]. Additionally, there is evidence for increased somatization, harm avoidance, hypervigilance, and catastrophizing [13,14,16]. Vulvodynia patients perceive themselves as having little control over their symptoms and are afraid that their symptoms will persist [4]. Several studies have found that the quality of life for patients with vulvodynia is decreased in comparison to controls [10].

Patients with vulvodynia may have lower levels of sexual desire, arousal, and frequency of intercourse [4,13,14]. One study found these patients to also have lower scores on lubrication, orgasm, and sexual satisfaction scales [17].

Vulvodynia patients score significantly less well in the areas of relationship issues and emotional function than do women with other chronic vulvovaginal disorders [18]. They may have more difficulty in forming and maintaining social relationships [10], though one study found their relationships to be within population norms [19].

Though controversial, childhood physical and sexual abuse is a possible risk factor for the subsequent development of vulvodynia [13,14]. There is also highly controversial evidence of dysfunctional interpersonal relationships, especially in sexual partnerships [13,14].

The important question is: "*Does psychological, sexual and/or social dysfunction stem from the presence of vulvodynia or does it play an etiologic role?*" One of the authors of this chapter (LE) sides with the majority of clinicians who believe that psychosocial and sexual dysfunction occurs as the result of chronic pain, whereas the other (PJL) favors the view that these dysfunctions pre-exist and lead to the onset of vulvodynia [13]. Desrochers *et al.* [14] has suggested the answer is not either-or.

Treatment

There have been very few controlled studies and even fewer randomized controlled studies regarding the management of patients with vulvodynia. As a result, treatment recommendations are mostly based on clinician experience and/or published guidelines [20,21]. Moreover, a rather high placebo response rate has been found in most of the controlled vulvodynia studies [22]. Ideally, patients should be treated in a psychodermatology multidisciplinary team (pMDT) along with gynecologists.

Therapy begins with patient education (using handouts and often referral to the website of the National Vulvodynia Association), psychological counseling, and, for patients with provoked vulvodynia, sexual counseling. The second, and equally important, step is referral (especially of those patients with provoked vulvodynia) to an experienced physical therapist for pelvic floor evaluation and appropriate physical therapy if dysfunction is found. Pain clearance rates with such therapy are as high as with most medical therapies [20,21].

There is a limited role for topical therapy but lidocaine (2% jelly or 5% ointment) either alone or mixed with prilocaine (EMLA cream®) can give some degree of short-term pain relief [9]. Most patients will require systemic therapy, usually with oral medications known to be effective for peripheral neuropathies. The first line of treatment is usually a tricyclic antidepressant, such as amitriptyline or nortriptyline, starting at a low, nightly dose of 5 or 10 mg and gradually increasing to the point of either acceptable pain relief or a maximum dose of 150 mg [20,21]. If there is failure or intolerance to these agents, combined reuptake inhibitors (venlafaxine or duloxetine; see Chapter 3) or anticonvulsants (gabapentin or pregabalin; see Chapter 19) can be tried [21]. As a last resort, patients with provoked vestibulodynia can consider surgery (vestibulectomy), but not all patients will obtain relief from this [22].

Of note, psychotherapy (primarily cognitive-behavioral therapy) has been reported to be as effective as the pharmacologic treatments discussed above [9,16,23].

Vulvodynia is a chronic disease, and data on long-term prognosis is scarce. The Michigan Women's Health Group noted a 17% remission rate over a mean duration of 12.5 years. Most clinicians believe that with the modalities discussed above, a clinically satisfying degree of improvement can be achieved.

Penodynia and scrotodynia

The first publication regarding idiopathic, chronic mucocutaneous male genital pain occurred in 1981 [24]. The perceived rarity of this condition is probably inaccurate. It is likely that patients with peno-scrotodynia (PSD) have been subsumed under the diagnosis of "chronic prostatitis/chronic pelvic pain syndrome" (CP/CPPS). Supporting this belief is the observation that approximately 90% of patients with a diagnosis of CP/CPPS have burning pain of the penis (especially the glans) and alterations in sensory perception similar to those occurring in other chronic pain syndromes [25,26].

Defining features and assessment

By definition, this is an idiopathic disorder. Thus, all recognizable causes of penile and scrotal pain (including pudendal neuropathy) must be eliminated, leaving PSD as a diagnosis of exclusion (Table 20.1). Historically, patients describe their pain as "burning," but other terms such as those noted for vulvodynia are sometimes used. Itching is rarely present. The pain has often been present for several years. The discomfort may occur on the glans penis, on the scrotal wall, or at both sites. It less commonly involves the shaft of the penis. Occasionally, there is extension of the pain to the perineum, the perianal area, or down the legs. Usually there is a background of low-grade constant pain with exacerbations of acute, more severe pain with sexual activity, exercise, sweating, and contact with tight clothing [27].

Nearly all patients believe that redness has developed or worsened since the pain began (Figure 20.2). This is particularly likely when the anterior wall of the scrotum is involved. In this latter setting, the term "red scrotum

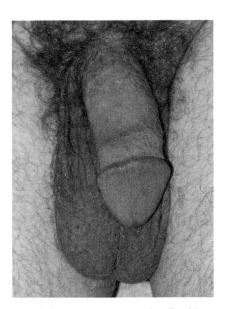

Figure 20.2 Red color on the scrotal wall – this within the normal spectrum for scrotal color change. When present in a man with scrotodynia, it is not indicative of pathologic inflammation and therefore cannot be considered as an explanation for the pain that is present (Reproduced with permission of Libby Edwards, 2013).

syndrome" is often used [28,29]. Rarely, when the glans is involved, there will be a dusky blue hue. In our opinion these color changes do not represent abnormalities, but fall within the range of color encountered in individuals without PSD.

Patients with scrotal wall involvement have often previously been treated with potent topical steroids because the redness was presumed to be inflammatory. Since long-term use of these agents may be associated with discomfort, increased redness, atrophy, and telangiectasia, all such therapy must be discontinued.

Pathogenesis

Although there is no evidence, it is likely that PSD represents a neuropathic pain syndrome much like vulvodynia, with concomitant hypersensitivity, allodynia, and pain at extragenital sites. It is likely that abnormalities in central sensitization are present.

Psychological, social, and sexual aspects

Patients with CP/CPPS frequently have psychological, sexual, and social dysfunction similar to that we have encountered in patients with PSD. For this reason, data from patients with CP/CPPS are included below.

A controlled study of CP/CPPS patients found odds ratios compared to controls of 3.6 for any mental health diagnosis, 4.3 for panic syndrome, and 4.5 for depression. One recently published paper describes patients with CP/CPPS as having a functional somatic syndrome [30]. A high prevalence of sexual dysfunction in CP/CPPS has been noted. In a controlled study of 38 men, patients with CP/CPPS had significantly higher levels of sexual dysfunction in domains such as decreased desire, erectile problems, impaired orgasm, and decreased sexual satisfaction [31]. We have found sexual dysfunction in most of our younger patients, with several stating that the pain prevented intercourse [27]. One of us (PJL) also found a decreased level of sexual activity in older patients [27]. Both authors of this chapter have noted that PSD frequently begins shortly after an, often non-marital, sexual encounter [32].

In the experience of both authors, there seems to be a lower than expected frequency of marriage in patients (11 of 24), and of those who are not married, most had never been in a long-term heterosexual relationship [27].

As is true for vulvodynia, one of us (LE) believes it is mostly the presence of chronic pain that leads to psychosocial and sexual

dysfunction, whereas the other (PJL) believes that pre-existing dysfunction is the most common cause of PSD.

Treatment and prognosis

Amitriptyline in doses as described for vulvodynia is often the first-line therapy. Gabapentin, pregabalin, and venlafaxine may be second line. Most clinicians would consider a referral for psychological, and where appropriate, sexual counseling. However, some patients may be unreceptive to this approach. There are no data available regarding the long-term prognosis for patients with PSF.

PRACTICAL TIPS

- Consider a diagnosis of vulvodynia, penodynia or scrotodynia when patients tell you they have experienced constant or intermittent pain in the vulva, penis or scrotal wall, respectively.

- It is however critically important to exclude pain due to infectious, inflammatory, neoplastic, and neurologic disorders before confirming the diagnosis of one of these idiopathic pain conditions.

- In excluding these other conditions, be aware that patients (and even other clinicians) may have the perception that the presence of red or violaceous color signifies the existence of underlying physical disease. However, in these situations, the color almost always falls within the spectrum of normal for these tissues and thus has no special meaning.

- In addition to pain, many of these patients have psychological, social, and sexual distress. There is controversy as to whether these factors cause, or are the result of, the patient's pain. Either way, these factors, if present, must be addressed, preferably by referral to psychological and/or sexual consultants.

- The primary therapy for vulvodynia is the administration of a tricyclic antidepressant (most often amitriptyline) and referral to a physical therapist for evaluation and treatment of the pelvic floor musculature dysfunction that is almost always present.

- First-line therapy for penodynia and scrotodynia is likewise the administration of a tricyclic antidepressant such as amitriptyline.

- Second-line therapies for all three disorders include venlafaxine, duloxetine, gabapentin, and pregabalin. All of these agents have been widely used in the treatment of painful neuropathies.

References

1. Moyal-Barracco M, Lynch PJ. ISSVD terminology and classification of vulvodynia. A historical perspective. *J Reprod Med* 2003; 49: 772–777.
2. Reed BD *et al.* Prevalence and demographic characteristics of vulvodynia in a population-based sample. *Am J Obstet Gynecol* 2012; 206: 170e1–9.
3. Reed BD *et al.* Urogenital symptoms and pain history as precursors of vulvodynia: a longitudinal study. *J Women's Health* 2012; 21: 1139–1143.
4. Piper CK *et al.* Experience of symptoms, sexual function, and attitudes towards counseling of women newly diagnosed with vulvodynia. *J Lower Genital Tract Dis* 2012; 16: 447–453.
5. Reed BD *et al.* Relationship between vulvodynia and chronic comorbid pain conditions. *Obstet Gynecol* 2012; 120: 145–151.

6. Danby CS, Margesson LJ. Approach to the diagnosis and treatment of vulvar pain. *Dermatol Ther* 2010; 23: 485–504.

7. Nunns D, Murphy R. Assessment and management of vulval pain. *BMJ* 2012; 344: e1723.

8. Bohm-Starke N. Medical and physical predictors of localized provoked vulvodynia. *Acta Obstet Gynecol* 2010; 89: 1504–1510.

9. Damstead-Petersen C *et al.* Current perspectives in vulvodynia. *Women's Health* 2009; 5: 423–436.

10. Ponte M *et al.* Effects of vulvodynia on quality of life. *J Am Acad Dermatol* 2009; 80: 70–76.

11. Ventolini G. Vulvar pain: Anatomic and recent pathophysiologic considerations. *Clin Anat* 2013; 26: 130–133.

12. Zhang Z *et al.* Altered central sensitization in subgroups of women with vulvodynia. *Clin J Pain* 2011; 27: 755–763.

13. Lynch PJ. Vulvodynia as a somatoform disorder. *J Reprod Med* 2008; 53: 390–396.

14. Desrochers G *et al.* Do psychosexual factors play a role in the etiology of provoked vestibulodynia? A critical review. *J Sex Marital Ther* 2008; 34: 198–226.

15. Khandker M *et al.* The influence of depression and anxiety on risk of adult onset vulvodynia. *J Women's Health* 2011; 20: 1445–1451.

16. Desrochers G *et al.* Fear avoidance and self-efficacy in relation to pain and sexual impairment in women with provoked vestibulodynia. *Clin J Pain* 2009; 25: 520–527.

17. Giraldo PC *et al.* Evaluation of sexual function in Brazilian women with recurrent vulvovaginal candidiasis and localized provoked vulvodynia. *J Sex Med* 2012; 9: 805–811.

18. Jelovsek JE *et al.* Psychosocial impact of chronic vulvovaginal conditions. *J Reprod Med* 2008; 53: 75–82.

19. Desrosiers M *et al.* Psychosexual characteristics of vestibulodynia couples: partner solicitousness and hostility are associated with pain. *J Sex Med* 2008; 5: 418–427.

20. Nunns D *et al.* Guidelines for the management of vulvodynia. *Br J Dermatol* 2010; 162: 1180–1185.

21. Cox KJ, Neville CE. Assessment and management options for women with vulvodynia. *J Midwifery Women's Health* 2012; 57: 231–240.

22. Andrews JC. Vulvodynia interventions – systematic review and evidence grading. *Obstet Gynecol Surv* 2011; 66: 299–315.

23. Desrochers G *et al.* Provoked vestibulodynia: psychological predictors of topical and cognitive-behavioral treatment outcome. *Behav Res Ther* 2010; 48: 106–115.

24. Cotteril JA. Dermatological non-disease: a common and potentially fatal disturbance of cutaneous body image. *Br J Dermatol* 1981; 104: 611–619

25. Anderson RU *et al.* Painful myofascial trigger points and pain sites in men with chronic prostatitis/chronic pelvic pain syndrome. *J Urol* 2009; 182: 2753–2758.

26. Naim M, Ende D. A new approach to the treatment of non-specific male genital pain. *BJU* 2011; 107 (Suppl 3): 34–37.

27. Lynch PJ. Anogenital pain. In: Lynch PJ, Edwards L (eds) *Genital Dermatology.* New York: Churchill Livingstone, 1994, pp. 237–249.

28. Fisher BK. Inflammatory lesions of the penis. In: Fisher BK, Margesson LJ. *Genital Skin Disorders. Diagnosis and Treatment.* St. Louis: Mosby, 1998, pp. 41–64.

29. Wollina U. Red scrotum syndrome. *J Dermatol Case Rep* 2011; 3: 38–41.

30. Potts JM, Payne CK. Urologic chronic pelvic pain. *Pain* 2012; 153: 755–758.

31. Smith KB *et al.* Sexual and relationship functioning in men with chronic prostatitis/chronic pelvic pain syndrome and their partners. *Arch Sex Behav* 2007; 36: 301–311.

32. Edwards L, Lynch PJ. Genital pain syndromes. In: Edwards L, Lynch PJ (eds) *Genital Dermatology Atlas.* Philadelphia: Wolters Kluwer/Lippincott Williams & Wilkins, 2011, pp. 46–56.

CHAPTER 21

Burning mouth syndrome

Alison Bruce, Rochelle R. Torgerson, Cooper C. Wriston and Tania M. Gonzalez Santiago

Department of Dermatology, Mayo Clinic, Rochester, MN, USA

Burning mouth syndrome (BMS) is a chronic pain disorder typically presenting as spontaneously occurring intraoral pain of any character in peri- or post-menopausal women in the absence of explanative organic disease. Symptoms last more than 4–6 months, frequently involve the lips or tongue, and often occur with xerostomia and dysgeusia. There may be associated psychosocial stressors, mood or personality disorders [1,2]. Fully characterizing the spectrum of clinical presentation is complicated by the varied terminology describing BMS in the literature. BMS may encompass conditions previously described as glossodynia, glossopyrosis, glossalgia, scalded mouth syndrome, estomatoporosis, stomatodynia, and oropyrosis [3].

Classically, BMS has been classified as primary or secondary. In the primary disorder, clinical and laboratory abnormalities are absent. As the "secondary" disorder describes common symptoms of unrelated conditions, the designation "secondary burning mouth syndrome" should be abandoned. Other explanative causes of intraoral burning pain include local, systemic, and psychological conditions (Table 21.1). If any associated condition is encountered during the clinical evaluation, it should be excluded as a cause of symptoms.

The identification and treatment of BMS has become increasingly important as the extent of its impact has been recognized. Patients with BMS report a significantly negative impact on quality of life. Patients with BMS experience a clinical burden similar to that from other chronic pain disorders. The mean duration of BMS has been reported to be 30 months, ranging from 1.5 months to 17 years. While some authors report clinical improvement over time, the prognosis may vary greatly, often depending directly on the extent of the supportive nature of the patient–physician relationship.

Limited data on the prevalence of BMS exist. Some groups have estimated between 0.7% and 7.9% of the adult population have experienced BMS [8]. A National Institutes of Health (NIH) survey estimated there are nearly 1 million burning mouth sufferers in the US.

Defining features

The pain of BMS is often persistent, bilateral, and symmetric. Pain can extend throughout the oral mucosa to involve the gingiva, the lips, and rarely the throat. Symptoms rarely correspond to a single nerve distribution. Most patients describe the pain as moderate to marked in intensity and worsening throughout the day, despite rarely waking them from sleep. Patients may report associated xerostomia and dysgeusia, although these are not consistent features. Patients may have a co-morbid mood disorder.

Practical Psychodermatology, First Edition. Anthony Bewley, Ruth E. Taylor, Jason S. Reichenberg and Michelle Magid.
© 2014 John Wiley & Sons, Ltd. Published 2014 by John Wiley & Sons, Ltd.

Table 21.1 Secondary causes of intraoral burning

Causes of oral pain	Indications for additional testing	Screening tests
Medication	History of efavirenz, fluoxetine, sertraline, clonazepam, venlafaxine, enalapril, captopril, lisinopril, candesartan, eprosartan, omeprazole, topiramate, clindamycin, or hormone replacement therapy [4,5]	Elimination and rechallenge
Allergic contact stomatitis (fragrance mix, cinnamic aldehyde, gold, myroxylon, benzoic acid, nickel, gallate, cobalt, sorbic acid, nicotinic acid, propylene glycol, menthol, tartrazine) [4,6]	Suggestive history, known triggers, intermittent symptoms, oral exam findings, regular use of certain dentifrices	Epicutaneous patch testing
Dentistry	Oral prostheses, dental procedures, poor dentition	Dental consultation, imaging
Microbial (*Candida, Herpes viridae*, bacteria)	Immunosuppression, recent antibiotics, functional oral pain, oral exam findings	Culture or PCR
Primary dermatosis (lichen planus, immunobullous disease, aphthosis, lingua plicata, geographic tongue) [7]	Oral exam findings, suggestive history	Biopsy for routine histology, direct immunofluorescence, serologic testing
Parafunctional habits	History of bruxism, tongue thrusting, cheek biting, oral exam findings	Elimination
Neoplastic	Oral exam findings, dysphagia, odynophagia, adenopathy	Biopsy for routine histology, advanced imaging (if indicated)
Xerostomia (Sjögren syndrome, rheumatoid arthritis, hyposalivation, medication-induced)	Oral exam findings, suggestive history	Evaluation for autoimmune disease (ANA, ENA, RF), medication review
Endocrinopathy (diabetes, thyroid disease, hypogonadism)	Weight change, bowel/bladder habits, fatigue, cold intolerance, alopecia	TSH, fasting glucose, glycated hemoglobin, endocrinology consultation
Gastroesophageal reflux	Heartburn, regurgitation, dysphagia, nausea, increased salivation	Gastroenterology consultation
Primary neurologic (trigeminal neuralgia, glossopharyngeal neuralgia, Parkinson's disease)	Dysesthesia, dysgeusia, ataxia, apraxia	Neurology consultation
Nutritional deficiency (iron, B vitamins, folate, zinc) [7]	Glossitis, cheilitis, suggestive history (alcoholism, homelessness, eating disorder, chronic enteritis or colitis)	CBC, ferritin, screening for micronutrient deficiency
Mood disorders	Dysthymia, anxiety, illicit drug use	Psychiatry consultation

PCR, polymerase chain reaction; ANA, antinuclear antibody; ENA, extractable nuclear antigen; RF, rheumatoid factor; TSH, thyroid stimulating hormone; CBC, complete blood count

BMS remains a clinical diagnosis. Diagnostic guidelines have been suggested by the International Headache Society as:
- pain in the mouth present daily and persisting for most of the day;
- oral mucosa of normal appearance;
- the exclusion of local and systemic disease.

Pathogenesis

The pathogenesis of BMS remains elusive, although increasing evidence implicates neuropathic factors. Some authors have proposed classifying BMS as an oral dysesthesia or painful neuropathy [9]. Proposed mechanisms for BMS include:
- dysfunction of the chorda tympani;
- small afferent fiber atrophy;
- upregulated transient receptor potential vanilloid type 1 (TRPV1).

Also, patients with BMS have been found to have a lower density of epithelial nerve fibers on the anterior two-thirds of the tongue. Histologic examination of lingual biopsies have shown epithelial and sub-papillary nerve fibers reflecting axonal degeneration, suggesting a trigeminal small-fiber sensory neuropathy in the etiopathogenesis. Further, central neuropathic mechanisms have been implicated in BMS, including alterations of glossopharyngeal nerve activity [10] and changes in central dopamine levels.

Assessment

As BMS is a diagnosis of exclusion, evaluation should distinguish secondary causes of oral burning pain. To differentiate these causes, a thorough history, review of systems, physical examination, assessment of mental health, and laboratory evaluation are required. Cost-effective laboratory testing on an initial evaluation can be guided by health history and symptoms. Second opinion evaluations at tertiary care facilities may necessitate broader screening for hypothyroidism, connective tissue disease, or nutritional deficiencies.

The history should assess the quality of oral symptoms, including onset, duration, frequency, location, character, radiation, severity, and precipitating and relieving factors of pain. A history should also be obtained for dentistry; medication, tobacco and alcohol use; dentifrice usage; parafunctional behaviors such as bruxism, tongue thrusting and cheek biting; mood and psychological symptoms; and past medial history. A review of symptoms should evaluate for headache, fatigue, gastrointestinal and genitourinary symptoms, insomnia, dysthymia, anxiety, and irritability.

A thorough examination of the head, neck, oral aperture, teeth, and oral mucosa is required, though usually, as in Figure 21.1A–D, there are no physical signs in primary BMS. Oral appliances should be removed and patients should point to symptomatic areas. Oral findings such as erosions, ulcerations, erythema, white patches, lingua plicata, atrophic glossitis, xerostomia, angular cheilitis, and poor dentition suggest secondary causes of oral burning pain. Direct examination or culture for *Candida* may be helpful in the setting of functional oral pain or as directed by the physical examination. Biopsy for routine histology, direct immunofluorescence, epicutaneous patch testing, herpes (simplex and zoster) culture, and bacterial culture may be useful if suggested by examination findings. Focused laboratory testing as suggested by other elements of the history or examination may occasionally be useful (Table 21.1). A thorough neurologic examination of the cranial nerves, assessment for lymphadenopathy, and evaluation of the mandible should be performed.

Treatment

Secondary causes of oral pain should be sought and corrected (Table 21.2). Every patient should

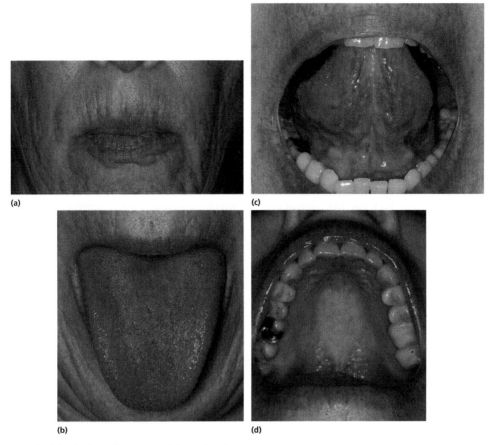

Figure 21.1 (a–d) Normal structure of the oral cavity.

Table 21.2 Treatments for secondary causes of intraoral burning (Source: Lebwohl, 2010 [4]. Reproduced with permission of Elsevier.)

Cause of oral pain	Intervention
Medication	Eliminate or change causative medications if possible
Allergic and irritant contact stomatitis	Avoid irritants (alcohol-based rinses, flavored dentifrices, acidic foods), avoid identified allergic contactants, remove or change dental appliances/prostheses, elimination diet (nickel)
Dentistry	Refit dental appliances/prostheses, revise structural causes
Candidosis	Nystatin swish and swallow, clotrimazole troche, oral fluconazole
Primary dermatosis	As directed by underlying dermatosis
Maladaptive parafunctional habits	Educational intervention, cognitive-behavioral therapy
Xerostomia	Sialogogues, oral lubricants, as directed by underlying autoimmune disease
Endocrinopathy	As directed by underlying endocrinopathy
Gastroesophageal reflux	Behavioral intervention, medical intervention (famotidine, omeprazole, etc.)
Nutritional deficiency	Micronutrient replacement (thiamine, riboflavin, pyridoxine, folate, cobalamin, iron, zinc, ascorbic acid, magnesium), address secondary causes
Mood disorders	Co-management with psychologist or psychiatrist as indicated

have his/her symptoms and experiences validated, and be reassured that the symptoms are not life-threatening. Despite the availability of multiple medical, behavioral, and educational interventions, a consistently effective treatment for BMS remains elusive.

Pharmacologic interventions may be topical or systemic. Clonazepam and capsaicin are the only topical therapies found to be effective for BMS in double-blind, randomized, placebo-controlled studies. "Suck and spit" clonazepam (1 mg) three times daily was found to be superior to placebo in controlling pain after 2 weeks of use. Topical capsaicin rinse (0.02%) three times daily resulted in improved pain scores compared to placebo, although cumulative adverse effects (gastric pain) limited its use [11]. Topical clonazepam has been shown to be cost-effective in the treatment of BMS compared to other systemic medications.

Effective systemic interventions include clonazepam, doxepin, duloxetine, milnacipran, and paroxetine. A stratified, double-blind controlled trial found clonazepam (0.5 mg once daily) to be superior to placebo in controlling oral pain after 9 weeks of use [12]. Another study reported that patients with fewer psychological symptoms, greater pain, xerostomia or dysgeusia may preferentially benefit from oral clonazepam. Paroxetine (10–30 mg daily) and duloxetine (20–40 mg daily) were found to be effective in the treatment of BMS and chronic non-organic orofacial pain (BMS and atypical odontalgia) in respective non-comparative studies. Milnacipran, a serotonin–norepinephrine reuptake inhibitor used in the clinical treatment of depression and fibromyalgia, has been found to be helpful for BMS. A non-comparative study of 30–90 mg daily showed efficacy in pain control for BMS with few dose-dependent adverse effects, though this may have been mostly due to the effect on depression. Of note, this drug is only approved for fibromyalgia in the US, and is not currently available in the UK. Randomized trials of alpha-lipoic acid have been disappointing, while reports of gabapentin efficacy and zinc replacement are conflicting or the studies poorly designed.

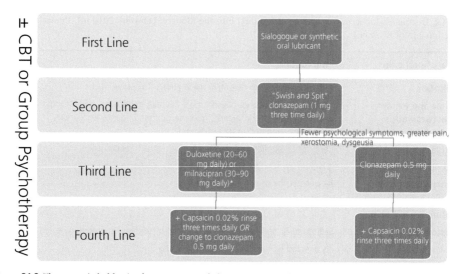

Figure 21.2 Therapeutic ladder in the treatment of chronic pain syndrome. Milnacipran is not available in the UK. If duloxetine is not helpful, other serotonin-specific reuptake inhibitors may be tried (e.g. paroxetine). CBT, cognitive-behavioral therapy.

Psychiatric interventions have been successful as monotherapy or in combination with other treatments for BMS. Cognitive therapy was effective for resistant BMS in a randomized trial comparing it with an attention program [13]. A randomized study of group psychotherapy compared to placebo capsules found efficacy in pain intensity for patients with BMS [14].

BMS can be challenging for patients and providers alike. A practical framework to identify and treat secondary causes of oral pain is important. As no treatment has been shown to be universally effective in the treatment of BMS and individual responses may vary significantly, we have suggested a therapeutic ladder in the treatment of this chronic pain syndrome (Figure 21.2). Psychiatric interventions may be used alone or adjunctively with other medical therapies. Validation of the condition and opportunity to meet other sufferers is extremely reassuring as most primary care physicians have never encountered a patient with this syndrome. Much research is needed to better understand and treat BMS.

PRACTICAL TIPS

- Evaluation of BMS includes looking for secondary causes such as nutritional deficiency, endocrinopathy, and connective tissue disease.
- Helpful treatments for BMS include clonazepam, doxepin, duloxetine, milnacipran, and paroxetine, though no treatment has been shown to be universally accepted.
- Psychiatric interventions have been successful as monotherapy or in combination with other treatments for BMS.

References

1. Abetz LM, Savage NW. Burning mouth syndrome and psychological disorders. *Aust Dent J* 2009; 54(2): 84–93; quiz 173.
2. Maina G *et al.* Personality disorders in patients with burning mouth syndrome. *J Pers Disord* 2005; 19(1): 84–93.
3. Crow HC, Gonzalez Y. Burning mouth syndrome. *Oral Maxillofac Surg Clin North Am* 2013; 25(1): 67–76.
4. Lebwohl M. *Treatment of Skin Disease: Comprehensive Therapeutic Strategies*, 3rd edn. Edinburgh: Saunders, 2010.
5. Rosen S *et al.* Probable clindamycin-induced ageusia, xerostomia, and burning mouth syndrome. *Ann Pharmacother* 2012; 46(7–8): 1119–1120.
6. Steele JC *et al.* Clinically relevant patch test results in patients with burning mouth syndrome. *Dermatitis* 2012; 23(2): 61–70.
7. Torgerson RR. Burning mouth syndrome. *Dermatol Ther* 2010; 23(3): 291–298.
8. Ship JA *et al.* Burning mouth syndrome: an update. *J Am Dent Assoc* 1995; 126(7): 842–853.
9. Jaaskelainen SK. Pathophysiology of primary burning mouth syndrome. *Clin Neurophysiol* 2012; 123(1): 71–77.
10. Grushka M *et al.* Burning mouth syndrome and other oral sensory disorders: a unifying hypothesis. *Pain Res Manag* 2003; 8(3): 133–135.
11. Silvestre FJ *et al.* Application of a capsaicin rinse in the treatment of burning mouth syndrome. *Med Oral Patol Oral Cir Bucal* 2012; 17(1): e1–4.
12. Heckmann SM *et al.* A double-blind study on clonazepam in patients with burning mouth syndrome. *Laryngoscope* 2012; 122(4): 813–816.
13. Bergdahl J *et al.* Cognitive therapy in the treatment of patients with resistant burning mouth syndrome: a controlled study. *J Oral Pathol Med.* 1995; 24(5): 213–215.
14. Miziara ID *et al.* Group psychotherapy: an additional approach to burning mouth syndrome. *J Psychosom Res* 2009; 67(5): 443–448.

CHAPTER 22

Nodular prurigo

Wei Sheng Tan, Hong Liang Tey and Mark B.Y. Tang

National Skin Centre, Singapore

Nodular prurigo or prurigo nodularis was first reported in 1909 to describe the multiple, extremely pruritic hyperkeratotic nodules found on the extensor aspect of the lower legs of middle-aged females. This condition is now well recognized and known to affect all ages and sexes, although there still appears to be a predilection for females and the elderly. The most commonly affected age group are patients in their 50s and 60s. It is an extremely chronic condition and most patients have had their lesions for a mean duration of 6.4–8.7 years [1,2].

Clinical features

Prurigo nodules are characterized by typical hyperkeratotic dome-shaped papulonodules that are usually excoriated or crusted centrally (Figure 22.1). They can range from a few lesions to a few hundred in number (Figure 22.2). The lesions are often symmetrically distributed. The limbs are the most commonly affected sites, especially over the distal areas. The extensor surfaces are also more extensively affected compared to the flexor surfaces. The nodules are usually distributed in a linear or follicular pattern, along the "lines of scratching." The face, palms, and soles are usually spared. In addition, the inability for patients to reach and scratch their mid upper back may lead to the characteristic "butterfly sign" (Figure 22.3), where there is a clear demarcation and sparing

of that "protected" area over the mid upper back.

The nodules are often surrounded by secondary pigmentary changes. Post-inflammatory hyperpigmentation is often seen in those of Asian or African descent, and paradoxical hypopigmentation or even depigmentation may also occur in chronic lesions, due to repeated trauma causing permanent pigment loss.

Occasionally, the lesions become secondarily infected, leading to crusting, tenderness, and abscess formation. Significant scarring, hyperpigmented or, less commonly, hypopigmented macules may be found after lesion resolution.

Pathogenesis

The aetiology of prurigo nodules is generally attributed to a repeated, vicious cycle of scratching or picking the skin, most commonly triggered by underlying dermatological or systemic illnesses.

A diverse range of dermatological, psychological, and systemic diseases has been reported to be associated with the condition (Table 22.1). Patients may have a single disease underlying their nodular prurigo, or a combination of both dermatological and systemic diseases. In up to 59% of patients, multifactorial causes may be found [1]. This supports the concept that nodular prurigo is a secondary phenomenon that develops due to chronic, recalcitrant

Practical Psychodermatology, First Edition. Anthony Bewley, Ruth E. Taylor, Jason S. Reichenberg and Michelle Magid.
© 2014 John Wiley & Sons, Ltd. Published 2014 by John Wiley & Sons, Ltd.

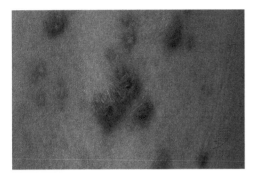

Figure 22.1 Multiple hyperkeratotic prurigo nodules with excoriated and slightly crusted central areas. Note how the older lesions have resolved as hyperpigmented and hypopigmented macules.

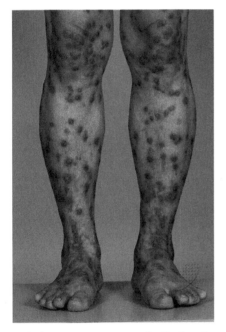

Figure 22.2 Extensive, symmetrically distributed prurigo nodules over the extensor aspects of the lower limbs, the most commonly affected site in patients.

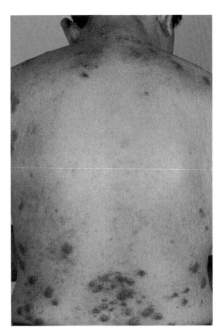

Figure 22.3 A patient with the "butterfly sign" showing sparing of the upper and mid back. Note the multiple prurigo nodules at the periphery of the spared area.

pruritus and recurrent scratching, and not a specific disease entity in itself.

Our study of extensive prurigo nodularis in 37 Asian patients at the National Skin Centre Singapore showed that all patients had identifiable underlying co-factors, with atopic eczema being the predominant aetiology in patients with both monofactorial and multifactorial disease. A third of all patients had an underlying systemic disease. Another study [1] found that an underlying disease could be identified in 87% of the 108 patients, with atopic diathesis also being the commonest association in 46.3% of patients. The atopic predisposition may predict for an earlier median age of onset of 19 years, compared to 48 years in non-atopic patients [2]. Associated systemic diseases are shown in Table 22.1.

Finally, psychological conditions have been associated with the development of prurigo nodularis [2]. Psychiatric co-morbidities, such as depression, anxiety, and obsessive-compulsive disorder, may be found as a primary cause or secondary to the severe pruritus [3]. Furthermore, psychological symptoms of anxiety and

Table 22.1 Dermatological, systemic and psychological conditions reported in association with nodular prurigo [2,6]

Dermatological	Systemic	Psychological
Atopic dermatitis	**Endocrine:**	Anxiety
Stasis dermatitis	Hyperthyroidism	Depression
Allergic contact dermatitis	Hypothyroidism	Delusional infestations
Cutaneous lymphoma	Diabetes mellitus	
Dermatitis herpetiformis	**Haematological:**	
Lichen planus	Iron-deficiency anaemia	
Grover's disease	Polycythemia rubra vera	
Insect bite reaction	Lymphoma	
Recurrent folliculitis	Leukaemia	
	Porphyria	
	Renal:	
	Chronic renal failure	
	Gastrointestinal:	
	Gluten sensitive enteropathy	
	Gastrointestinal malignancy	
	Obstructive biliary disease	
	Lactose intolerance	
	Sorbitol intolerance	
	α1-antitrypsin deficiency	
	Infections:	
	HIV	
	Hepatitis B	
	Hepatitis C	
	Mycobacterium infection (*M. tuberculosis*, *M. avium intracellulare*)	
	Helicobactor pylori infection	
	Neurological:	
	Brachioradial pruritus	
	Chronic pain syndrome	

depression are also more frequently reported in nodular prurigo patients compared to controls [4]. This underscores the importance of predisposing psychological or personality traits that, in combination with underlying systemic or dermatological conditions, may initiate and perpetuate the intense, recalcitrant scratching behaviour that causes this chronic condition.

Clinical assessment

A careful history and full physical examination is essential in the clinical evaluation of the patient (Box 22.1). In particular, a personal and family history of atopy and eczema must be elicited. A thorough skin examination is paramount to look for predisposing skin diseases. A practical tip is to carefully examine the intervening skin between prurigo nodules, looking for features of eczema, xerosis, and flexural lichenification, which may indicate the presence of atopic dermatitis. Palmar hyperlinearity, ichthyotic scaling, and keratosis pilaris may also suggest an underlying filaggrin mutation, which is the strongest genetic risk factor for atopic dermatitis. Systemic review for weight loss, intermittent fever, night sweats, lymphadenopathy, and organomegaly may indicate

Box 22.1 Clinical assessment

- Skin – thorough dermatological assessment, including of the intervening "unaffected" skin
- Full systemic review and examination, particularly for renal, liver, and thyroid disease
- Psychological assessment – consider referral to a multidisciplinary clinic, psychiatrist or psychologist
- Systemic work-up for causes of generalized pruritus:
  - Full blood count
  - Electrolytes and renal function test
  - Liver function test
  - Thyroid function tests
  - Chest X-ray
  - Other relevant investigations, such as HIV serology and CT scan for malignancies, depending on the clinical indications

an underlying haematological malignancy. Medication-induced itch may need to be excluded in patients with multiple co-morbidities with polypharmacy.

In addition, psychological screening and assessment is also vital in the holistic assessment of patients, especially in those with symptoms of depression and anxiety. The severity of the itch and details of the scratching behaviour should be carefully documented to identify external cues and triggers.

Differential diagnosis

The differential diagnoses for itchy papulonodules are varied. Acquired perforating dermatosis, thought to be a distinctive clinical entity, is currently considered to result from chronic scratching, similar to prurigo nodules. Nodular scabies may also manifest as intensely pruritic excoriated nodules, which are often located on the genitalia, scrotum or axilla.

Hypertrophic lichen planus can present similarly with keratotic nodules and plaques, but the lesions are often more heavily hyperpigmented or purplish in colour, with findings of typical lichenoid lesions elsewhere or in the oral mucosa. A predominant photodistribution of lesions should prompt the exclusion of photosensitive dermatoses, such as actinic prurigo, and one of the porphyrias. Other less common differential diagnoses include dystrophic epidermolysis bullosa pruriginosa, pemphigus nodularis, multiple keratoacanthoma, and lymphomatoid papulosis. Finally, psychodermatological conditions such as delusional infestations may also manifest as multiple excoriated lesions on the body and limbs (see Chapter 14).

Clinical and laboratory investigations

Lesional skin biopsies for histology are often not routinely required as the diagnosis of nodular prurigo can often be made on clinical grounds. However, in atypical or recalcitrant cases, skin biopsies may be indicated to exclude other differential diagnoses, such as malignancy, which can mimic nodular prurigo. Histological findings of prurigo nodules include marked compact hyperkeratosis with focal parakeratosis, irregular epidermal hyperplasia or pseudoepitheliomatous hyperplasia with vertically streaked collagen fibres in the papillary dermis. Hypertrophy and increased proliferation of sub-epidermal and dermal nerves, known as neuronal hyperplasia, have been noted in prurigo nodules, but are not a constant feature [2,5].

Management

Given the multifaceted aetiology of nodular prurigo, a team approach is fundamental in its

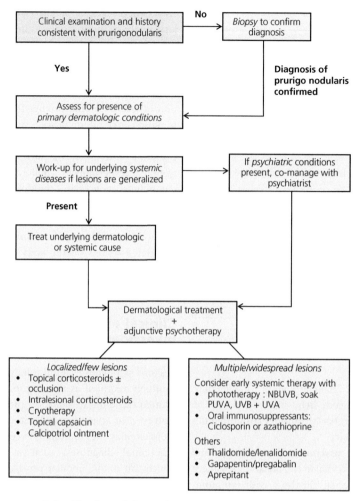

Figure 22.4 Management algorithm for nodular prurigo.
NBUVB, narrowband ultraviolet B; PUVA, psoralen ultraviolet A; UVA, ultraviolet A.

management. A psychodermatology multidisciplinary team clinic, such as the multidisciplinary Itch Clinic at our centre, comprising a dermatologist, psychiatrist, psychologist, and nurse, has been helpful in ensuring a holistic evaluation and management of severe cases of nodular prurigo. Patient education, psychological support, and close follow-up are critical to ensuring patient adherence and optimal outcome of treatment. A summary of the approach to a

patient with nodular prurigo is presented in Figure 22.4.

The mainstay of therapy should be targeted at the underlying dermatological or systemic disease.

As atopic dermatitis is the most commonly associated dermatosis, aggressive treatment using skin barrier repair and anti-inflammatory agents is paramount. In patients with extensive lesions, skin directed therapies such as phototherapy or escalation to systemic immunosuppressive agents, such as short tapering courses of oral corticosteroids, azathioprine or ciclosporin, may improve both the eczema and nodular prurigo. Since most patients with atopic eczema are colonized with *Staphylococcal aureus*, judicious use of antibiotics or antiseptics may be indicated to treat secondarily infected lesions or for maintenance decolonization. Sedative antihistamines may help minimize nocturnal scratching.

The following therapeutic ladder may be considered for the treatment of nodular prurigo [6].

First-line treatment options

- *Topical corticosteroids* – the use of potent topical corticosteroids with or without the use of occlusion has been found to be effective in a small paired randomized controlled trial [7]. Combination corticosteroid creams with salicylic acid or antibiotics, such as fusidic acid, may be helpful in thick or superficially infected lesions, respectively. In addition, intralesional corticosteroids can be administered to very thick lesions. The perilesional skin should be examined for skin atrophy in patients with prolonged use of topical or intralesional corticosteroids.
- *Liquid nitrogen cryotherapy* – this may be effective as a physical method to debulk and flatten thick lesions. Repeated sessions are needed and patients should be warned of the risk of dyspigmentation.
- *Topical capsaicin cream* – this has been reported to be effective, with relatively rapid relief of pruritus[8]. This has been attributed to the depletion of substance P in dermal nerves.
- *Topical calcipotriol ointment* – this vitamin D analogue was shown to be more effective than 0.1% beta-methasone valerate ointment in a small randomized, double blind right/left study [9], with a more rapid onset of action, and larger reduction in lesion size and lesion count after 8 weeks of treatment. Calcipotriol

may be useful as a non-steroid alternative for patients.

Second-line treatment options

The early use of these treatment options should be considered in patients with extensive or recalcitrant lesions.

- *Phototherapy* – whole body or localized phototherapy with various light sources, such as monochromatic excimer light (308 nm), broadband UVB, narrow-band UVB, UVA-1, and oral and bath PUVA, have been used to treat nodular prurigo. The mechanism of action of phototherapy is through its postulated immunomodulatory and anti-inflammatory effects, leading to itch reduction or improvement of the underlying dermatitis. Even though UVA penetrates deeper into the dermis compared to UVB radiation and in view of the marked epidermal hyperplasia in nodular prurigo, clear evidence that UVA therapy is more efficacious than UVB treatment is lacking. Our experience is that a combination of narrow-band UVB and broad-band UVA therapy appears to produce significant improvement for our patients.
- *Oral immunosuppressant agents* – systemic anti-inflammatory agents such as oral ciclosporin and azathioprine have been used successfully in small case series. Both drugs induced partial remission, but there was a rapid recurrence of lesions upon cessation of medication.

Newer/third-line treatment options

- Thalidomide/lenalidomide – there has been renewed interest in the use of these agents in treating refractory prurigo. The mechanism of action of thalidomide is attributed to its immunomodulatory effects, central sedative effect, and attenuation of peripheral itch perception. The dose of thalidomide used ranges from 200 mg to 400 mg/day. In the largest case series of 42 patients treated with thalidomide [10], the majority (76.1%) improved with treatment. Pooled data suggest that relief of pruritus occurred within 2–3 weeks of initiating treatment and lesion reduction or clearance occurred after 3–5 months. It has also been used in sequential combination with UVB phototherapy with a high response rate [5]. A prospective study [11] in HIV patients with prurigo nodularis showed that half the patients given thalidomide 33–200 mg/day had a 50% reduction in itch and skin involvement. Regular neurological assessments must be carried out to detect peripheral neuropathy, a dose dependent side effect that mostly occurs at doses greater than 200 mg/day. HIV-infected patients are also at greater risk of thalidomide-induced peripheral neuropathy. Lenalidomide, a derivative of thalidomide, may have a lower risk of peripheral neuropathy and has been successfully used in one patient with prurigo nodularis who had thalidomide-induced peripheral neuropathy. The teratogenic side effect limits the use of these agents in women of childbearing age.

* *Gabapentin* – this was reported to be effective in a small case series of five patients [12], whilst the use of pregabalin (75 mg/day) achieved complete response in 76% of 30 patients in another study [13]. These agents are thought to minimize the sensation of itch through a mechanism similar to the attenuation of neuropathic pain.
* *Aprepitant* – elevated substance P in nodular prurigo lesions has prompted the use of aprepitant, a substance P antagonist that blocks the binding of substance P to its receptor, neurokinin-1, to treat this condition. In a small pilot study of 20 patients with chronic pruritus treated with aprepitant 80 mg daily for 1 week, 13 of the 20 patients had a significant reduction in pruritus intensity (by 48.5%), which led to clinical improvement in their lesions [14].
* *Antipsychotics/antidepressants* – in patients with associated psychiatric co-morbidities, psychiatric medications may be indicated. Olanzapine, an atypical antipsychotic, was used to treat five patients with concurrent depression and neuroticism with marked improvement of pruritus and lesional count [15].
* Naltrexone – the opioid antagonist naltrexone was reported to be effective in a small trial of 17 nodular prurigo patients, with nine patients having a 50% or greater reduction in pruritus intensity and lesion count [16]. The onset of pruritus reduction also occurred rapidly within 2–8 days.

Psychological and behavioural therapy

Psychological and behavioural therapy in nodular prurigo may be helpful in allowing patients to gain insight and manage their scratching behaviour to break the scratch–itch cycle.

A study on the impact of a psychological assessment and management in patients with chronic intractable skin diseases, including atopic dermatitis and nodular prurigo, demonstrated that 68% of patients had a significant life event associated with the onset of their skin condition. Psychological intervention led to a good outcome in the majority of patents, including eight of the 10 patients with nodular prurigo [17].

Habit reversal therapy (see Chapter 8), which aims to modify the patient's incessant scratching behaviour by introducing another competing response to the itch stimulus, may be a useful adjunctive treatment option. A small study of six nodular prurigo patients managed by dermatology nurses trained in habit reversal therapy, together with close follow-up visits, found that this form of behavioural therapy was helpful [18].

Future research

Nodular prurigo remains a challenging dermatological condition to manage given its diverse pathogenic factors. It is clear that larger clinical trials are needed to determine the most appropriate evidence-based treatment for patients. However, given the heterogeneity of clinical presentation and different causes in daily

practice, management needs to be holistic and individualized for patients. Newer antipruritic strategies, such as anti-interleukin 31 agents, may hold promise in the future for patients afflicted with this distressing skin condition.

PRACTICAL TIPS

- Detailed and repeated skin examinations should be performed in patients with nodular prurigo; the interlesional skin may reveal the presence of underlying primary dermatoses.
- Patients without an obvious dermatological cause should be screened for underlying systemic diseases (see Box 22.1).
- Treatment should be directed at the underlying cause and in accordance with the extent and severity of lesions.
- Adjunctive psychotherapy can be very useful in selected patients.

References

1. Iking A et al. Prurigo as a symptom of atopic and non-atopic diseases: aetiological survey in a consecutive cohort of 108 patients. *J Eur Acad Dermatol Venereol* 2013; 27(5): 550–557
2. Rowland Payne CME et al. Nodular prurigo—a clinicopathological study of 46 patients. *Br J Dermatol* 1985; 113: 431–439.
3. Tanaka M et al. Prurigo nodularis consists of two distinct forms: early-onset atopic and late-onset non-atopic. *Dermatology* 1995; 190: 269–276.
4. Dazzi C et al. Psychological factors involved in prurigo nodularis: A pilot study. *J Dermatol Treat* 2011; 22: 211–214.
5. Lee MR et al. Prurigo nodularis: a review. *Australas J Dermatol* 2005; 46: 211–218.
6. Fostini AC et al. Prurigo nodularis: an update on etiopathogenesis and therapy. *J Dermatol Treat* Epub 2013 Jun 14.
7. Saraceno R et al. An occlusive dressing containing betamethasone valerate 0.1% for the treatment of prurigonodularis. *J Dermatol Treat* 2010; 21: 363–366.
8. Ständer S et al. Treatment of prurigo nodularis with topical capsaicin. *J Am Acad Dermatol* 2001; 44: 471–478.
9. Wong SS, Goh CL. Double-blind, right/left comparison of calcipotriol ointment and betamethasone ointment in the treatment of prurigo nodularis. *Arch Dermatol* 2000; 136: 807–808.
10. Andersen TP, Fogh K. Thalidomide in 42 patients with prurigo nodularis. *Dermatology* 2011; 223: 107–112.
11. Maurer T et al. Thalidomide treatment for prurigo nodularis in human immunodeficiency virus-infected subjects: efficacy and risk of neuropathy. *Arch Dermatol* 2004; 140: 845–849.
12. Gencoglan G et al. Therapeutic hotline: Treatment of prurigo nodularis and lichen simplex chronicus with gabapentin. *Dermatol Ther* 2010; 23: 194–198.
13. Mazza M et al. Treatment of prurigonodularis with pregabalin. *J Clin Pharm Ther* 2013; 38: 16–18.
14. Ständer S et al. Targeting the neurokinin receptor 1 with aprepitant: a novel antipruritic strategy. *PLoS One* 2010; 5: e10968.
15. Hyun J et al. Olanzapine therapy for subacute prurigo. *Clin Exp Dermatol* 2006; 31: 464–465.
16. Metze D et al. Efficacy and safety of naltrexone, an oral opiate receptor antagonist, in the treatment of pruritus in internal and dermatological diseases. *J Am Acad Dermatol* 1999; 41: 533–539.
17. Capoore HS et al. Does psychological intervention help chronic skin conditions? *Postgrad Med J* 1998; 74:662–4.
18. Grillo M et al. Habit reversal training for the itch-scratch cycle associated with pruritic skin conditions. *Dermatol Nurs* 2007; 19: 243–248.

SECTION 6

Special populations and situations

CHAPTER 23

Child and adolescent psychodermatology

Birgit Westphal[1] and Osman Malik[2]

[1] Barts and The London Children's Hospital, Royal London Hospital, London, UK
[2] Newham Child and Family Consultation Service, London, UK

Paediatricians often point out that paediatrics is not "just general medicine in little people". This statement could equally be applied to child and adolescent psychiatry. In adults, we find variations in adjustment to illness determined by bio-psycho-social factors, which shape development and contribute to the formation of the personality. In adult mental health, we see the end result of this process and assess well-established modes of functioning, which are part of an individual's personal make-up and identity. In children and adolescents who are continuously learning and adapting to the environment, clinicians have an opportunity and responsibility to assess the impact of illness on development and to intervene where necessary in order to reduce the development of maladaptive coping strategies.

Classification and clinical presentations

The literature highlights various ways in which paediatric psychodermatological conditions can be classified. For the purposes of this chapter, which focuses on practical approaches to assessment and intervention, we organize the classification according to three main groups:

- skin disorders that cause psychological problems;
- skin disorders that are exacerbated by stress and psychosocial factors;
- skin disorders that are manifestations of psychiatric illness.

Paediatric skin disorders that cause psychological problems

Paediatric skin disorders are associated with a range of psychological effects. We focus on those conditions that appear to be the most researched and common in paediatric psychodermatology practice: atopic dermatitis, psoriasis, acne vulgaris, vitiligo, burns and alopecia areata. This is not, of course, an exhaustive list.

Psychological effects resulting from skin disorders may be related either to physical symptoms/impairment or to negative self-perception and stigmatization. In some cases, there may be overlapping symptoms of both (Table 23.1). In broad terms, comparing psychological morbidity in the two groups suggests that behaviour-related disorders are more common in the "physical symptoms group", whereas mood-related disorders are more common in the "appearance-stigmatization group".

Atopic dermatitis is the most common condition in the "physical symptoms group", with a

Practical Psychodermatology, First Edition. Anthony Bewley, Ruth E. Taylor, Jason S. Reichenberg and Michelle Magid.
© 2014 John Wiley & Sons, Ltd. Published 2014 by John Wiley & Sons, Ltd.

Table 23.1 Main cause of psychological distress in dermatological disorders

Physical symptoms	Appearance/ stigmatization
• Atopic dermatitis • Psoriasis • Burns	• Acne vulgaris • Psoriasis • Burns • Vitiligo • Alopecia areata

prevalence in children of 10–20%. UK data suggest that atopic dermatitis affects around 16.5% of children aged 1–5 years old [1]. This chronic skin disorder is characterized by pruritus and inflammation, which results in a vicious cycle of itching and scratching leading to pain and discomfort. Functional impairment, sleep disturbance and attention/concentration problems are all well-known effects. The child may become clingy and find it difficult to separate beyond an age when this is developmentally appropriate. The skin care routine needed to manage the condition can impact on family life, as parents often feel exhausted. These factors combined may result in impaired quality of life (QoL). It is notable in this regard that atopic dermatitis has been found to have a greater impact on the QoL of children than many other chronic paediatric illnesses [2]. Similar effects have been found in children with psoriasis.

Teasing, bullying and stigmatization are common causes of psychological morbidity in the "appearance-related group". Disfigurement reduces self-esteem and this may affect self-perception, both of which may impede peer integration. When affected areas are visible to others, psychological distress is more pronounced. Acne is one such disorder associated with low self-esteem and depression. Another is alopecia areata where psychiatric morbidity is observed in about 75% of sufferers. In a recent study of 75 young people with alopecia areata, 16% fulfilled criteria for major depressive disorder and 13% for generalized anxiety disorder [3].

In vitiligo, age, gender and location of the lesions affect the degree of psychological morbidity and QoL. However, the child's perception of the lesions is the most significant determining factor. Early onset may be protective as there is somewhat less focus on physical appearance prior to the onset of puberty and the child has longer to adjust to illness [4]. However, children are inevitably affected by how others perceive them, which may have an impact on their developing sense of self.

Skin disorders affecting both physical functioning and appearance are most complex in terms of psychological morbidity. In burn patients, psychological morbidity results on the one hand from functional impairment and pain and, on the other, from disfigurement and symptoms of post-traumatic stress. However, scarring has been found to have a greater impact on QoL compared to functional impairment [5].

Skin disorders that are exacerbated by stress and other psychosocial factors

Stress generates physiological responses that influence local immune and inflammatory functions of the skin, resulting in exacerbations of inflammatory skin disorders like atopic dermatitis and psoriasis. In individuals who are constitutionally predisposed, stress acts as a trigger. Scratching behaviour often increases in response to stress and the child may learn to use scratching behaviour to seek attention from parents. Parental stress may reduce meticulous skin care and result in worsening of the skin condition. Therefore, identification and treatment of stress and psychological morbidity are key in controlling and reducing relapses in certain chronic skin disorders.

Skin disorders presenting as manifestations of psychiatric illness

Some skin disorders are manifestations of an underlying psychiatric disorder, either as

Table 23.2 Psychiatric disorders underlying skin disorders

Psychiatric disorder	Skin disorder
Obsessive compulsive and related disorders	Trichotillomania (hair-pulling) Neurotic excoriation (compulsive skin picking and scratching) Onychophagia (nail biting)
Anxiety disorders	Trichotillomania (hair pulling) Neurotic excoriation (compulsive skin picking and scratching) Onychophagia (nail biting)
Learning disability/ autism	Skin self-injury, picking, and biting
Personality disorder (>16 years) or traits if younger	Self-injury
Factitious disorder (or by proxy)	Dermatitis artefacta
Psychosis	Delusional skin picking

a sole symptom or as part of a constellation of symptoms. We describe skin disorders here according to their underlying psychopathology (Table 23.2).

In obsessive-compulsive related disorders (OCRDs), the dermatological manifestation may take the form of hair pulling, skin picking (neurotic excoriations) and nail biting. In children these conditions are often under-recognized and under-diagnosed. They can co-exist with each other and are co-morbid with other psychiatric diagnoses like anxiety disorders. *Trichotillomania or hair pulling* is a long-term problem that usually starts in childhood or early adolescence. It was classified as an impulse-control disorder in the DSM-IV, but was reclassified as an OCRD in DSM-5 (see Chapter 10 and Chapter 16). Children who present with trichotillomania are often vulnerable to developing anxiety. Whilst they may be distressed by their condition, hair pulling is commonly

concealed from parents, unless the eyebrows or eyelashes are affected, and children often deny the behaviour. Eating the pulled hair (trichophagia) may result in the formation of hair casts in the gut accompanied by gastrointestinal symptoms. In younger children, trichotillomania is more often considered to be a habit, while in adolescents it is often found to be a formal mental illness [6].

Onychophagia or nail biting is very common in children and may be more prevalent than available data suggest. Nail biting can present with other impulse-control and body-focused repetitive behaviour disorders. For example, a study by Ghanizadeh [7] found a frequent occurrence of nail biting in children referred to a child and adolescent mental health clinic, with the most common co-morbid psychiatric diagnoses being attention deficit hyperactivity disorder (ADHD) (74.6%), oppositional defiant disorder (36%) and separation anxiety disorder (20.6%). Enuresis, tic disorder and OCD were also represented. A significant proportion (>50%) of the parents were found to have at least one psychiatric diagnosis, most commonly major depression.

Skin picking and self-induced skin lesions can be of varying types and aetiology. *Neurotic excoriations* in childhood are linked with psychosocial stressors, poor impulse control and psychiatric morbidity. Usually an initial skin insult – a minor scratch or insect bite – triggers picking and scratching behaviours. Parental factors should be considered as the child may use the behaviour to seek parental attention. In OCRDs, skin picking functions to relieve the anxiety resulting from not acting on the obsessional thoughts to skin pick. This is seen in middle childhood and adolescence, sometimes associated with a tic disorder.

Dermatitis artefacta is classified as a factitious disorder and is discussed in detail in Chapter 17. The literature on factitious disorder suggests inadequate care giving, unresolved psychological dilemmas, emotional distress and unstable personality features as possible underlying factors. When questioned about the skin problem, the young person denies his/her role and any psychological distress. In rare cases, where a parent is suspected of inducing skin lesions in a child or exaggerating the severity of an existing condition, fabricated or induced illness (FII) should be considered – "factitious disorder imposed on another" (previously called "factitious disorder by proxy;" FDP or FDbP) in the US – as listed under 300.19 Factitious disorder in DSM-5. In these cases, the parent has a need for the child to be recognized as unwell in order to obtain attention. In the past, such parental behaviour was described as "Münchausen syndrome by proxy" (MSbP or MBP), which is a controversial term for this paediatric diagnosis, as it refers to an adult disorder and does not describe the actual finding in the child who is experiencing abuse.

Skin mutilation (self-harm) is typically found as a maladaptive coping mechanism in adolescents with (emerging) personality disorders. Past history of abuse (physical, emotional, sexual) can be a precipitating factor. Self-punishment or "the urge to feel something" in the context of emotional numbness are common motivations. Copy-cat behaviour (school, family, internet) should be considered. The behaviour – if not addressed – can become chronic.

Repetitive behaviour in autism and learning disability can manifest as skin biting or skin picking. The function of habitual behaviours is to self-soothe or self-stimulate, and often are more frequent with distress or boredom. It is important to understand this function when planning an intervention. Children with high functioning autism (HFA) can present with sensory sensitivities, being hyper- or hypo-sensitive to touch (and texture), smells and noise. This must not be dismissed or confused with cutaneous dysesthesia, which is a burning sensation or sensation of pain on touch often associated with peripheral neuropathy, or which can be psychosomatic. The features of HFA are subtle and may be missed; it is important to recognize the spectrum of autistic spectrum disorder (ASD) and mild learning disability.

Developmental perspective

Children and adolescents face age-specific challenges throughout development. These need to be successfully negotiated in order for development to progress. For children presenting with psychodermatological disorders, development may be affected at any point by:
- psychological effects of living with a skin disorder;
- repeated exacerbations due to stress and psychosocial factors;
- psychiatric illness for which the skin disorder is the manifestation.

The extent to which development is impeded, however, will depend upon child intrinsic factors (nature) and family/wider environmental factors (nurture). Assessment of interacting nature and nurture influences is essential to clarify whether intervention is needed in order to promote a favourable developmental outcome. In an audit of adherence in patients with atopic eczema, for instance, Devereux *et al.* found that whilst physicians consistently assessed physical severity of the skin condition, less emphasis was placed on monitoring everyday activities, sleep and psychosocial well-being [8]. Since the child's social environment can contribute significantly to disease exacerbation and associated co-morbidity, all factors relating to the child should be monitored routinely (Figure 23.1).

When assessing a child presenting with a psychodermatological problem, it is useful to start by asking the following question: "*Why does this child with these interacting nature–nurture influences present with a psychodermatological disorder at this particular point in time?*" To answer this, a thorough history giving consideration to all of the above can then be organized according to the bio-psycho-social model (Table 23.3). This conceptual model will assist in developing a formulation by clarifying which factors can be addressed and which cannot be changed. It will also facilitate assessment of the impact of illness on development and QoL.

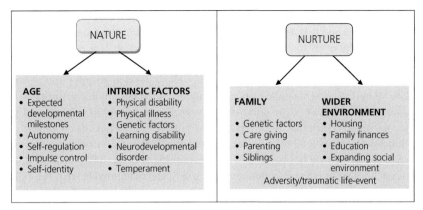

Figure 23.1 Relevant factors in psychiatric and developmental assessment of a child illness.

Table 23.3 Sample formulation in a bio-psycho-social framework

Factor	Biological	Psychological	Social
Predisposing	• Family history of mental illness		• No permanent housing
Trigger	• Exacerbation of eczema	• Bullied at school	• Family moved house • New area, no friends
Maintaining		• Parent with mental illness	
Protective		• Supportive wider family	• Supportive aunt who lives close

This is important because caring for a child with a skin disease presents the family with a number of challenges. Parents may experience a range of emotional responses to their child's skin condition: initial shock, embarrassment, guilt and disappointment are all observed responses in our clinical practice. Questions about the cause of the condition and attribution of blame related to a perception of having failed to produce a healthy child are also common.

Several age groups are particularly relevant in paediatric psychodermatology.

Infancy (age 0–1 years)

In infancy, parent–infant interactions, which in normal circumstances promote development, may be painful and distressing. The infant may resist physical comfort, which can lead to parents feeling rejected and inadequate. Together with parental stress, fatigue and anxiety this can impact adversely on bonding.

Lack of bonding is associated with insecure attachment, which will over time negatively impact on development if not addressed.

Early middle–childhood (age 6–8 years)

Social integration and focus on learning are key developmental challenges of middle childhood. Negative peer group responses are a common source of distress and the child's experience of being perceived negatively by peers may impact on self-esteem and peer integration. Attention problems caused by itching and physical discomfort commonly affect learning, as may anxiety, low mood and irritability.

Parental over-protection may limit the child's exposure to new experiences, or parents may fail to set boundaries for behaviour which, if not addressed, can prevent the child from developing age-appropriate impulse control and the ability to cope with frustration.

Many parents are exhausted by the demands of the skin care routine and may feel that their child is developmentally ready to take on some responsibility in this regard. However, whilst most children of this age have well-developed self-care skills, they lack understanding about the necessity of rigid adherence to the skin care routine, and motivation is poor due to the physical discomfort associated with it. This can lead to parent–child conflict, which has been shown to increase scratch behaviour in young children. A decline in skin care resulting in exacerbation of the skin condition is also common.

Adolescence (age 12–18 years)

As children develop, they become increasingly aware of the attitudes and responses of peers. Their developing sense of self, identity and self-esteem can all be affected, particularly in adolescence when the physical changes associated with the onset of puberty engender intense focus on the body. Concerns about self-image and appearance are often associated with shame and embarrassment. Heightened sensitivity to peer responses to appearance can impact on peer group integration and the formation of meaningful relationships outside the family.

In order to develop adaptive coping strategies, children with skin conditions need good quality physical care, emotional support and parental validation throughout development. Family vulnerabilities and stressors impacting on family functioning will inevitably make it more difficult for parents to provide what the child needs in these regards. This may affect long-term prognosis and developmental outcome (Figure 23.2).

Any assessment of a child should consider the wider question of safeguarding and risk.

Treatment

There is limited evidence for the effectiveness of psychological interventions for management of psychodermatology conditions in children and adolescents. This is due to a lack of good quality research evidence. A more effective

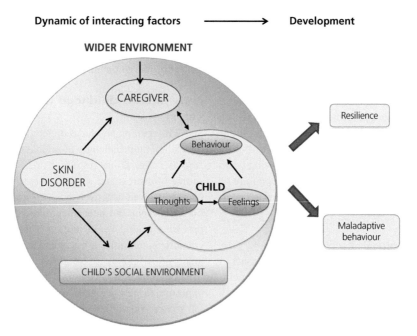

Figure 23.2 Interacting factors that contribute to the outcome of a child's development.

Table 23.4 Treatment approaches to psychiatric and psychological issues

Problems identified	Suggested intervention
Issues of care in infancy	Parent–child interaction work
Inappropriate parental developmental expectations	Parent–child interaction work
Low self-esteem, low mood, poor adaptive coping strategies, social anxiety, non-adherence	CBT, problem-solving therapy, parent–child interaction work
Axis-1 psychiatric diagnosis	Psychiatric management
Learning disability/ developmental disorder/ ADHD	Multimodal approaches
Parental mental health issues	Psychological support for parent and family
Family dysfunction	Family therapy/ intervention

ADHD, attention deficit hyperactivity disorder; CBT, cognitive-behavioural therapy

approach can be developed when interventions are connected to individual assessment of needs using the conceptual bio-psychosocial model considering risk and resilience (Table 23.4).

Part 1: Interventions for psychological problems caused by a skin disorder, and stress and psychosocial factors exacerbating a skin disorder

General principles of parenting a child who is ill and in distress

The way physical illness symptoms are managed by parents depends on their attitudes to and anxiety about illness. Generally the child will cope better if the parents:
- have a clear, realistic understanding of the child's illness, treatment and prognosis;
- are able to explain this in an age-appropriate way to the child;
- contain the child's anxiety and promote coping strategies;

- give a consistent response to any behaviours associated with the illness and agree a similar approach with any other adults involved in the child's care.

Better control of the skin disorder and management of physical symptoms to improve psychological outcome and reduce stress

The recommendation here is to treat the cause of distress. If the primary cause is the skin condition itself, treatment should be aimed at reducing physical symptoms in order to improve physical and psychological outcome. In acne for instance, treatment with isotretinoin or antibiotics reduces psychological impairment by improving the skin condition, which is the cause of distress and depression.

Adolescents with acne who were treated with isotretinoin have been reported to be at a higher risk for depression and suicidal ideation. This was previously thought to be a side effect of the medication, but larger studies have not found a causative relationship [9]. It is likely that patients with severe acne requiring isotretinoin have secondary depression. There is controversy over the exact mechanism of action and relationship between isotretinoin and suicidal thoughts, so it is important for the prescriber to monitor mood and refer high-risk patients to a child and adolescent psychiatrist.

A Cochrane review in 2012 examined the effectiveness of psychological therapies for parents of children/adolescents with chronic illness (including skin disorders) [10]. The authors found that psychological therapies that included parents significantly reduced the child's reported pain. Cognitive-behavioural therapy (CBT) for the child significantly improved symptoms, while problem-solving therapy for the parents significantly improved parent behaviour and mental health. The treatment of atopic dermatitis in children has received particular attention and several studies have shown the effectiveness of educational interventions (Table 23.5) and habit reversal (see Chapter 8).

Table 23.5 Educational interventions in paediatric atopic dermatitis

Treatment programme	Approach	Outcome	Location
Eczema Education Programme	Nurse-led education of parents of children with atopic dermatitis	Improved child QoL and improved parent confidence (and self-efficacy)	UK, 2012
German Atopic Dermatitis Intervention Study	Educational programme for parental management of atopic dermatitis in children and self-management in adolescents	Improved disease control	Germany, 2009
Parent Education Programme	Six meetings of 90 minutes each at weekly intervals with a paediatric allergist, dermatologist and psychologist	Lower levels of anxiety in parents and improved QoL at the end of the programme, but low cost-effectiveness	Italy, 2009

Part 2: Specific child and adolescent approaches to primary psychiatric skin disorders

Early intervention in trichotillomania and other OCRDs is recommended. Habit modification and habit reversal techniques are most helpful when the parent is involved in treatment by actively encouraging the child to practise alternative responses and anxiety-reduction procedures [11]. Parents should also reward desired behaviour. Similar techniques apply to neurotic skin picking and nail biting. One study differentiated a group of young people whose hair pulling was found to be obsessional in nature, suggesting that treatment is in accordance with OCD. In some cases, reducing an unrelated behaviour or habit (like thumb sucking, called a co-morbid behaviour) reduces the frequency of the index behaviour [12]. More severe cases can be referred to a child and adolescent psychiatrist for management, especially as some patients may benefit from selective serotonin reuptake inhibitors (SSRIs), which need specialist monitoring [6]. Finally, any co-morbid psychiatric disorder and familial disturbances identified should be referred to a child and adolescent mental health clinician for treatment.

Patients with learning disability or autism can present with features of skin biting and occasionally skin picking. The repeated self-injury is done either to self-soothe or to self-stimulate. If the self-injury worsens in situations that the child finds stressful, it is likely to be a form of self-soothing and can improve with stress reduction. If the self-injury arises when the child is bored, it is more likely to be self-stimulating and can be managed by distracting the child with alternative sensory stimulation. Child and adolescent mental health services with expertise in neurodevelopmental disorders can help with a behavioural analysis to differentiate between these causes.

Young people with dermatitis artefacta usually resist psychological intervention and involvement of their parents is helpful. However, parents may find it difficult to accept that lesions are self-induced and may also feel they are being blamed for having a role in their child's self-injury. The approach to these patients is discussed in Chapter 17. In the rare circumstances when the dermatologist suspects a parental role in fabrication or induction of a skin disorder, this becomes a safeguarding issue that requires multidisciplinary collaboration between child mental health and social services. An assessment of parental capacity to change beliefs and behaviours towards the child should be considered. The parent may have an underlying personality or psychiatric disorder that requires treatment. Statutory intervention may be required to protect the child.

PRACTICAL TIPS

- Paediatric skin disorders are associated with a range of psychological effects, which are more likely to be behaviour related in patients with physical symptoms/impairment (atopic dermatitis or psoriasis) and mood related in patients with experience of negative self-perception (vitiligo, acne or alopecia areata). In patients with burns or psoriasis, overlapping symptoms of both may feature.

- Identifying the child's developmental stage and needs helps in planning his/her management.

- Discussing diagnosis or difficulties with the caregiver first – without the child present – can help with containment, lower anxiety and improve adherence by allowing time to create an age-appropriate narrative for the child.

References

1. Emerson RM *et al*. Severity distribution of atopic dermatitis in the community and its relationship to secondary referral. *Br J Dermatol* 1998; 139: 73–76.

2. Beattie PE *et al*. A comparative study of impairment of quality of life in children with skin disease and children with other chronic diseases. *Br J Dermatol* 2006; 155: 145–151.

3. Yuksel D *et al*. Psychiatric evaluation of children and adolescents with alopecia areata. *Eur J Pediatr Dermatol* 2012; 22: 37–38.

4. Prcic S *et al*. Some psychological characteristics of children and adolescents with vitiligo. *Medicinski pregled* 2006; 59: 265–269.

5. Lohmeyer JA *et al*. Psychological and behavioural impairment following thermal injury in childhood. *Handchirurgie Mikrochirurgie Plastische Chirurgie* 2007; 39: 333–337.

6. Franklin ME *et al*. Trichotillomania and its treatment: a review and recommendations. *Expert Rev Neurother* 2011; 11: 1165–1174.

7. Ghanizadeh A. Association of nail biting and psychiatric disorders in children and their parents in a psychiatrically referred sample of children. *Child Adolesc Psychiatry Mental Health* 2008; 2: 1753–2000.

8. Devereux C *et al*. An audit of adherence to the National Institute for Health and Clinical Excellence (NICE) guidelines on the management of atopic eczema in children. *Br J Dermatol* 2010; 163: 128–129.

9. Misery L *et al*. Isotretinoin and adolescent depression. *Annal Dermatol Venereol* 2012; 139: 118–23.

10. Eccleston C *et al*. Psychological interventions for parents of children and adolescents with chronic illness. *Cochrane Database Syst Rev* 2012; 8: CD009660.

11. Vitulano LA *et al*. Behavioral treatment of children and adolescents with trichotillomania. *J Am Acad Child Adolesc Psychiatry* 1992; 31: 139–146.

12. Watson TS *et al*. Elimination of thumb-sucking as a treatment for severe trichotillomania. *J Am Acad Child Adolesc Psychiatry* 1993; 32: 830–834

CHAPTER 24

Psychodermato-oncology: psychological reactions to skin cancer

Andrew G. Affleck[1] and Lesley Howells[2]

[1] Department of Dermatology, Ninewells Hospital and Medical School, Dundee, UK
[2] Maggie's Centre, Ninewells Hospital, Dundee, UK

Patients with skin cancer make up a heterogeneous group. Practitioners often focus on differences in tumour biology, but may overlook the variety of patient beliefs, and feelings that inform their illness experience. People and their families, faced with a sudden life change such as a diagnosis of a potentially serious form of skin cancer, may experience a series of intense emotions as they cope with the challenges the cancer creates for their home and working life, their sense of self, and the possible loss of the future they had assumed for themselves (Figure 24.1).

The vast majority of skin cancers are keratinocytic in origin (basal and squamous cell carcinomas); these are locally invasive but curable by surgical excision. Of all skin cancers, approximately 10% are melanomas but melanomas are the cause of 80% of deaths due to skin cancer. Overall, one-quarter of people diagnosed with invasive melanoma will develop local recurrence or metastases (spread of cancer to another body part).

skin tumours as well as in those with life-threatening clinical scenarios (Box 24.1).

Psychodermato-oncology, a branch of psycho-oncology, may be defined as "psychosocial, emotional, and behavioural factors associated with the diagnosis of skin cancer and its treatment". The benefits of high quality psychological care in a cancer setting have been reported in many publications [1] and recommendations are made in many national guidelines [2,3] (Box 24.2 and Table 24.1). About one in five people will be at least moderately distressed when diagnosed with skin cancer, and in patients with malignant melanoma the number rises to one in three. The emotional impact of cancer may be overwhelming to some people – it compromises their ability to function on a day-to-day basis, and affects their capacity to hear, retain, understand and act on information; they feel a loss of control, isolation and helplessness; they struggle with uncertainty and fears about their future and life expectancy.

Defining features

Distress, with emotions intensifying or appearing unexpectedly, can occur at any stage of a patient's cancer "journey" and can be found in patients with objectively "mild" locally invasive

Assessment

Health professionals should have good relational skills and be confident in talking with and listening to patients who may be confused, scared and ashamed of their beliefs and feelings.

Practical Psychodermatology, First Edition. Anthony Bewley, Ruth E. Taylor, Jason S. Reichenberg and Michelle Magid.
© 2014 John Wiley & Sons, Ltd. Published 2014 by John Wiley & Sons, Ltd.

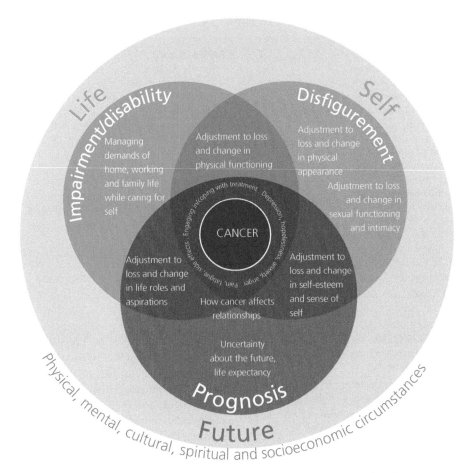

Figure 24.1 Psychosocial challenges of cancer. (Source Paijmans R. (2010) Background to the Cancer Psychology Referral Guidelines. Pan-Birmingham Cancer Network. Reproduced with permission.)

Active consideration regarding choice of words and phrases is needed.

Routine screening for distress by the medical team is widely advocated to identify vulnerable patients and to allow support to be tailored to the patient's needs [4]. A baseline assessment of the patient's mood, ideas and expectations regarding his/her skin cancer is desirable. Screening for distress and difficulty coping related to skin cancer can be done using key questions, simple visual analogue scales and, when needed, validated symptom assessment tools. These tools include the "Distress thermometer", an ultra-short measure of

psychological and practical distress; the "Skin Cancer Index" [5,6], a skin cancer-specific screening tool; and the "Hospital Anxiety and Depression Scale", which provides useful clinical cut-off points (see Appendix A4, A12, and A13). However, as a rule of thumb, any patient who shows distress and experiences difficulties in daily life related to cancer, especially in the context of a low level of social support, should be offered psychological input, regardless of whether or not they have a diagnosed psychological disorder.

Distress is frequently undisclosed to the person's medical team, so potentially alleviating

Box 24.1 Psychological factors along the skin cancer journey

- **Preoperatively:**
  - Unrealistic expectations
  - Unsubstantiated illness beliefs
  - High cosmetic need (more concerned about aesthetic outcome than removing the cancer)
  - Needle phobia
  - Extreme anxiety/catastrophizing
  - Abnormal illness behaviour – denial/neglect of tumour
- **Perioperatively:**
  - Anxiety and panic – fleeting vs. specific
  - Fear of pain
  - Fear that cancer will not be completely removed
  - Fear that the functional or aesthetic outcome will be poor

- **Postoperatively:**
  - Psychological morbidity – feelings of abandonment, social anxiety
  - Financial worry (cost of procedure, time off from work)
  - Adjustment to being visibly different
  - Fear of cancer recurrence
  - Post-traumatic stress disorder
  - "Survivorship" – late physical and psychological hurdles to overcome when striving to regain a sense of normality
- **Advanced metastatic disease and palliative care:**
  - Anticipatory grief
  - Fear of death
  - Family psychological support (e.g. communicating with children about death)

Box 24.2 National Institute for Health and Care Excellence (NICE) recommendations on psychosocial factors and skin cancer

- During follow-up of patients treated for skin cancer, there should be provision of psychological and emotional support to patient, caregiver and family
- Those who are directly involved in treating patients should receive specific training in communication and breaking bad news. They have a responsibility to provide good communication with patients and carers
- Skin cancer patients should have access to psychological support services
- There should be at least one skin cancer clinical nurse specialist (CNS) who will play a leading role in supporting patients and caregivers
- Skin cancer CNSs who have received training will be better equipped to identify and assist with the management of patients with psychosocial needs
- All people with cancer should be offered access to timely and tailored psychosocial support

psychosocial support is not provided. It is important to note that the level of psychological distress does not necessarily relate to the need perceived by the patient, so patients may not accept help at first even if offered. Repeated recommendation is vital to ensure help is available when the person sees the need.

Psychological morbidity

With surgery for skin cancer

Some degree of anxiety and stress is common in any individual having skin surgery; it would appear that only a minority are extremely anxious. Tips to help reduce anxiety and make the patient's experience of surgery as positive as possible have been described [7].

Larger surgical defects require more complex reconstructions. Most patients achieve satisfactory aesthetic outcomes, but certain procedures are more likely to result in significant disfigurement, including large excisions on the nose or lip (Figure 24.2A–C) or procedures requiring split-thickness skin graft repair (Figure 24.3A). How closely the actual size of the scar matches

Table 24.1 NICE guidance four-level model of psychological assessment and intervention (Source: National Institute for Health and Care Excellence. *Cancer Service Guidance: Improving Supportive and Palliative Care for Adults with Cancer.* London: NICE, 2009. Available from http://guidance.nice.org.uk, with permission)

Level	Group	Assessment	Intervention
1	All health and social care professionals	Recognition of psychological needs	Effective information giving, compassionate communication and general psychological support
2	Health and social care professionals with additional experience	Screening of psychological distress	Psychological techniques such as problem solving
3	Trained and accredited professionals	Assessment of psychological distress and diagnosis of some psychopathology	Counselling and specific psychological interventions such as anxiety management and solution focused therapy, delivered according to an explicit theoretical framework
4	Mental health specialists	Diagnosis of psychopathology	Specialist psychological and psychiatric interventions such as psychotherapy, including cognitive behavioural therapy (CBT)

presurgery expectations is associated with the resultant emotional distress. However, even small surgical excisions with apparent good aesthetic outcomes as judged objectively by the surgeon can cause the individual patient quite marked subjective distress. Use of skin camouflage can improve aesthetic outcome and may improve coping (Figure 24.3B). Adjustment to becoming visibly different is reviewed in Chapter 12 and by Thomson & Kent [8].

After skin cancer

Knowledge about patients' subjective experience of having skin cancer enables health professionals to relate to patients better and have productive discussions. The emotions experienced by patients and techniques that specifically focus on assessing and providing nursing support for these patients are discussed in Chapter 9.

The vast majority of patients with skin cancer do cope and adjust well over time, putting the experience behind them and continuing with their lives without lasting psychological consequences. In response to the challenges of skin cancer, people differ in their coping style,

resilience to adversity and previous potentially debilitating life experience. People with pre-existing chronic disease, poor mental health and lack of strong social support may be at greater risk.

The nature of supportive care will vary with the patient's level of distress. The National Institute for Health and Care Excellence (NICE) in the UK emphasizes the importance for all professionals involved in the person's treatment to appreciate their role in enhancing psychological well-being (Table 24.1). Most people can be adequately supported with the medical team's crucial emphasis on high quality communication (NICE Level 1), through which concerns are elicited, listened to and acknowledged, and complex information offered in a paced and understandable form; anxieties displayed during surgical procedure are managed; and additional cancer support services are signposted. Level 2 support from allied health professionals can involve cancer-related problem solving, coaching in lifestyle change post-cancer, and guidance on the choice and use of psychological self-help materials [e.g. those produced by Macmillan Cancer Support (Figure 24.4) and groups such

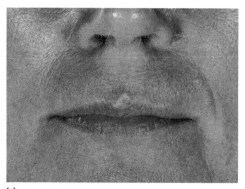

(a)

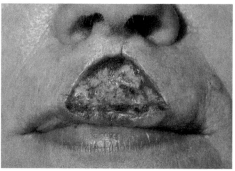

(b)

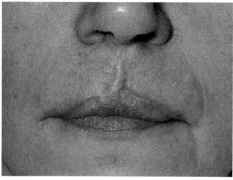

(c)

Figure 24.2 (a) Basal cell carcinoma of the upper lip. (b) Defect after clearance of tumour with Mohs' surgery. (c) Aesthetic outcome 4 months after local flap reconstruction under general anaesthetic – revision procedure being considered (courtesy of Mr Sean Laverick, Consultant Maxillo-Facial Surgeon, NHS Tayside).

as Changing Faces for support in coping with disfigurement (www.changingfaces.org; see Chapter 12). Maggie's Cancer Centres in the UK have the advantage of offering all the NICE recommended levels of emotional, social and practical support under one roof adjacent to NHS cancer treatment centres and on a drop-in basis (www.maggiescentres.org). Patients identified through screening as particularly vulnerable should be referred for prompt assessment in partnership with a psychological specialist (NICE Level 4) to gauge the level of intervention required and determine whether psychotropic medication is indicated.

Studies following patients with surgical excision of facial skin cancer find that although female and younger patients were more vulnerable to anxiety preoperatively, surgical excision of facial skin cancers improved social, emotional and aesthetic well-being. The extent of disease was a factor in quality of life scores; lesions requiring less extensive reconstruction (e.g. direct closure) were associated with a more positive outlook. This might be explained by the patient's perception that less complex surgery meant less serious disease.

Coping strategies (see also Chapter 5 and Chapter 7)

Coping strategies can be described as the thinking styles and behaviours a person uses when faced with a threat. Strategies can be categorized into three main styles:

- *problem-focused coping* (e.g. active planning, seeking information and assistance);
- *emotion-focused coping* (e.g. emotional expression, venting, avoidance through alcohol or drugs, denial);
- *meaning-focused coping* (e.g. let go of untenable goals and replace them with acceptable substitute goals; reprioritize our efforts to reflect what we really value most).

Problem-focused coping is generally considered more effective in promoting adjustment

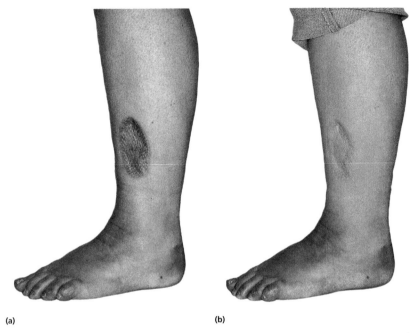

(a)   (b)

Figure 24.3 (a) 2-year aesthetic result of split-thickness skin graft after a 2-cm wide local excision of an intermediate thickness melanoma on the leg. (b) Improved appearance after use of skin camouflage.

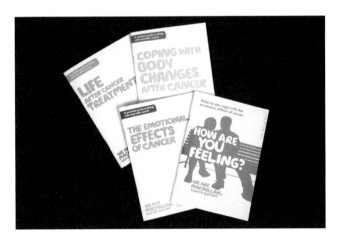

Figure 24.4 Information leaflets produced by Macmillan Cancer Support.

and reducing distress when the stressor can be influenced or changed, but most people use a combination of styles when faced with the loss of control and uncertainty inherent within the cancer experience.

Positive outcomes after skin cancer treatment include improved self-examination, vigilant sun-protective measures and the need to "spread the word", a need to "live life to the fullest", strengthening of emotional relationships with family and friends, more empathy with friends who have had cancer, deepening of spirituality and coming to terms with mortality [9]. Some patients initially (and a few long-term) have unhelpful feelings (e.g. guilt, anger, resentment, helplessness, and anxiety

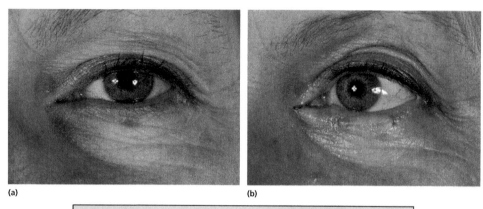

(a)   (b)

"Hate, Terrified, Nervous, Ugly, Unattractive, Shock, Angry, Hellish, Falling apart, Emotional, Miserable, Wobbly, Weepy, No confidence, Low self-esteem, Wary, Scary, Fragile, Freak, Bad, Self-conscious"

(c)

Figure 24.5 (a) Primary basal cell carcinoma of the lower eyelid associated with cancer phobia – "Terrified it might be skin cancer." (b) Aesthetic outcome 3 months after surgical defect repaired with a full-thickness skin graft – associated adjustment disorder. (c) Extracts from patient diary after skin cancer surgery.

about "not being in control"). Some adopt extreme measures that are disproportionate and unhelpful, contributing to decreased life quality (e.g. stop going on sunny holidays, constantly check skin). Ideally, hope, optimism and self-esteem should be maintained with a sensible concern for future safety and the right balance in terms of feelings and behavioural adaptations. Positive active change should be encouraged when desirable and acceptance when controllability of outcomes is low.

Maladaptive coping is associated with adjustment disorder and can be seen after skin cancer surgery. A 60-year-old woman with a basal cell carcinoma (BCC) on the lower eye-lid was "terrified that she may have cancer". After excision and full-thickness graft reconstruction she kept an emotional disclosure diary, which shows her distress and difficulty coping (Figure 24.5A,B). Denial of illness as a coping mechanism is not uncommon. This can lead to neglect of a skin cancer with delay in treatment and so potential adverse outcome. A 44-year-old single woman

presented with a large ulcerated BCC on her scalp. She had used cognitive and behavioural escape/avoidance as a coping style for several years (Figure 24.6).

Specific forms of psychosocial support

It is seldom that a person has a distinct diagnosable psychological disorder in response to his/her skin cancer diagnosis. Since many cancer fears have a rational basis, many traditional psychological approaches have been successfully adapted for this population. Each approach can be tailored to the individual and his/her family's needs and delivered in a group or individual format.

Psychoeducation groups
Open disclosure of negative feelings can be therapeutic and normalization of these feelings can help patients with all forms of skin cancer.

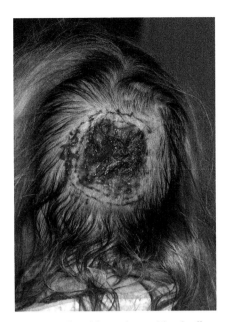

Figure 24.6 Neglected large ulcerated basal cell carcinoma of the scalp.

Box 24.3 Framework for a psychoeducation group at diagnosis

- Health education specific to skin cancer diagnosis
- Stress management techniques (e.g. understanding stress, relaxation, mindfulness techniques)
- How to use problem-focused coping strategies (e.g. managing relationships at home and work, and with your medical team)

Box 24.4 Framework for a psychoeducation group at the end of active treatment

- Practical and experiential introduction to exercise, nutrition, and stress management
- Managing risk behaviour such as sun exposure.
- Cognitive behavioural therapy techniques to help live with uncertainty and fears of cancer recurrence, and to look afresh at work, home life and relationships, and to accommodate changed priorities
- Training in how to build and utilize effective post-treatment partnerships with medical teams to enable smooth communication to enhance the monitoring of disease recurrence and late effects of treatment

Psychoeducation is particularly successful in a group format, as the participants become a natural therapeutic support network. Ideally, the group is facilitated by a psychological specialist in skin cancer and has a different theme each week (Box 24.3 and Box 24.4) with open discussion. Hand-outs and online resources can be offered at key transition points in the cancer journey (e.g. at diagnosis and when active treatment is completed). There are some excellent self-help books available [10].

Cancer phobia

There are patients who have either been previously diagnosed with a cancer or are so terrified of receiving a diagnosis of cancer that the sole focus of their life is the prospect of getting cancer. Some patients' beliefs are so fixed that they fall into the delusional spectrum of disorders (referred to as "delusional disorder, somatic type" or "monosymptomatic delusional hypochondriasis"). Others may present with an obsessional, anxious quality to their irrational fears, and are instead diagnosed with "body dysmorphic disorder". Most have an ongoing anxiety disorder, which may be very severe. Many will catastrophize every symptom or sign that they experience, and many have a concomitant somatic symptom disorder (which makes treatment with psychotropic medication difficult as they experience most of the side effects of the medication and so abandon it). Regardless of the ultimate psychiatric diagnosis, patients with cancer phobia are not exclusive to dermatology and many patients who are fearful of skin cancer are fearful of other cancers too. In assessing patients, the usual rules apply (see Chapter 6) for assessment of suicidal ideation and risk. Similarly if a delusional disorder is identified, treatment via a psychiatrist and/or psychodermatology clinic is essential. Many patients with an anxiety disorder and cancer phobia will benefit from antidepressants and cognitive-behavioural therapy (CBT) (see Chapter 3 and Chapter 13). It needs to be understood that for the patient the fear is very real. Nursing staff and patient advocacy groups (see Chapter 7 and Chapters 9) may have a particular role to play in facilitating management of this group of patients.

Cognitive-behavioural techniques

There is an established evidence base for the use of CBT in managing cancer distress, particularly anxiety, depression and post-traumatic stress disorder (PTSD). These techniques are discussed in detail in Chapter 5, with a nursing-specific framework in Chapter 9. Regarding cancer phobic patients specifically, their thoughts may be catastrophic in nature (e.g. assuming all skin marks are now cancer), they are often overly self-critical and they can make negative assumptions rather than rational conclusions based on fact. Strategies to challenge these thoughts and find an alternative but also realistic perspective are used.

Fears of recurrence can be addressed through disease education, relaxation or mindfulness meditation, and learning how to reframe catastrophizing thoughts.

Future research

Though clinical practice guidelines emphasize the necessity of a multidisciplinary approach and tailored psychosocial support for people with skin cancer, this is often not made available to patients [1]. Future research is required to evaluate not just the effectiveness of psychosocial screening and support, but also the efficacy, cost-effectiveness and feasibility of delivery.

The main areas of research are:
- role of stress and emotion in the development of skin cancer – evidence from both laboratory and animal studies;
- behavioural factors affecting the development of skin cancer (e.g. sun-bed addiction, neglect/denial of cancer);
- psychosocial factors experienced during or after skin cancer surgery;
- influence of psychosocial factors on prognosis;
- influence of psychosocial interventions on prognosis.

The evidence has been appraised in a recent systematic review [3].

PRACTICAL TIPS

- Discuss and address feelings of uncertainty and being overwhelmed.
- Encourage patients to share their feelings with family or with others who have been through similar experiences.
- Encourage patients to focus on their strengths, look at what resources they have and how they have coped in the past with adversity.
- Challenge patients' catastrophic thoughts and help them to distinguish facts from thoughts and feelings (e.g. encourage them to see the positive side of mortality statistics rather than focusing on the negative).
- If patients are being hard on themselves, self-critical or self-blaming, reflect this back to them. Encourage them to be kind to themselves. A useful question may be: *"What would you tell your best friend if she were in this situation and had these thoughts?"*

References

1. Kasparian NA. Psychological stress and melanoma: Are we meeting our patients' psychological needs? *Clin Dermatol* 2013; 31: 41–46.
2. National Institute for Health and Care Excellence. Guidance on cancer services: Improving outcomes for people with skin tumours including melanoma. 2006. Available at http://www.nice.org.uk/nice media/live/10901/28906/28906.pdf.
3. Clinical Practice Guidelines for the Management of Melanoma in Australia and New Zealand. Chapter 16 Psychosocial issues in melanoma, 2008, pp. 101–111. Available at http://www .nhmrc.gov.au/_files_nhmrc/publications/attach ments/cp111.pdf.
4. Carlson LE *et al.* Screening for distress and unmet needs in patients with cancer: review and recommendations. *J Clin Oncol* 2012; 30: 1160–1177.
5. Rhee JJS *et al.* The skin cancer index: Clinical responsiveness and predictors of quality of life. *Laryngoscope* 2007; 117: 399–405.
6. Cormier JN *et al.* Health-related quality of life in patients with melanoma: overview of instruments and outcomes. *Dermatol Clin* 2012; 30: 245–254.
7. Shenefelt PD. Relaxation strategies for patients during dermatologic surgery. *J Drugs Dermatol* 2010; 9: 795–799.
8. Thompson A, Kent G. Adjusting to disfigurement: processes involved in dealing with being visibly different. *Clin Psychol Rev* 2001; 21: 663–682.
9. Burden-Jones D *et al.* Quality of life issues in non-metastatic skin cancer. *Br J Dermatol* 2010; 162; 147–151.
10. Owen R. *Facing the Storm. Using CBT, Mindfulness and Acceptance to Build Resilience when your World's Falling Apart.* Hove: Routledge, 2011.

CHAPTER 25

Botulinum toxin treatment in depression

M. Axel Wollmer,[1] Michelle Magid[2] and Tillmann H.C. Kruger[3]

[1] Asklepios Clinic North – Ochsenzoll, Hamburg, Germany
[2] Department of Psychiatry, University of Texas Southwestern, Austin, TX, USA
[3] Center of Mental Health, Hannover Medical School (MHH), Hannover, Germany

Beyond the mere cosmetic benefits, treatment of glabellar (forehead) frown lines with botulinum toxin may enhance emotional well-being and counteract negative emotions like fear and sadness. Based on these observations, botulinum toxin is being studied in the treatment of depression. To date, the results of two open case series [1,2] and three randomized controlled trials [3–5] consistently showed that adjunctive, but also sole, injection of botulinum toxin into the glabellar region can improve symptoms of unipolar depression, even if the condition has been chronic and previously treatment resistant.

Theory and pathogenesis

The simultaneous contraction of the frontalis muscle and the corrugator muscles in the forehead region can cause an appearance of grief or sadness. This expression is often referred to as the omega sign, as the dynamic wrinkles from this anguished look often resemble the Greek letter omega, Ω (Figure 25.1A).

The facial musculature has the communicative function of expressing emotions. Thus, *feeling* depressed leads to *looking* depressed. However, the reverse may be true as well – *looking* depressed leads to *feeling* depressed. There are two main theories for this:

- *Behavioral theory* – behavioral psychologists believe people who naturally appear angry or depressed are received more negatively (e.g. avoiding, angry, rude) by those they encounter. In turn, these people respond negatively. Over time, this vicious cycle leads to heightened negative emotional states, as well as feelings of worthlessness, simply due to exhibiting a less welcoming facial expression.

- *Facial feedback hypothesis* – this hypothesis was first described in the 19th century by James Williams and Charles Darwin. It states that facial expression can influence emotional perception. For example, smiling at a party will make the party seem more enjoyable. Conversely, the more we frown, the sadder we feel, and the sadder we feel, the more we frown.

Modern neuroscience has shown that the simple act of frowning may in and of itself, influence brain activity in a way that can lead to negative emotional states. In depression there may be increased contraction of the muscles in the glabellar region of the forehead. These contracted muscles provide proprioceptive feedback to the brain and this feedback may

Practical Psychodermatology, First Edition. Anthony Bewley, Ruth E. Taylor, Jason S. Reichenberg and Michelle Magid.
© 2014 John Wiley & Sons, Ltd. Published 2014 by John Wiley & Sons, Ltd.

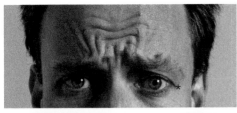
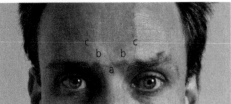

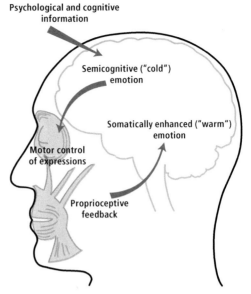

Figure 25.1 Facial features of depression and botulinum toxin injection scheme. Top: Facial features like the omega melancholicum, the Ω-shaped wrinkle pattern of the forehead, and Veraguth's folds that span the diagonals between the lateral corners of the eyes and the medial end of the eyebrows (*) are associated with agitation in depression. Bottom: Glabellar injection sites used in studies of onabotulinumtoxinA in the treatment of depression: procerus muscle are injected with 7 U in women and 9 U in men (a); medial corrugator muscles are bilaterally injected with 6 U in women and 8 U in men (b); lateral corrugator muscles are bilaterally injected with 5 U in women and 7 U in men (c).

Figure 25.2 The facial feedback theory. Proprioceptive afferences from the musculature activated during facial expression of emotional states feed back to the brain and intensify the experience of these emotions to make them felt as "warm." In other words, if the brain "feels" depressed there is a signal to contract the respective muscles in the face. The muscle contraction is fed back to the brain which then "feels" increasingly depressed (Source: Al Abdulmohsen and Kruger, 2011 [6]. Reproduced with permission of Elsevier.)

contribute to the maintenance and enhancement of depression (Figure 25.2). Disrupting this vicious circle (i.e. stopping a patient from frowning) may attenuate negative emotions and alleviate depression [7,8] .

Treatment

Botulinum toxin A (also known as Botox©) is a commercially made version of the toxin that is produced by the bacterium *Clostridium botulinum*. While dangerous at high doses, it can be diluted significantly and injected directly into skin muscles to prevent them from contracting. It has uses in muscle spasms and overactive bladder, but is most commonly known for its ability to decrease the appearance of wrinkles

in the face. There is minimal systemic absorption, and the excellent safety record of the commercially-available product has been proven over 20 years of skin treatments.

Recent studies [3,4] have shown that treatment with botulinum toxin A may improve depressive symptoms, and may be another option for patients who have not responded to medications and/or psychotherapy. Botulinum toxin A [3,4] was injected at five points in the glabellar region. Women received 29 units and men 39 units (to account for their higher muscle mass). In these studies, onabotulinumtoxinA was the specific preparation used (produced by Allergan under the brand name Allergan©). The injection scheme is summarized in Figure 25.1B). More than half of the participants who received botulinum toxin experienced a $\geq$50% reduction in their symptoms, and about one-third attained remission of depression within 6 weeks after the treatment. Alleviation of depression can be expected about 2 weeks after the intervention and may continue to improve over the period the paralytic effect is present. Depression may reappear in some cases when the paralytic effect wears off, but improvement or remission can be restored by reinjection of botulinum toxin.

As botulinum toxin is still off-label for depression, it should be used primarily in difficult treatment situations when established methods have not been successful. In our experience, botulinum toxin treatment is effective in patients with chronic, severe, and treatment resistant depression. The probability of response may be increased in those with strong activation of the glabellar musculature (e.g. expression of the Ω sign). This is frequently the case in patients who demonstrate a more agitated depression.

Future research

It is possible that a more personalized dosage may lead to even better results. Other muscles involved in sad facial expression, such as the frown muscles around the mouth, may be targeted.

One study has already shown that the use of botulinum toxin A for the treatment of depression is comparable in cost to standard psychopharmacologic treatment [9]. Further studies are indicated to look at the safety and cost-effectiveness of long-term treatment regimens.

According to the facial feedback theory and the observation of mood-lifting effect in healthy subjects, glabellar injection of botulinum toxin does not specifically treat depression, but rather attenuates the experience of negative emotions that occur in the majority of psychiatric disorders. Therefore, application in psychiatry may expand far beyond depression in the future.

PRACTICAL TIPS

- Facial feedback mechanisms may be involved in the pathogenesis of depression and may be a new target in its treatment.
- Injection of botulinum toxin in the glabellar (forehead) region is a new off-label treatment in the management of depression supported by a series of studies (Ib evidence level).
- In the future, it may be considered as an adjunctive or alternative treatment for patients who have not responded sufficiently to established psychiatric interventions.

References

1. Finzi E, Wasserman E. Treatment of depression with botulinum toxin A: a case series. *Dermatol Surg* 2006; 32: 645–649.
2. Hexsel D *et al.* Evaluation of self-esteem and depression symptoms in depressed and nondepressed subjects treated with onabotulinumtoxinA for glabellar lines. *Dermatol Surg* 2013; 39(7): 1088–1096.
3. Wollmer MA *et al.* Facing depression with botulinum toxin: a randomized controlled trial. *J Psychiatr Res* 2012; 46: 574–581.
4. Finzi E, Rosenthal N. Treatment of depression with botulinum toxin A: A randomized, double-blind, placebo controlled trial *Neuropsychopharmacology* 2012; 38: 316.
5. Magid M *et al.* ClinicalTrials.gov Identifier: NCT01392963, unpublished data.
6. Al Abdulmohsen T, Kruger TH. The contribution of muscular and auditory pathologies to the

symptomatology of autism. *Med Hypoth* 2011; 77: 1038–1047.

7. Alam M *et al*. Botulinum toxin and the facial feedback hypothesis: can looking better make you feel happier? *J Am Acad Dermatol* 2008; 58: 1061–1072.

8. Finzi E. *The Face of Emotion: How Botox Affects Our Moods and Relationships*. New York: Palgrave Macmillan, 2013.

9. Beer K. Cost effectiveness of botulinum toxins for the treatment of depression: preliminary observations. *J Drugs Dermatol* 2010; 9: 27–30.

CHAPTER 26

The Morgellons debate

Jason S. Reichenberg and Michelle Magid

University of Texas Southwestern, Austin, TX, USA

Proponents of Morgellons disease define it as illness in which thread-like fibers (Figure 26.1) under the skin cause crawling sensations, skin changes (Figure 26.2), fatigue, pain, and "brain fog." The term is not widely accepted by the medical community, who mostly believe it is a form of delusional infestation or somatic symptom disorder. In this chapter, we discuss the history and current debate of this highly-controversial topic.

In 1674, physician Sir Thomas Browne wrote about a disease afflicting children in the Languedoc area of France called *"the Morgellons . . . wherein they critically break out with harsh hairs on their backs, which . . . delivers them from coughs and convulsions."* In 2001, Mary Leitao discovered the article by Browne when trying to find a medical explanation for the "fibers" growing underneath her 2-year-old son's skin, which she visualized using a microscope. The term "Morgellons disease" found its modern use when Leitao established the Morgellons Research Foundation in 2002. Although some believed that Leitao suffered from a psychological disorder, others with similar stories believed there was finally a medical answer to their suffering [1].

Morgellons disease is now a highly sensationalized topic, with much debate about whether or not it even exists. At the time of this publication, a Google search for "Morgellons" resulted in 694 000 hits; whereas a Google search for "delusions of parasitosis"

resulted in 44 000 hits. The Charles E. Holman Foundation (CEHF) runs an annual Morgellons meeting, hosts a busy website (http://www.thecehf.org/), and has a medical and scientific advisory panel.

Defining features and pathogenesis

Proponents of Morgellons disease have provided diagnostic criteria to make the diagnosis (Box 26.1), though certainly the presence of fibers visualized by patients is the most characteristic feature [2].

The dermatology and psychiatry community has been hesitant to embrace the term Morgellons disease to explain the symptoms of these patients [3], with most physicians arguing it is a form of delusional infestation. Some have suggested that the term "Morgellons" should be used by physicians to develop a therapeutic relationship with patients who present with fibers [4], but others caution that patient-derived diagnostic terms should not be used to describe unconfirmed medical conditions. Furthermore, the CEHF website stresses the use of antibiotics/antiparasitics as the mainstay of treatment. Other websites have suggested that misdiagnosed patients may consider litigation in the future [5]. Desperate patients may try to self-treat using medications bought from the Internet, without medical supervision.

Practical Psychodermatology, First Edition. Anthony Bewley, Ruth E. Taylor, Jason S. Reichenberg and Michelle Magid.
© 2014 John Wiley & Sons, Ltd. Published 2014 by John Wiley & Sons, Ltd.

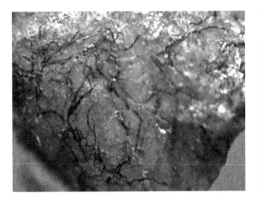

Figure 26.1 Example of Morgellons fibers in the skin at 100× magnification (courtesy of the Charles E. Holman Foundation).

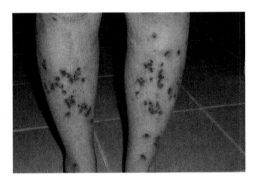

Figure 26.2 Example of common skin findings in patients with Morgellons disease. This 42-year-old female had a history of lesions on her legs, arms and buttocks (courtesy of the Charles E. Holman Foundation).

In 2012, the Centers for Disease Control and Prevention published a large prospective study of 115 patients with Morgellons disease. The study was not able to conclude whether these patients had a new condition or wider recognition of an existing condition such as delusional infestation. The skin materials studied were found to be composed of cellulose (from plants or clothing material). Of the patients studied, 63% had evidence of clinically significant somatic complaints, and in 50% drugs of abuse were detected in hair samples [6]. The article was criticized due to its patient selection, which was limited to a specific geographic area and

Box 26.1 Case Definition for Morgellons Disease as listed by the Morgellons Research Foundation

- Skin lesions accompanied by intense itching
- Crawling sensations on and under the skin, often compared to insects moving, stinging, or biting (cutaneous dysethesia)
- Colored fibers in and on the lesions (or "fuzz balls" or "black specks")
- Fatigue significant enough to interfere with daily activity
- Musculoskeletal pain
- Inability to concentrate and difficulty with short term memory "brain fog"
- Behavioral changes

(adapted from Savely VR, Stricker, RB. Morgellons Disease: the mystery unfolds. *Expert Reviews in Dermatology* 2007; 2(5): 585–591)

excluded patients whose symptoms had existed for greater than 3 months. Of the 115 patients, 90% were found by a search of medical records with terms including "delusions, parasitosis." Furthermore, the Morgellons Research Foundation was not invited to participate in the study, nor to refer patients for evaluation.

There have been attempts to elucidate a cause for Morgellons disease. The disease has similarities to a cattle-born spirochete infection, and polymerase chain reaction techniques have detected material from spirochetes (borrelial species) in the tissue of patients with Morgellons disease [7]. The Morgellons community has embraced these findings as evidence that the disease may be related to (or triggered by) chronic Lyme disease. However, the concept of chronic Lyme disease is not acknowledged by most infectious disease experts in the US, with a recent consensus statement refuting its existence altogether [8].

One recent study proposed that patients presenting with a chief complaint of "fibers" may be different than those presenting with "bugs" [9]. "Fiber" patients were more likely to have a somatic symptom disorder with features of both chronic pain (dysesthetic syndrome) and health anxiety (see Chapter 18 and Chapter 19). These patients are sometimes compared to the princess in the fable *The Princess and the Pea* due to their hypersensitivity to insignificant stimuli (e.g. debris in the air or on clothes), which most people are able to ignore. "Bug" patients were more likely to have classic delusional symptoms and to receive a final diagnosis of "delusional infestation" (as described in Chapter 14).

Assessment and treatment

The Morgellons community suggests that patients who visualize fibers should be tested for concomitant infection with bacteria/spirochetes, though the laboratories referenced do not all have FDA approval for commercial use. Treatment is then initiated depending on the results, with a focus on the use of long-term antibiotics and antiparasitics. There is no focus on psychiatric medication.

There are reports of patients with Morgellons disease having been successfully treated with pimozide and olanzapine [10], drugs commonly used in patients with delusional disorders. One recent report suggests using antidepressants such as citalopram, as these medications have been beneficial in treating somatic preoccupation, depression, and anxiety [11]. This approach focuses less on "how to get rid of" the fibers and more on "how to live with" the fibers by improving quality of life and reducing patient distress. It is important to test for and address concomitant substance use disorders when present.

Though the diagnosis of Morgellons disease is controversial, it is clear that these patients are suffering greatly and would benefit from a holistic approach to treatment that addresses their medical, psychiatric, and social needs.

PRACTICAL TIPS

- There is controversy as to whether Morgellons disease is a distinct physical disease, or a renaming of a previously-described psychiatric disease.
- Regardless of the cause of symptoms, these patients are extremely disabled by their disease, and many have co-morbid psychiatric disease.
- When patients present with crawling sensations, fatigue, pain, and "brain fog," it is important to rule out a treatable cause.
- If no treatable cause is found, an easy cure may not be possible. Treatment should often be tailored to the patient's specific clinical picture, with a focus on improving quality of life.

References

1. Harlan C. Mom fights for answers on what's wrong with her son. *Pittsburgh Post-Gazette* July 23 2006. Available at http://www.post-gazette.com/stories/news/health/mom-fights-for-answers-on-whats-wrong-with-her-son-443228/#ixzz2TPjH7Bg7.
2. Savely VR, Stricker RB. Morgellons disease: the mystery unfolds. *Exp Rev Dermatol* 2007; 2(5): 585–591.
3. Koblenzer C. The challenge of Morgellons disease. *J Am Acad Dermatol* 2006; 55: 920–922.
4. Murase JE, Wu JJ, Koo J. Morgellons disease: a rapport enhancing term for delusions of parasitosis. *J Am Acad Dermatol* 2006; 55: 913–914.
5. http://www.thecehf.org/appointment-tips-for-morgellons-patients.html (last accessed 11 December 2013).
6. Pearson ML *et al.* Clinical, epidemiologic, histopathologic and molecular features of an

unexplained dermopathy. *PLoS ONE* 2012; 7(1): e29908.

7. Middelveen MJ *et al.* Association of spirochetal infection with Morgellons disease. *F1000 Res* 2013; 2(25).

8. Feder H *et al.* A critical appraisal of "chronic Lyme disease". *N Engl J Med* 2007; 357: 1422–1430.

9. Reichenberg JS *et al.* Patients labeled with delusions of parasitosis compose a heterogenous group: A retrospective study from a referral center. *J Am Acad Dermatol* 2013; 68(1): 41–46 .e2.

10. Koblenzer CS. Pimozide at least as safe and perhaps more effective than olanzapine for treatment of Morgellons disease. *Arch Dermatol* 2006; 142(10): 1364.

11. Delacerda A, Reichenberg J, Magid M. Successful treatment of patients previously labeled as having delusions of parasitosis with antidepressant therapy. *J Drugs Dermatol* 2012; 11(12): 1506–1507.

CHAPTER 27

Substance misuse and the dermatology patient

Alexander Verner

Tower Hamlets Specialist Addictions Service (SAU), East London Foundation NHS Trust, London, UK

Substance use disorder is common, and so is highly likely to be present in some patients with psychodermatological conditions. Some addictions are of direct relevance to dermatological conditions (e.g. smoking and psoriasis) and many addictions will produce a range of dermatological signs, either directly (e.g. the track marks produced by intravenous drug use) or indirectly (e.g. signs of liver disease in alcoholic cirrhosis). Substance misuse, if not addressed, can lead to profound morbidity or premature death.

The range of substances used and misused is vast, with most being depressants, stimulants, hallucinogens or a combination of the three. In addition to its direct psychiatric effects, substance misuse can have indirect effects that persist even after the cessation of the drug.

Approximately half of the world's adult population consumes alcohol, which causes 4.4% of the global net burden of disease. Tobacco smoking continues to account for approximately five million deaths worldwide per year and is the "single greatest reversible risk factor" for morbidity and mortality [1]. Illicit drugs are used by an estimated 185 million adults worldwide; the morbidity and mortality is well described for these substances. There are also drugs with variable legality, differing between countries and over time (e.g. cannabis and khat).

A further category of misuse concerns drugs that are legally prescribed to the patient (e.g. oxycodone or benzodiazepines) but are taken improperly, or drugs prescribed to someone else and diverted to your patient (either by misguided good intent or for financial gain). Most drugs liable to be abused have a short time-to-peak plasma concentration and a short half-life. These may include sleeping agents, such as zopiclone, zaleplon, and zolpidem (the "Z" drugs), which dermatologists may be asked to prescribe to patients with sleeping problems due to skin itching.

Multiple "newer" drugs are available from the internet, which are sometimes misleadingly described as "legal highs" – customers think legal means "safe", which it does not (e.g. the cannabinoid "Spice" or the synthetic stimulant mephedrone). These can produce a range of psychiatric symptoms, including intoxication, psychosis and acute lowering of mood following the cessation of use. Deaths have occurred due to perturbed physiology and by precipitating abnormal mental states (e.g. suicide by violent means after mephedrone use).

Substance misuse is present in half of all patients with schizophrenia or bipolar affective disorder, approximately one-third of those with anxiety or depression and four-fifths of those with antisocial personality disorder. Conversely, of those patients seen for substance misuse,

Practical Psychodermatology, First Edition. Anthony Bewley, Ruth E. Taylor, Jason S. Reichenberg and Michelle Magid.
© 2014 John Wiley & Sons, Ltd. Published 2014 by John Wiley & Sons, Ltd.

approximately 70% will have another co-morbid mental illness.

The prevalence of substance misuse in patients suffering dermatological conditions is not known. However, there are some pathophysiological links between some substances and some dermatological conditions, such as exacerbation of psoriasis by tobacco and alcohol, or the link between smoking/nicotine and ulcerative colitis.

Defining features

If ever there was a disease that exists on a continuum, then substance misuse is it. Use may wax and wane over time; one patient may also be severely dependent upon one substance (e.g. cigarettes) but use other substances (e.g. alcohol and caffeine) non-problematically.

The DSM-5 criteria list 11 defining symptoms for substance use disorder, two of which must be present to make a diagnosis of a disorder and occurring within a 12-month period (Box 27.1). The disorder should be further specified as "mild" (two to three symptoms present), "moderate" (four to five symptoms), or severe (six or more symptoms).

Although tolerance and withdrawal can occur for almost any substance, marked physiological dependence usually only occurs with sedative drugs (e.g. alcohol, opiates, benzodiazepines, and barbiturates).

Pathogenesis

Substance misuse is unique among mental illnesses in that it requires the presence of a consumable product for its genesis and maintenance. Assuming that the substance is available, there are a number of biological, psychological and social factors that may lead an individual towards a substance use disorder (Box 27.2).

Many of the human activities that satisfy a physiological urge result in the release of dopamine in the nucleus accumbens. Almost all drugs liable to be misused release dopamine to

Box 27.1 DSM-5 criteria for substance use disorder

- Tolerance: an increased amount of the substance is required to produce the same effect
- Experiencing withdrawal and getting relief from withdrawal symptoms by consumption of the substance
- Taking larger amounts over a longer period than was intended
- Unsuccessful efforts to cut down or control use
- Important social, occupational or recreational activities are given up or reduced due to substance use
- Recurrent use despite interpersonal problems caused by the substance
- Recurrent use resulting in a failure to fulfil obligations
- Recurrent use in situations in which it is physically hazardous
- Continuing to use despite knowing it is causing physical or psychological problems
- Spending a great deal of time trying to obtain the substance
- Craving the substance

Box 27.2 Some reasons for substance use disorder

- Heritable predisposition to disordered use (especially alcohol)
- Use of prescribed analgesia for a painful condition
- Attempt to counteract the effects of subjectively unpalatable antipsychotic medication
- Depressed/anxious patient wishing to alter his/her mood state
- Patients with mental illness who have a very limited range of ways of experiencing pleasure
- A wish to change appearance (anabolic steroids/tanning)
- Boredom
- Lonely people befriended by drug dealer/user/misuser
- To deal with ever-present awful life circumstances (e.g. prostitution)

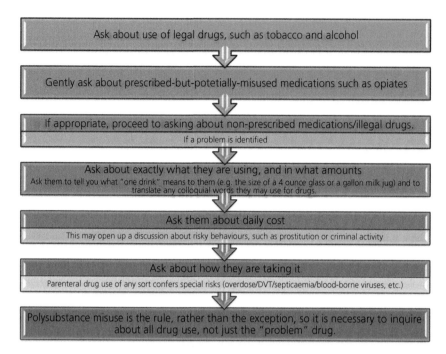

Figure 27.1 Taking a substance misuse history.

levels far in excess of what would be produced by satisfying appetite for food or sexual pleasure. The reward system can be said to have been "hijacked" by the drug, and patients may indulge in drug use to the exclusion of other rewarding activities, as they subjectively experience this behaviour as intensely pleasurable.

Assessment

In a non-addiction medical setting, the most valuable thing to do is to ask the right questions to establish whether there is a substance use disorder, and if there is, to refer on accordingly. It is important to approach patients suspected of drug misuse without passing judgement on them. A recommended schema for questioning is offered in Figure 27.1.

Patients presenting to a psychodermatology clinic may be anywhere on the continuum of "no problem" to "severely dependent" on their misused substance. Some patients may be in treatment; others may have never considered or accessed treatment; and others may have made a number of attempts at treatment without success (so far).

Formal screening questionnaires include the Alcohol: World Health Organization: Alcohol Use Disorders Identification Test (AUDIT; see Appendix A16), a 10-item questionnaire, and the Drugs and alcohol: World Health Organization: Alcohol, Smoking and Substance Involvement Screening Test (ASSIST; see Appendix A17) version 3. For the busy practitioner, the CAGE questionnaire is often used (see Appendix A1). Although it was devised for alcohol screening, CAGE can be useful for any substance. It comprises four questions asking about the need to **C**ut down, if people have **A**nnoyed you about your use, if you feel **G**uilty about your use, and if you have needed an **E**ye opener in the morning to help with withdrawal. Answering "yes" to two or more of these questions has a 71% sensitivity and 90% specificity for an alcohol misuse disorder [2].

When performing the physical examination, it is important to look for signs of substance

Table 27.1 Cutaneous signs associated with substance misuse

Sign	Substance
Yellowing of fingers	Tobacco, cannabis
Scratch marks	Stimulant drugs can cause pruritus and formication (a sensation of insects crawling underneath the skin) Opiates cause histamine release and pruritus Liver disease (of any cause) can induce pruritus
Signs of liver disease – jaundice (yellow skin/sclera) (Figure 27.2), ascites (enlarged belly), "paper money" skin, telangiectasia (spider veins), clubbing of fingernails, signs of porphyria (Figure 27.3)	Alcoholic cirrhosis; intravenous drug use leading to hepatitis B/C
Bruxism (teeth grinding)	Stimulants
Poor dentition	Frequent correlate of substance misuse of any sort, especially methamphetamine
Premalignant and malignant lesions in the oropharynx (back of mouth)	Tobacco, alcohol, dental neglect Consider human papillomavirus
Track marks	Sign of venous injecting of drugs – can be anywhere on the body, including the neck and groin
Cutaneous granulomas	Due to adulterants/diluents in an injected drug or its solvent
Intranasal granulomas, septal necrosis	Nasally inhaled cocaine
Skin infections including necrotizing fasciitis	Injecting drugs or as a consequence of trauma to skin due to excoriation
Signs of infective endocarditis	Injecting drugs
Signs of HIV	May have been acquired from injecting drugs
Skin ulceration	Injecting drugs. Often difficult to heal
Purple plaques or skin necrosis on ears or extremities	Levamisole toxicity related to cocaine use (Figure 27.4)

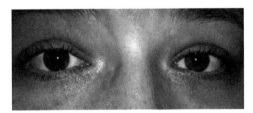

Figure 27.2 Scleral icterus is often seen in patients with liver problems. These problems may be due to chronic hepatitis infections or the effect of chronic alcohol use (courtesy of Dr J. Reichenberg).

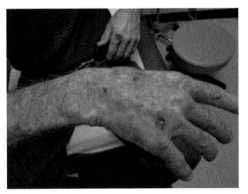

Figure 27.3 Superficial erosions on sun-exposed skin of the backs of the hands is classic for porphyria cutanea tarda. This can be a result of chronic hepatitis and is often exacerbated by alcohol misuse (courtesy of Dr J. Reichenberg).

misuse. Cutaneous manifestations may be the "first noticeable consequence" [3]; much of the organ damage caused by substance misuse may be hidden from view and asymptomatic (Table 27.1).

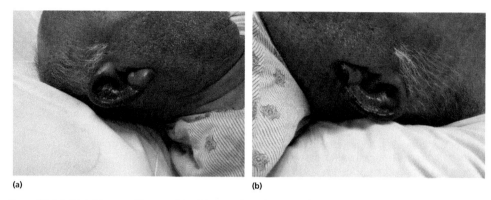

(a)   (b)

Figure 27.4 (a,b) A 56-year-old man with a history of cocaine use. The patient developed dusky purpura and necrosis of the bilateral ears. Levamisole is an antiparasitic medication often used as a cutting agent in cocaine, and can cause vasculitis, characteristically on the pinna of the ears and the cheeks (courtesy of Dr J. Reichenberg).

Table 27.2 Laboratory assessment of patients with suspected substance misuse

Recommended test	Interpretation
Urine drug screen	Unexpected results should be interpreted by contacting the laboratory, repeat testing and further discussion with the patient/collateral
Breath alcohol levels	May not be practical in a non-addiction setting. Remember a frequent alcohol user may have a high blood alcohol concentration and appear perfectly sober
Complete blood count	Alcohol misuse can produce anaemia, thrombocytopenia, macrocytosis and leucopaenia
Serum electrolytes	Renal disease can occur in injecting drug users by a variety of mechanisms
Liver function tests (including gamma-GT)	Elevated values could be due to hepatitis/cirrhosis of alcoholic or non-alcoholic cause
Testing for hepatitis B and C, and HIV	Especially important if the patient has ever injected him/herself with any drug Consider referral for sexual health screening
Pregnancy test	Recommended for any suspected substance misuse in women of child-bearing age If pregnant, discuss fetal risks of exposure

LFT, liver function test; GT, glutamyl transferase

Laboratory investigations are important in the screening process (Table 27.2).

Treatment

Treatment should be tailored according to where the patient is in his/her addiction journey [4]. For some patients, one-off psychosocial education is adequate to reduce, for example, drinking to safe levels. For others, more intensive work is required.

Although medication has a role, it is a relatively small one; the mainstay of treatment is psychosocial (usually cognitive-behavioural therapy, motivational interviewing or programmes based around the Twelve Steps of Alcoholics Anonymous). The evidence suggests that the modality of treatment is less important than the quality of the therapeutic relationship. It should also be remembered that, for the entrenched substance misuser, epiphanies are extremely rare [5] and a single episode of detox/rehab is unlikely to provide a cure.

The non-specialist should restrict him/herself to asking the right questions, possibly offering brief interventions (dependent upon competencies), and referring to relevant treatment agencies. In the UK, public services can be identified by contacting Public Health England, formerly known as the National Treatment Agency for Substance Misuse (NTA) (http://www.nta.nhs.uk/). In the US, help can be found by contacting the Substance Abuse and Mental Health Services Administration (SAMHSA) (http://www.samhsa.gov/).

You may come across patients being maintained or treated with drugs to enable abstinence (Table 27.3).

Emergency situations

If you suspect *opiate overdose* (respiratory depression, pinpoint pupils, unresponsive), then administer 400 µg of naloxone, preferably intravenously, and transfer to hospital. You may need to repeat the dose, as it is short-acting; its half-life is much shorter than that of opiates.

Acute alcohol withdrawal needs immediate specialist assessment and treatment. If untreated, delirium tremens can supervene,

Table 27.3 Drugs used in the treatment of substance misuse

Drug	Used to treat	Notes
Methadone	Illicit opiates like heroin	Full opioid agonist, and carries a risk of opiate overdose; it also can prolong the QTc
Buprenorphine	Illicit opiates like heroin	As it is a partial opioid agonist, it is safer in overdose, and can protect the patient using heroin "on top" from overdosing
Naloxone	Illicit opiates like heroin	Short-acting opiate antagonist given parenterally to patients suspected of opiate overdose
Buprenorphine/naloxone (Suboxone)	Illicit opiates like heroin	As above. Prescribed to reduce the chance of the patient crushing up the tablet and injecting him/herself with it
Naltrexone/nalmefene	Illicit opiates like heroin; alcohol dependence	Opiate receptor antagonists with half-lives longer than that of naloxone. The oral preparation works best in the highly motivated patient who has a partner who can encourage the taking of it
Disulfiram	Alcohol misuse	Inhibits acetylaldehyde dehydrogenase; if the patient takes alcohol, acetylaldehyde builds up and makes the patient feel very unwell
Acamprosate	Alcohol misuse	GABA agonist; works to reduce a patient's craving for alcohol
Nicotine patches/chewing gum	Nicotine replacement therapy	Can cause irritant or contact dermatitis to skin or mucosa
Varenicline	Nicotine cessation	Partial agonist of nicotine receptor. Can cause agitation and suicidal thoughts
Buproprion	Nicotine cessation	Also an antidepressant

with significant mortality; Wernicke's encephalopathy can develop, with a risk of Korsakoff's psychosis (not a psychosis but an irreversible amnesia if left untreated).

Pregnant patients who misuse substances require specialist assessment and treatment, and prebirth counselling. Many pregnancies are unplanned in the general population; this is equally true in the population who misuse substances.

PRACTICAL TIPS

- Ask about substance misuse; do so sensitively and non-judgementally.
- Be aware that substance misuse can be the cause, consequence or both of other psychiatric and dermatological conditions.
- Unless addressed, patients are unlikely to make improvements in their well-being.
- Polysubstance misuse is the rule, not the exception.
- Substance misuse is a chronic relapsing condition with high morbidity and mortality.
- Remain aware of your own limitations in assessing and treating substance misuse; familiarize yourself with your local resources and refer out when appropriate.

References

1. Latt N *et al. Addiction Medicine*. Oxford: Oxford University Press, 2009.
2. Schorling JB. Review: sensitivity of the CAGE questionnaire for the DSM diagnosis of alcohol abuse and dependence in general clinical populations was 71% at cut points 2. *Evidence Based Med* 2005; 10(1): 26–26.
3. Lui SW *et al*. The effects of alcohol and drug abuse on the skin. *Clin Dermatol* 2010; 28: 391–399.
4. Marshall EJ *et al. The Treatment of Drinking Problems: A Guide to the Helping Professions*. Cambridge: Cambridge University Press, 2010.
5. Sellman D. The 10 most important things known about addiction. *Addiction* 2009; 105: 6–13.

Glossary

Acne A disease of the pilosebaceous unit, which generally presents in adolescence with seborrhea, comodones, papules, pustules, cysts and scarring

Acne excoriée A condition in which the person picks at acne-related skin blemishes, resulting in a worsening of the skin blemishes, further urges to pick, and a vicious cycle that is difficult to stop

Action planning A behavior change technique that helps patients to achieve agreed health goals. The planning is the (usually joint) formulation of the highly specified stages or processes by which the person will achieve that goal

Adherence and non-adherence The degree to which a patient follows medical advice, including following a prescribed course of medication, following lifestyle advice, hospital attendance, etc. Use of neutral adjectives such as "high" or "low" adherence rather than "good" or "poor" is viewed as good practice

Adjustment disorder A symptom complex that occurs when an individual is having difficulty adjusting to or coping with a particular life stressor, i.e. being diagnosed with skin cancer

Affect Observable behavior (e.g. irritable, labile, flat, inappropriate) that represents the expression of a subjectively experienced emotion

Agitated depression Depression with increased psychomotor activity

Agoraphobia Anxiety and fear of going out of the house or being in wide open spaces

Akathisia A movement disorder characterized by an unpleasant sensation of inner restlessness that manifests itself with an inability to sit still

Alexithymia Inability to identify and describe emotions

Allodynia Pain that is experienced as a result of a stimulus that does not ordinarily cause pain

Alopecia Hair loss from any cause

Alopecia areata An autoimmune hair loss disorder in which the patient's immune system attacks the hairs and makes them fall out

Alopecia totalis Alopecia areata when all scalp hair is lost

Alopecia universalis Alopecia areata when all scalp and body hair is lost

American Psychiatric Association (APA) The largest professional group for psychiatrists in the US

Anhedonia Inability to experience pleasure

Antidepressants Medications designed to treat depressive symptoms

Antipsychotics A class of drugs designed to treat psychotic, delusional, and hallucinatory symptoms

Anxiety A clinical syndrome in which (often irrational) fears and restlessness override the normal day-to-day functioning of the individual

Approved mental health professional (AMHP) The professional with the role of assessing and deciding whether there are grounds to detain a person under the UK Mental Health Act 1983, amended 2007, if they meet the statutory criteria

Atopic dermatitis Eczema (dry, scaly, weepy, itchy skin) associated with atopy

Atopy A genetic predisposition towards the development of IgE and delayed hypersensitivity reactions (usually associated with other atopic disease, e.g. asthma and hay fever) to environmental antigens

Attachment A child's psychosocial ability to bond, securely or insecurely, with parents or a caregiver

Attentional biases A prior tendency to focus attention on a particular target. This may include focusing on own body image and feelings (e.g. "*I feel ugly*") rather than on the external world (e.g. what a conversational partner is saying)

Attention deficit hyperactivity disorder (ADHD) A neurodevelopmental disorder marked by significant inattention, hyperactivity, and impulsivity

Atypical antipsychotics Second-generation antipsychotic medications thought to be less likely to cause extrapyramidal (movement) side effects

Autism or autism spectrum disorder (ASD) A neurodevelopmental disorder marked by impairment in reciprocal social interaction and difficulties

Practical Psychodermatology, First Edition. Anthony Bewley, Ruth E. Taylor, Jason S. Reichenberg and Michelle Magid.
© 2014 John Wiley & Sons, Ltd. Published 2014 by John Wiley & Sons, Ltd.

in social communication, and by restricted, repetitive, or stereotyped behaviors and interests

Basal cell carcinoma (BCC) The most common and usually most benign skin cancer

Basic talk therapies Therapies based on directed dialogues between a healthcare professional and a patient

Benzodiazepine A class of psychiatric medications that enhances action at the GABA receptor, which produces anxiolytic, sedative, and hypnotic effects

Bibliotherapy A form of guided self-help using a structured book as a treatment for depression

Bipolar affective disorder A mood disorder characterized by episodes of mania and depression, and, if severe, psychotic symptoms in both

Black box warning In the US, a warning on prescription drugs that indicates significant risk or life-threatening adverse effects. This is the strongest warning issued by the Food and Drug Administration (FDA)

Body dysmorphic disorder (BDD) A preoccupation with an imagined or greatly exaggerated physical flaw or imperfection which causes significant distress

Borderline personality disorder One of several "personality disorders," characterized by instability of affect and relationships, uncertain self-image, and impulsivity, with high levels of self-harm and suicidality

Botulinum toxin A Bacterial toxin that inhibits cholinergic neurotransmission at the motor end plate. When used in medicine, it is often known by the brand name "Botox©"

Bruxism Teeth grinding

Cacosmia The imagining of smelling foul odors

Care programme approach (CPA) A UK system to deliver mental health and social care in the community, first used in 1991 and modified in 1999. Key elements are a written care plan, care coordinator allocation, risk assessment, and regular reviews

Catastrophizing A cognitive distortion in which a person is prone to always expect the worst of all possible outcomes/futures

Central sensitization The situation wherein neurons in the brain, previously activated by a noxious stimulus, become sensitized and as a result become hyper-responsive to the same or similar stimuli when encountered again

Child and Adolescent Mental Health Services (CAMHS) A service for Children and Adolescents provided by the National Health Service in the UK

Chronic prostatitis/chronic pelvic pain syndrome (CP/CPPS) This term is used for unexplained chronic pain in any part of the male genitourinary system and the surrounding mucocutaneous tissue

Cognitive-behavioral therapy (CBT) Treatment grounded in replacing distorted thoughts about ourselves and the world with more accurate, evidence-based thoughts, which can positively influence the way we think, feel, and behave

Cognitive processes Thinking styles and thought processes

Common sense–self- regulatory model A dynamic, "information-processing" model that helps to explain people's emotional and behavioral responses to the perception of symptoms or the diagnosis of an illness

Compliance The extent to which a patient's behavior matches the prescriber's recommendation. This term has negative connotation, placing blame on the patient for not following advice, and has been largely replaced by the term adherence

Compulsions Urges to perform overt physical (e.g. checking, washing) or mental (e.g. praying) rituals according to certain rules that are designed to neutralize or prevent obsessional fears and reduce anxiety

Concordance A partnership between the patient and the provider where negotiation takes place and an agreement is reached that respects the patient's needs and beliefs concerning taking (or not taking) a medication

Conversion disorder A condition in which psychological distress unconsciously manifests itself as an impairment in motor or sensory neurologic function (e.g. blindness)

Coping Constructive and adaptive strategies used to reduce stress and manage conflict

Delirium Temporary state of disorientation and cognitive dysfunction, often caused by a medical condition or substance

Delirium tremens An acute and potentially fatal episode of delirium and autonomic instability seen in alcohol dependence, caused by sudden withdrawal from alcohol

Delusional disorder A psychiatric disorder in which an individual holds a fixed, false belief that is outside the individual's cultural normality

Delusional infestation (previously delusions of parasitosis, Ekbom's syndrome, and parasitophobia) A person's delusional belief that they are infested with insects, mites, bacteria, viruses or similar materials

Dementia Persistent decline in cognitive function and/or social abilities; often seen in the older population

Depression A clinical syndrome in which mood is lowered and life is unenjoyable

Dermabrasion A technique in which a mechanical device is used to remove the top layers of a patient's skin. When the skin heals, it may have an improved texture

Dermafiller An injected aesthetic; usually a synthetic skin filler that makes the skin appear fuller or less wrinkled.

Dermatitis artefacta A form of factitious disorder in which a patient creates his/her own skin disease and denies responsibility for his/her actions

Dermatitis simulata A type of dermatitis artefacta in which the patient does not cause significant skin damage, but rather uses paints, adhesives, or make-up to feign skin disease

Detached mindfulness The practice of observing thoughts and feelings as events without evaluating them, and allowing them to come and go without engaging with them or responding to them

Discontinuation syndrome Recrudescence of clinical symptoms on decreasing or abruptly stopping an antidepressant

Disfigurement A visible mark or blemish to appearance that is generally considered to deviate from normative appearance. Also known as visible difference

Drug reaction with eosinophilia and systemic symptoms (DRESS) A rare drug reaction characterized by a skin rash and internal organ involvement, often caused by antiseizure medications

DSM-5 Diagnostic and Statistical Manual of Mental Disorders Version Five. Published in 2013 by the American Psychiatric Association. A classification system for diagnosing mental illness.

DSM-IV-TR Diagnostic and Statistical Manual of Mental Disorders Version Four, text revision. Published in 2000 by the American Psychiatric Association. This is a classification system for diagnosing mental illness.

Dysesthesia From the Greek "dys" (abnormal) and "aesthesia" (sensation). An abnormal, unusual, and unpleasant sensation within the skin, which may be spontaneous or evoked

Dysgeusia Altered taste

Dystonia A movement disorder characterized by sustained muscle contractions, which produce twisting and abnormal postures

Eczema A pruritic skin disorder with erythema, edema, excoriations (superficial skin tears), and lichenification (epidermal thickening). Compared to contact dermatitis which usually implies an external cause

Electrocardiogram (ECG or EKG) A test that measures the electrical activity of the heart from sensors placed on the skin, and produces a graphic tracing

Electrolysis A technique of hair removal in which a fine needle is introduced into each hair follicle and an electrical current is passed through the tissue

Erythromelalgia Bilateral red, burning, painful extremities secondary to small fiber neuropathy

Excoriations Superficial skin tears

Exposure and response prevention A behavioral intervention, often used in obsessive-compulsive disorder, which involves entering feared situations and waiting for the fear response to subside naturally rather than responding with anxiety-reducing behaviors

Extrapyramidal syndrome A cluster of movement disorders, such as acute dystonia, akathisia, parkinsonism, or tardive dyskinesia, caused by dopamine blockers, such as antipsychotic medication

Eye movement desensitization and reprocessing (EMDR) A newer type of therapy combining eye movements with traumatic events in an attempt to dampen negative emotionally charged memories

Factitious disorder A psychological disorder in which the patient induces physical or psychological symptoms in order to assume the sick role

Folie à deux (trois, quatre, etc.) Shared delusional beliefs between two (or more) people. The person who originally developed the belief is called the inducer

General anxiety disorder (GAD) Persistent unremitting anxiety disorder, usually with persistent unremitting worries and anxiety thoughts

Genodermatoses Any truly and directly identifiable genetic disorder of the skin

Glabellar Referring to the glabella, the lower middle forehead between the eyebrows

Glossodynia Tongue pain

Goal setting A collaborative process of agreeing to an outcome (usually behavioral), such as weight loss or improved adherence which the patient wants to achieve (see action planning).

Good faith Honesty and sincere intention to deal fairly with others. May not be a sufficient protection in a medical malpractice lawsuit

Granuloma An area of chronic inflammation in the tissue characterized by giant cells

Habit reversal A behavioral treatment involving becoming more aware of an undesirable behavior, and practicing alternative and competing responses in place of that behavior

Harm avoidance A personality trait that includes excessive worrying, fearfulness, shyness, and doubtfulness

Health anxiety A preoccupation with acquiring or having a serious illness, despite medical evidence to the contrary. Also known as hypochondriasis or illness anxiety disorder

Hirsutism Excess hair in women in areas that are under androgen control, e.g. beard, moustache, chest

Hyperalgesia The experience of greater pain than would be expected from a mildly painful stimulus

Hypochondriasis See health anxiety

ICD-10 The 10th revision of the International Statistical Classification of Diseases and Related Health Problems (ICD), a medical classification list by the World Health Organization

Illness beliefs Beliefs about the nature of an illness or symptoms (terms frequently used interchangeably with illness cognitions, illness perceptions or illness representations)

Immune privilege A biologic state in certain tissues, such as the brain, eye, and hair follicle, where there is a relative tolerance to antigens without leading to inflammation. Loss of the immune privilege has been implicated in the pathology of alopecia areata and primary scarring alopecia

Impulse control disorders Psychiatric disorders characterized by a strong impulse to engage in a behavior that is harmful to self or others. Resisting the impulse creates a feeling of discomfort, which is temporarily relieved by engaging in the behavior

Isotretinoin A retinoid medication that is a derivative of vitamin A; primarily used in an oral formulation for treating acne

Khat An African flowering plant that has stimulant-like effects when chewed

KOH preparation A potassium hydroxide preparation from a skin swab or scraping used to recognize fungi, yeasts, and some other organisms

Laser resurfacing A technique in which a laser is used to precisely burn off the top layers of a patient's skin. When the skin heals, it may have an improved texture

Leukopenia Abnormally low white blood cell count

Lichenification Skin thickening

Lichen simplex chronicus The cutaneous manifestation of thickened skin caused by repeated rubbing at one site

Macrocytosis Enlargement of red blood cells, as evidenced by an abnormally high mean corpuscular volume

Medically unexplained cutaneous symptoms (MUS) Symptoms in the absence of an organic cause

Melanoma A malignant, easy to spread skin cancer arising from pigment-producing cells

Mental Health Act (UK) (1983, 2007) A 1983 Act of UK Parliament, amended in 2007, which legislates for people diagnosed with a mental disorder to be detained in hospital, against their wishes, for assessment and treatment of their mental disorder

Mephedrone A synthetic stimulant

Meralgia paresthetica Numbness, tingling, or pruritus of the lateral thigh(s) due to injury or impingement of the lateral cutaneous femoral nerve

Metabolic syndrome A group of medical disorders that, if found concurrently, are associated with an increased risk of cardiovascular disease and diabetes. These include obesity, lipid abnormalities, increased blood pressure, and elevated blood sugar

Metastatic Spread of a cancer to a different site from the primary, e.g. from skin to lymph nodes or internal organs

Mindfulness The focusing of attention and awareness, based on the concept of mindfulness in Buddhist meditation. It differs from traditional CBT approaches in that the aim is not to challenge or modify beliefs but to limit the influence that they may have on behavior

Miniaturization A term used to describe hair fibres becoming smaller with successive hair cycles and is the characteristic feature of genetic hair loss

Minoxidil A medication that is commonly used in a topical form to promote hair growth. Originally marketed as an oral antihypertensive agent

National Institute for Health and Care Excellence (NICE) A UK public body of the Department of Health, set up in 1999 to publish evidence-based clinical guidelines

Negative intrusive imagery Distressing and unwanted mental images, especially visual, but which may occur in any sensory modality

Neuralgia Pain in the distribution of a nerve

Neuropathy Pathology and/or change in function of a nerve

Neurotic excoriations A condition in which self-induced skin lesions are produced by excessive scratching, picking, or other manipulation of the skin

Neurolinguistic programming (NLP) A type of therapy focusing on changing the connection between neurologic processes ("neuro"), language ("linguistic"), and behavioral patterns learned through experience ("programming") to achieve specific life goals

Nodular prurigo (i.e. prurigo nodularis, picker's nodules, neurodermatitis) A chronic dermatitis characterized by multiple thickened nodules or papules which arise from chronic scratching or picking

Noradrenergic and specific serotonergic antidepressant (NASSA) A class of antidepressant medications believed to exert its therapeutic effect by antagonizing the α2-adrenergic receptor and specific serotonin receptors

Norepinephrine-dopamine reuptake inhibitor (NDRI) A class of antidepressant medications believed to exert its therapeutic effect by increasing the availability of norepinephrine and dopamine. Commonly used to treat depression when poor energy is a main component

Normalizing A technique where the therapist helps the client to see his/her experience as "normal" for someone in his/her position

Notalgia paresthetica Burning or itching of the scapular region, often unilateral, and due to neuropathy of spinal nerve(s) T2–T6.

Obsessions Intrusive thoughts, images or impulses that the person experiences as unwanted, senseless, or disturbing, and that lead to anxiety

Obsessive-compulsive disorder (OCD) A psychiatric disorder in which obsessions or compulsions create significant distress

Olfactory delusion The delusional hallucination of smelling odors. If the odor is unpleasant, it is also known as cacosmia

Olfactory reference syndrome A delusional condition in which an individual erroneously believes they smell bad (e.g. foul body odor or bad breath)

Onychophagia Habitual nail biting

Panic disorder Anxiety disorder characterized by fears with added panic attacks or GAD (see above)

Paradoxical intervention A type of therapeutic intervention in which the therapist instructs the patient to continue the harmful behavior instead of stopping it. The intended outcome is that the patient has more insight and control over what they are doing, which can then lead to change

Paraesthesia An abnormal sensation

Parkinsonism A movement disorder characterized by tremor, moving slowly, rigidity, and postural instability, often caused by antipsychotic medications

Pathologic skin picking Engaging in recurrent and repetitive picking of the skin that results in noticeable tissue damage and/or psychological distress. Also known as skin picking disorder

Penodynia Chronic, idiopathic pain of the mucocutaneous tissue of the glans or shaft of the penis

Problem-solving therapy A psychological treatment that helps an individual to effectively manage the negative effects of stressful life events

Proxy Illness presentation in which a person presents another person, such as his/her child, to a doctor as being the person having the symptoms

Pruritus Itch

Psoriasis A partly inherited chronic, relapsing, inflammatory disease that can affect both skin and joints. Classical presentation is well-demarcated silvery plaques with a predilection for the elbows, knees, and scalp

Psychodermatology The field of medicine that concerns the overlapping areas of psychiatry, psychology, and dermatology. Also known as psychocutaneous medicine

Psychodermato-oncology Psychosocial, emotional, and behavioral factors associated with the diagnosis of skin cancer and its treatment

Psychoeducation Providing relevant information to the client or family about a diagnosis and prognosis

Psychogenic excoriation See neurotic excoriations

Psycho-oncology A field at the intersection of psychology and oncology concerned with aspects of cancer that go beyond medical treatment, including quality of life, and psychological and social aspects of cancer

Psychopharmacology The science of drugs and chemicals that affect the functioning of the brain

Psychosexual dysfunction Sexual dysfunction that is psychogenic in origin

Psychosis An abnormal state of mind resulting in distortion of reality, characterized by delusions, hallucinations, and disordered thinking

Psychosocial Relates to the interaction between a patient's psychological well-being and his/her social environment

Putamen A round structure located at the base of the forebrain, which functions to regulate movements and influence various types of learning

Red scrotum syndrome Sometimes use erroneously as a synonym for scrotodynia. It is erroneous because the perceived redness falls within the normal spectrum of scrotal redness

Rhinoplasty A surgical procedure in which the nose is modified in some way

Rosacea A disorder of the cutaneous (usually facial) microvasculature and pilosebacceous unit that is characterized by redness of the face or chest. Several types exist, some demonstrating broken blood vessels on the cheeks; others showing papules, pustules or facial swelling

Rumination Repetitive, negatively toned thinking that is non-productive and does not result in any solution

Scarring (cicatricial) alopecia The term used to represent physical destruction of the hair follicle growing apparatus, leading to permanent hair loss

Schizophrenia A psychotic disorder that affects cognition, behavior, and emotion, characterized by so-called "positive" symptoms (delusions, hallucinations) or "negative" symptoms (loss of interest, energy, and emotion)

Scrotodynia Chronic, idiopathic pain of the cutaneous tissue of the scrotum

Self-help The act of improving and educating yourself through self-guided resources, such as videos, books, and support groups

Self-monitoring The patient's own monitoring of symptoms. In relation to behaviors that the patient is trying to change, this might involve monitoring when the behavior occurs and its psychosocial or physiologic consequences

Self-regulation Refers to the efforts undertaken by an individual in order to alter his/her own beliefs, emotions or behavior

Serotonin norepinephrine reuptake inhibitor (SNRI) A class of antidepressant medications that is believed to exert their therapeutic effect by acting on the neurotransmitters serotonin and norepinephrine

Serotonin-specific reuptake Inhibitor (SSRI) A class of antidepressant medication that is believed to exert its therapeutic effect by increasing the availability of serotonin in the synaptic cleft

Socratic questioning Asking strategic, explorative questions to understand the client's perspectives and help him/her work out solutions to his/her problems

Somatic symptom and related disorders A category in the DSM-5 which includes psychiatric illnesses in which physical concerns are above and beyond what can be explained by examination and diagnostic testing. This term has replaced the term "somatoform disorders" used in the DSM-IV

Spice A drug that is composed of a wide variety of herbal mixtures, causing marijuana-like effects. Street names include K2, fake weed, Yucatan Fire, Skunk, and Moon Rocks

Stepped care A model of healthcare that seeks to ensure that patients have an appropriately increasing level of care according to clinical need

Stigma Disapproval of a person on the basis of a characteristic deemed to be undesirable

Stimulus control A psychological (behavioral) treatment technique used in the treatment of habit/impulse control problems, such as hair pulling and skin picking. It involves making the target behavior more difficult to perform and attenuates its reinforcing qualities

Stratified approach A clinical management approach that aims to match the best available therapy with individuals based upon assessment of those patient characteristics known to be associated with a positive treatment response. The term is used in contrast to a stepped approach in which all patients start on the lowest intensity therapy, only progressing to higher levels if they do not respond to the lower levels of intervention

Substance use disorders A group of disorders in which individuals misuse recreational or prescribed drugs and alcohol

Suicidal ideation Thinking about suicide

Tardive dyskinesia A movement disorder characterized by repetitive, involuntary, purposeless movements, including grimacing, tongue protrusion, lip smacking, puckering of the lips, and rapid eye blinking, often caused by long-term antipsychotic medication use

Terra firma-forme A condition of the skin where a patient develops brown, dirt-like plaques that can be completely removed by vigorous scrubbing with alcohol. The condition is often idiopathic, but if there is a history of inadequate cleaning, the condition is sometimes called dermatosis neglecta

Thrombocytopenia Abnormally low platelet count

Tinea versicolor Skin infection due to the yeast Malassezia that manifests as macules, papules, and plaques, with variations in color pigmentation of the skin and fine scale. Also known as pityriasis versicolor

Track marks The line of bruised needle holes and scarring, usually on the arms and legs, produced by intravenous drug users who "shoot up" at a slightly higher points each time, causing damage to the skin's connective tissues

Trichotillomania Recurrent psychogenic pulling out of (scalp and other) hair. Also known as hair pulling disorder

Tricyclic antidepressant (TCA) An older class of antidepressant medications (with a chemical three-ringed shape) used in different doses for anti-depressant and neuroleptic purposes

Trigeminal neuralgia Brief paroxysms of severe unilateral pain in the distribution of one or more branches of the trigeminal nerve

Trigeminal trophic syndrome Intractable neuropathic dysesthesia within the distribution of the trigeminal nerve that results in self-mutilation from chronic scratching, usually due to damage of the trigeminal nerve or its associated brain nuclei

Urticaria Red, itchy, short-lived (<24 hours) swellings of the skin

Vestibulectomy A surgical procedure rarely appropriate or necessary for refractory vestibulodynia. The painful, posterior half of the vestibular tissue is surgically removed and vaginal tissue is advanced to cover the defect

Vestibulitis An old and now inappropriate name for vestibulodynia. Current evidence does not demonstrate the presence of inflammation, which would be necessary for the use of the suffix "-itis"

Vestibulodynia Chronic idiopathic pain of the vulvar vestibule; it may occur spontaneously or be provoked by physical stimuli

Visible difference See disfigurement

Vitiligo Autoimmune or segmental depigmentation (lightening of color) of the skin

Vulvodynia Discomfort/pain/unpleasant sensations of the external female genitalia in the absence of inflammatory skin disease

Xerostomia Dry mouth

Appendix
Screening questionnaires and scales

A1 CAGE questionnaire

1. Have you ever felt you needed to **C**ut down on your drinking?
2. Have people **A**nnoyed you by criticizing your drinking?
3. Have you ever felt **G**uilty about drinking?
4. Have you ever felt you needed a drink first thing in the morning (**E**ye-opener) to steady your nerves or to get rid of a hangover?

Scoring
The CAGE questionnaire can identify alcohol problems over the lifetime. Two positive responses are considered a positive test and indicate if further assessment is warranted.

Practical Psychodermatology, First Edition. Anthony Bewley, Ruth E. Taylor, Jason S. Reichenberg and Michelle Magid.
© 2014 John Wiley & Sons, Ltd. Published 2014 by John Wiley & Sons, Ltd.

A2 Dermatology Life Quality Index (DLQI)

DERMATOLOGY LIFE QUALITY INDEX (DLQI)

Hospital No: ....   Date: ....

Name: ....   Score: ....

Address: ....   Diagnosis: ....

....

The aim of this questionnaire is to measure how much your skin problem has affected your life OVER THE LAST WEEK. Please tick (✓) one box for each question.

1. Over the last week, how **itchy, sore, painful** or **stinging** has your skin been?
    - Very much ☐
    - A lot ☐
    - A little ☐
    - Not at all ☐

2. Over the last week, how **embarrassed** or **self conscious** have you been because of your skin?
    - Very much ☐
    - A lot ☐
    - A little ☐
    - Not at all ☐

3. Over the last week, how much has your skin interfered with you going **shopping** or looking after your **home or garden**?
    - Very much ☐
    - A lot ☐
    - A little ☐
    - Not at all ☐   Not relevant ☐

4. Over the last week, how much has your skin influenced the **clothes** you wear?
    - Very much ☐
    - A lot ☐
    - A little ☐
    - Not at all ☐   Not relevant ☐

5. Over the last week, how much has your skin affected any **social** or **leisure** activities?
    - Very much ☐
    - A lot ☐
    - A little ☐
    - Not at all ☐   Not relevant ☐

6. Over the last week, how much has your skin made it difficult for you to do any **sport**?
    - Very much ☐
    - A lot ☐
    - A little ☐
    - Not at all ☐   Not relevant ☐

7. Over the last week, has your skin prevented you from **working** or **studying**?
    - Yes ☐
    - No ☐   Not relevant ☐

    If "No", over the last week how much has your skin been a problem at **work** or **studying**?
    - A lot ☐
    - A little ☐
    - Not at all ☐

8. Over the last week, how much has your skin created problems with your **partner** or any of your **close friends** or **relatives**?
    - Very much ☐
    - A lot ☐
    - A little ☐
    - Not at all ☐   Not relevant ☐

9. Over the last week, how much has your skin caused any **sexual difficulties**?
    - Very much ☐
    - A lot ☐
    - A little ☐
    - Not at all ☐   Not relevant ☐

10. Over the last week, how much of a problem has the **treatment** for your skin been, for example by making your home messy, or by taking up time?
    - Very much ☐
    - A lot ☐
    - A little ☐
    - Not at all ☐   Not relevant ☐

Please check you have answered EVERY question. Thank you.

Source: www.dermatology.org.uk. Reproduced with permission.

DERMATOLOGY LIFE QUALITY INDEX (DLQI) - INSTRUCTIONS FOR USE

The Dermatology Life Quality Index questionnaire is designed for use in adults, i.e. patients over the age of 16. It is self explanatory and can be simply handed to the patient who is asked to fill it in without the need for detailed explanation. It is usually completed in one or two minutes.

SCORING

The scoring of each question is as follows:

Very much	scored 3
A lot	scored 2
A little	scored 1
Not at all	scored 0
Not relevant	scored 0
Question 7, 'prevented work or studying'	scored 3

The DLQI is calculated by summing the score of each question resulting in a maximum of 30 and a minimum of 0. The higher the score, the more quality of life is impaired.

HOW TO INTERPRET MEANING OF DLQI SCORES

0 – 1	no effect at all on patient's life
2 – 5	small effect on patient's life
6 – 10	moderate effect on patient's life
11 – 20	very large effect on patient's life
21 – 30	extremely large effect on patient's life

REFERENCES

Finlay AY and Khan GK. Dermatology Life Quality Index (DLQI): a simple practical measure for routine clinical use. *Clin Exp Dermatol* 1994; **19**:210-216.

Basra MK, Fenech R, Gatt RM, Salek MS and Finlay AY. The Dermatology Life Quality Index 1994-2007: a comprehensive review of validation data and clinical results. *Br J Dermatol* 2008; **159**:997-1035.

Hongbo Y, Thomas CL, Harrison MA, Salek MS and Finlay AY. Translating the science of quality of life into practice: What do dermatology life quality index scores mean? *J Invest Dermatol* 2005; **125**:659-64.

There is more information about the DLQI, including over 85 translations, at www.dermatology.org.uk. The DLQI is copyright but may be used without seeking permission by clinicians for routine clinical purposes. For other purposes, please contact the copyright owners.

A3 EQ-5D-5L

Under each heading, please tick the **ONE** box that best describes your health **TODAY**

MOBILITY

I have no problems in walking about	❑
I have slight problems in walking about	❑
I have moderate problems in walking about	❑
I have severe problems in walking about	❑
I am unable to walk about	❑

SELF-CARE

I have no problems washing or dressing myself	❑
I have slight problems washing or dressing myself	❑
I have moderate problems washing or dressing myself	❑
I have severe problems washing or dressing myself	❑
I am unable to wash or dress myself	❑

USUAL ACTIVITIES *(e.g. work, study, housework, family or leisure activities)*

I have no problems doing my usual activities	❑
I have slight problems doing my usual activities	❑
I have moderate problems doing my usual activities	❑
I have severe problems doing my usual activities	❑
I am unable to do my usual activities	❑

PAIN / DISCOMFORT

I have no pain or discomfort	❑
I have slight pain or discomfort	❑
I have moderate pain or discomfort	❑
I have severe pain or discomfort	❑
I have extreme pain or discomfort	❑

ANXIETY / DEPRESSION

I am not anxious or depressed	❑
I am slightly anxious or depressed	❑
I am moderately anxious or depressed	❑
I am severely anxious or depressed	❑
I am extremely anxious or depressed	❑

- We would like to know how good or bad your health is **TODAY**.

- This scale is numbered from **0** to **100**.

- **100** means the <u>best</u> health you can imagine.
  0 means the <u>worst</u> health you can imagine.

- Mark an **X** on the scale to indicate how your health is **TODAY**.

- Now, please write the number you marked on the scale in the box below.

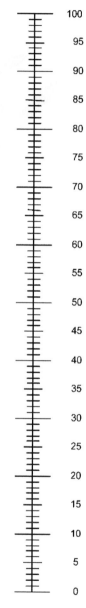

The best health
you can imagine

YOUR HEALTH TODAY =

The worst health
you can imagine

Grading

For grading instructions, please see the EQ-5D-5L user guide which can be downloaded at http://www.euroqol.org/fileadmin/user_upload/Documenten/PDF/Folders_Flyers/UserGuide_EQ-5D-5L_v2.0_October_2013.pdf

A4 Hospital Anxiety and Depression Scale

This questionnaire helps your physician to know how you are feeling. Read every sentence. Place an "X" on the answer that best describes how you have been feeling during the LAST WEEK. You do not have to think too much to answer. In this questionnaire, spontaneous answers are more important

A	I feel tense or 'wound up':	
	Most of the time	3
	A lot of the time	2
	From time to time (occ.)	1
	Not at all	0
D	**I still enjoy the things I used to enjoy:**	
	Definitely as much	0
	Not quite as much	1
	Only a little	2
	Hardly at all	3
A	**I get a sort of frightened feeling as if something awful is about to happen:**	
	Very definitely and quite badly	3
	Yes, but not too badly	2
	A little, but it doesn't worry me	1
	Not at all	0
D	**I can laugh and see the funny side of things:**	
	As much as I always could	0
	Not quite so much now	1
	Definitely not so much now	2
	Not at all	3
A	**Worrying thoughts go through my mind:**	
	A great deal of the time	3
	A lot of the time	2
	From time to time, but not often	1
	Only occasionally	0
D	**I feel cheerful:**	
	Not at all	3
	Not often	2
	Sometimes	1
	Most of the time	0
A	**I can sit at ease and feel relaxed:**	
	Definitely	0
	Usually	1
	Not often	2
	Not at all	3

D	I feel as if I am slowed down:	
	Nearly all the time	3
	Very often	2
	Sometimes	1
	Not at all	0
A	**I get a sort of frightened feeling like "butterflies" in the stomach:**	
	Not at all	0
	Occasionally	1
	Quite often	2
	Very often	3
D	**I have lost interest in my appearance:**	
	Definitely	3
	I don't take as much care as I should	2
	I may not take quite as much care	1
	I take just as much care	0
A	**I feel restless as I have to be on the move:**	
	Very much indeed	3
	Quite a lot	2
	Not very much	1
	Not at all	0
D	**I look forward with enjoyment to things:**	
	As much as I ever did	0
	Rather less than I used to	1
	Definitely less than I used to	2
	Hardly at all	3
A	**I get sudden feelings of panic:**	
	Very often indeed	3
	Quite often	2
	Not very often	1
	Not at all	0
D	**I can enjoy a good book or radio/TV program:**	
	Often	0
	Sometimes	1
	Not often	2
	Very seldom	3

Scoring

HADS has 14 items, seven of which are aimed at evaluating anxiety, marked by the letter A (HADS-A), and seven for depression, marked by the letter D (HADS-D). Each item receives a score that ranges from 0–3, achieving a maximal score of 21 points for each scale.

- HADS-A (Anxiety): 0–8 without anxiety, ≥9 with anxiety
- HADS-D (Depression): 0–8 without depression, ≥9 with depression

Source: Zigmond & Snaith, 1983. Acta Psychiatrica Scandinavica 67: 361–370. Reproduced with permission from Wiley.

A5 Mini Mental State Examination

Patient's Name: _____   Date: _____

Instructions: *Ask the questions in the order listed. Score one point for each correct response within each question or activity.*

Maximum Score	Patient's Score	Questions
5		"What is the year? Season? Date? Day of the week? Month?"
5		"Where are we now: State? County? Town/city? Hospital? Floor?"
3		The examiner names three unrelated objects clearly and slowly, then asks the patient to name all three of them. The patient's response is used for scoring. The examiner repeats them until patient learns all of them, if possible. Number of trials: _____
5		"I would like you to count backward from 100 by sevens." (93, 86, 79, 72, 65, ...) Stop after five answers. Alternative: "Spell WORLD backwards." (D-L-R-O-W)
3		"Earlier I told you the names of three things. Can you tell me what those were?"
2		Show the patient two simple objects, such as a wristwatch and a pencil, and ask the patient to name them.
1		"Repeat the phrase: 'No ifs, ands, or buts.'"
3		"Take the paper in your right hand, fold it in half, and put it on the floor." (The examiner gives the patient a piece of blank paper.)
1		"Please read this and do what it says." (Written instruction is "Close your eyes.")
1		"Make up and write a sentence about anything." (This sentence must contain a noun and a verb.)
1		"Please copy this picture." (The examiner gives the patient a blank piece of paper and asks him/her to draw the symbol below. All 10 angles must be present and two must intersect.)
30		TOTAL

Source: Folstein *et al.*, 1975. J Psychiatric Research 12: 189–98. Reproduced with permission from Elsevier.

Method	Score	Interpretation
Single Cutoff	<24	Abnormal
Range	<21	Increased odds of dementia
	>25	Decreased odds of dementia
Education	21	Abnormal for 8th grade education
	<23	Abnormal for high school education
	<24	Abnormal for college education
Severity	24-30	No cognitive impairment
	18-23	Mild cognitive impairment
	0-17	Severe cognitive impairment

A6 Patient Health Questionnaire (PHQ)

This questionnaire is an important part of providing you with the best health care possible. Your answers will help in understanding problems that you may have. Please answer every question to the best of your ability unless you are requested to skip over a question.

Name _____ Age _____ Sex: ☐ Female ☐ Male   Today's Date_____

1. During the <u>last 4 weeks</u>, how much have you been bothered by any of the following problems?	Not bothered	Bothered a little	Bothered a lot
a. Stomach pain	☐	☐	☐
b. Back pain	☐	☐	☐
c. Pain in your arms, legs, or joints (knees, hips, etc.)	☐	☐	☐
d. Menstrual cramps or other problems with your periods	☐	☐	☐
e. Pain or problems during sexual intercourse	☐	☐	☐
f. Headaches	☐	☐	☐
g. Chest pain	☐	☐	☐
h. Dizziness	☐	☐	☐
i. Fainting spells	☐	☐	☐
j. Feeling your heart pound or race	☐	☐	☐
k. Shortness of breath	☐	☐	☐
l. Constipation, loose bowels, or diarrhea	☐	☐	☐
m. Nausea, gas, or indigestion	☐	☐	☐

2. Over the <u>last 2 weeks</u>, how often have you been bothered by any of the following problems?	Not at all	Several days	More than half the days	Nearly every day
a. Little interest or pleasure in doing things	☐	☐	☐	☐
b. Feeling down, depressed, or hopeless	☐	☐	☐	☐
c. Trouble falling or staying asleep, or sleeping too much	☐	☐	☐	☐
d. Feeling tired or having little energy	☐	☐	☐	☐
e. Poor appetite or overeating	☐	☐	☐	☐
f. Feeling bad about yourself – or that you are a failure or have let yourself or your family down	☐	☐	☐	☐
g. Trouble concentrating on things, such as reading the newspaper or watching television	☐	☐	☐	☐
h. Moving or speaking so slowly that other people could have noticed? Or the opposite – being so fidgety or restless that you have been moving around a lot more than usual	☐	☐	☐	☐
i. Thoughts that you would be better off dead or of hurting yourself in some way	☐	☐	☐	☐

FOR OFFICE CODING: Som Dis if at least 3 of #1a–m are "a lot" and lack an adequate biol explanation.

Maj Dep Syn if answers to #2a or b and five or more of #2a–i are at least "More than half the days" (count #2i if present at all).

Other Dep Syn if #2a or b and two, three, or four of #2a–i are at least "More than half the days" (count #2i if present at all).

3. Questions about anxiety.	**NO**	**YES**
a. In the last 4 weeks, have you had an anxiety attack – suddenly feeling fear or panic?	☐	☐
If you checked "NO", go to question #5.		
b. Has this ever happened before?	☐	☐
c. Do some of these attacks come suddenly out of the blue – that is, in situations where you don't expect to be nervous or uncomfortable?	☐	☐
d. Do these attacks bother you a lot or are you worried about having another attack?	☐	☐

4. Think about your last bad anxiety attack.	**NO**	**YES**
a. Were you short of breath?	☐	☐
b. Did your heart race, pound, or skip?	☐	☐
c. Did you have chest pain or pressure?	☐	☐
d. Did you sweat?	☐	☐
e. Did you feel as if you were choking?	☐	☐
f. Did you have hot flashes or chills?	☐	☐
g. Did you have nausea or an upset stomach, or the feeling that you were going to have diarrhea?	☐	☐
h. Did you feel dizzy, unsteady, or faint?	☐	☐
i. Did you have tingling or numbness in parts of your body? . . .	☐	☐
j. Did you tremble or shake?	☐	☐
k. Were you afraid you were dying?	☐	☐

5. Over the last 4 weeks, how often have you been bothered by any of the following problems?	**Not at all**	**Several days**	**More than half the days**
a. Feeling nervous, anxious, on edge, or worrying a lot about different things.	☐	☐	☐
If you checked "Not at all", go to question #6.			
b. Feeling restless so that it is hard to sit still.	☐	☐	☐
c. Getting tired very easily.	☐	☐	☐
d. Muscle tension, aches, or soreness.	☐	☐	☐
e. Trouble falling asleep or staying asleep.	☐	☐	☐
f. Trouble concentrating on things, such as reading a book or watching TV.	☐	☐	☐
g. Becoming easily annoyed or irritable.	☐	☐	☐

FOR OFFICE CODING: Pan Syn if all of #3a-d are "YES" and four or more of #4a-k are "YES". Other Anx Syn if #5a and answers to three or more of #5b-g are "More than half the days".

6. Questions about eating.	NO	YES
a. Do you often feel that you can't control <u>what</u> or <u>how much</u> you eat?	☐	☐
b. Do you often eat, <u>within any 2-hour period</u>, what most people would regard as an unusually <u>large</u> amount of food?	☐	☐

If you checked "NO" to either #a or #b, go to question #9.

	NO	YES
c. Has this been as often, on average, as twice a week for the last 3 months?	☐	☐

7. In the last 3 months have you <u>often</u> done any of the following in order to avoid gaining weight?	NO	YES
a. Made yourself vomit?	☐	☐
b. Took more than twice the recommended dose of laxatives?	☐	☐
c. Fasted – not eaten anything at all for at least 24 hours?	☐	☐
d. Exercised for more than an hour specifically to avoid gaining weight after binge eating?	☐	☐

8. If you checked "YES" to any of these ways of avoiding gaining weight, were any as often, on average, as twice a week?	NO	YES
	☐	☐

9. Do you ever drink alcohol (including beer or wine)?	NO	YES
	☐	☐

If you checked "NO" go to question #11.

10. Have any of the following happened to you <u>more than once in the last 6 months</u>?	NO	YES
a. You drank alcohol even though a doctor suggested that you stop drinking because of a problem with your health.	☐	☐
b. You drank alcohol, were high from alcohol, or hung over while you were working, going to school, or taking care of children or other responsibilities.	☐	☐
c. You missed or were late for work, school, or other activities because you were drinking or hung over.	☐	☐
d. You had a problem getting along with other people while you were drinking.	☐	☐
e. You drove a car after having several drinks or after drinking too much.	☐	☐

11. If you checked off <u>any</u> problems on this questionnaire, how <u>difficult</u> have these problems made it for you to do your work, take care of things at home, or get along with other people?

Not difficult at all	Somewhat difficult	Very difficult	Extremely difficult
☐	☐	☐	☐

FOR OFFICE CODING: Bul Ner if #6a,b, and-c and #8 are all "YES"; Bin Eat Dis the same but #8 either "NO" or left blank. Alc Abu if any of #10a-e is "YES".

Source: www.phqscreeners.com

PHQ (depression, anxiety, somatic symptom, alcohol, eating disorder) questionnaire scoring

Page 1
- **Somatic symptom disorder:** ≥3 of #1 a–m bother the patient "a lot" and lack of an adequate biological explanation
- **Major depressive syndrome:** if #2a or b and ≥5 of #2a–i are at least "more than half the days"‖ (count #2i if present at all)
- **Other depressive syndrome:** if #2a or b and 2–4 of #2a–i are at least "more than half the days" (count #2i if present at all)

Note: the diagnoses of major depressive disorder and other depressive disorder requires ruling out normal bereavement (mild symptoms, duration <2 months), a history of a manic episode (bipolar disorder) and a physical disorder, medication or other drug as the biological cause of the depressive symptoms.

Page 2
- **Panic syndrome:** if # 3a–d are all "YES" and ≥4 of #4a–k are "YES"
- **Other anxiety syndrome:** if #5a and ≥3 of #5b–g are "more than half the days"

Note: The diagnoses of panic disorder and other anxiety disorder require ruling out a physical disorder, medication or other drug as the biological cause of the anxiety symptoms.

Page 3
- **Bulimia nervosa:** if #6a,b, and c, and #8 are "YES"
- **Binge eating disorder**: the same but #8 is either "NO" or left blank
- **Alcohol use disorder:** if any of #10 a–e are "YES"‖

A7 Patient Health Questionnaire-9 (PHQ-9)

Over the last 2 weeks, how often have you been bothered by any of the following problems? (Use "✓" to indicate your answer)	Not at all	Several days	More than half the days	Nearly every day
1. Little interest or pleasure in doing things	0	1	2	3
2. Feeling down, depressed, or hopeless	0	1	2	3
3. Trouble falling or staying asleep, or sleeping too much	0	1	2	3
4. Feeling tired or having little energy	0	1	2	3
5. Poor appetite or overeating	0	1	2	3
6. Feeling bad about yourself – or that you are a failure or have let yourself or your family down	0	1	2	3
7. Trouble concentrating on things, such as reading the newspaper or watching television	0	1	2	3
8. Moving or speaking so slowly that other people could have noticed? Or the opposite – being so fidgety or restless that you have been moving around a lot more than usual	0	1	2	3
9. Thoughts that you would be better off dead or of hurting yourself in some way	0	1	2	3

FOR OFFICE CODING 0 + _____ + _____ + _____

=Total Score: _____

If you checked off any problems, how **difficult** have these problems made it for you to do your work, take care of things at home, or get along with other people?

Not difficult at all	Somewhat difficult	Very difficult	Extremely difficult
☐	☐	☐	☐

Source: www.phqscreeners.com

PHQ-9 (depression) questionnaire scoring

PHQ-9 severity: This is calculated by assigning scores of 0, 1, 2, and 3 to the response categories of – not at all, – several days, – more than half the days, and – nearly every day, respectively. PHQ-9 total score for the nine items ranges from 0 to 27. Scores of 5, 10, 15, and 20 represent cut-off points for mild, moderate, moderately severe, and severe depression, respectively.

PHQ-9 scores and proposed treatment actions (reproduced from Kroenke K, Spitzer RL. *Psychiatr Ann* 2002; 32: 509–521).

PHQ-9 score	Depression severity	Proposed treatment actions
0–4	None–minimal	None
5–9	Mild	Watchful waiting; repeat PHQ-9 at follow-up
10–14	Moderate	Treatment plan, considering counseling, follow-up and/or pharmacotherapy
15–19	Moderately severe	Active treatment with pharmacotherapy and/or psychotherapy
20–27	Severe	Immediate initiation of pharmacotherapy and, if severe impairment or poor response to therapy, expedited referral to a mental health specialist for psychotherapy and/or collaborative management.

A8 Physical symptoms (PHQ-15)

During the <u>past 4 weeks</u>, how much have you been bothered by any of the following problems?

	Not bothered at all (0)	Bothered a little (1)	Bothered a lot (2)
a. Stomach pain	☐	☐	☐
b. Back pain	☐	☐	☐
c. Pain in your arms, legs, or joints (knees, hips, etc.)	☐	☐	☐
d. Menstrual cramps or other problems with your periods	☐	☐	☐
WOMEN ONLY			
e. Headaches	☐	☐	☐
f. Chest pain	☐	☐	☐
g. Dizziness	☐	☐	☐
h. Fainting spells	☐	☐	☐
i. Feeling your heart pound or race	☐	☐	☐
j. Shortness of breath	☐	☐	☐
k. Pain or problems during sexual intercourse	☐	☐	☐
l. Constipation, loose bowels, or diarrhea	☐	☐	☐
m. Nausea, gas, or indigestion	☐	☐	☐
n. Feeling tired or having low energy	☐	☐	☐
o. Trouble sleeping	☐	☐	☐

(For office coding: Total Score T_____ = _____ + _____)

Source: www.phqscreeners.com

PHQ-15 (somatic symptom) questionnaire scoring

PHQ-15 severity: This is calculated by assigning scores of 0, 1, and 2 to the response categories of – not bothered at all‖, – bothered a little, and – bothered a lot, for the 13 somatic symptoms and two depressive symptoms. PHQ-15 scores of 5, 10, and 15 represent cut-off points for low, medium, and high somatic symptom severity, respectively.

A9 Dimensional Obsessive-Compulsive Scale

This questionnaire asks you about 4 different types of concerns that you might or might not experience. For each type there is a description of the kinds of thoughts (sometimes called *obsessions*) and behaviors (sometimes called *rituals* or *compulsions*) that are typical of that particular concern, followed by 5 questions about your experiences with these thoughts and behaviors. Please read each description carefully and answer the questions for each category based on your experiences in the last month.

Category 1: Concerns about Germs and Contamination

Examples...

-Thoughts or feelings that you are contaminated because you came into contact with (or were nearby) a certain object or person.
-The feeling of being contaminated because you were in a certain place (such as a bathroom).
-Thoughts about germs, sickness, or the possibility of spreading contamination.
-Washing your hands, using hand sanitizer gels, showering, changing your clothes, or cleaning objects because of concerns about contamination.
-Following a certain routine (e.g., in the bathroom, getting dressed) because of contamination
-Avoiding certain people, objects, or places because of contamination.

The next questions ask about your experiences with thoughts and behaviors related to contamination <u>over the last month</u>. Keep in mind that your experiences might be different than the examples listed above. Please circle the number next to your answer:

1.   About how much time have you spent each day thinking about contamination and engaging in washing or cleaning behaviors because of contamination?

   0   None at all
   1   Less than 1 hour each day
   2   Between 1 and 3 hours each day
   3   Between 3 and 8 hours each day
   4   8 hours or more each day

2.   To what extent have you avoided situations in order to prevent concerns with contamination or having to spend time washing, cleaning, or showering?

   0   None at all
   1   A little avoidance
   2   A moderate amount of avoidance
   3   A great deal of avoidance
   4   Extreme avoidance of nearly all things

3.   If you had thoughts about contamination but could not wash, clean, or shower (or otherwise remove the contamination), how distressed or anxious did you become?

   0   Not at all distressed/anxious
   1   Mildly distressed/anxious
   2   Moderately distressed/anxious
   3   Severely distressed/anxious
   4   Extremely distressed/anxious

4.   To what extent has your daily routine (work, school, self-care, social life) been disrupted by contamination concerns and excessive washing, showering, cleaning, or avoidance behaviors?

   0   No disruption at all.
   1   A little disruption, but I mostly function well.
   2   Many things are disrupted, but I can still manage.
   3   My life is disrupted in many ways and I have trouble managing.
   4   My life is completely disrupted and I cannot function at all.

5.   How difficult is it for you to disregard thoughts about contamination and refrain from behaviors such as washing, showering, cleaning, and other decontamination routines when you try to do so?

   0   Not at all difficult
   1   A little difficult
   2   Moderately difficult
   3   Very difficult
   4   Extremely difficult   continued →

Category 2: Concerns about being Responsible for Harm, Injury, or Bad Luck

Examples…

-A doubt that you might have made a mistake that could cause something awful or harmful to happen.
-The thought that a terrible accident, disaster, injury, or other bad luck might have occurred and you weren't careful enough to prevent it.
-The thought that you could prevent harm or bad luck by doing things in a certain way, counting to certain numbers, or by avoiding certain "bad" numbers or words.
-Thought of losing something important that you are unlikely to lose (e.g., wallet, identify theft, papers).
-Checking things such as locks, switches, your wallet, etc. more often than is necessary.
-Repeatedly asking or checking for reassurance that something bad did not (or will not) happen.
-Mentally reviewing past events to make sure you didn't do anything wrong.
-The need to follow a special routine because it will prevent harm or disasters from occurring.
-The need to count to certain numbers, or avoid certain bad numbers, due to the fear of harm.

The next questions ask about your experiences with thoughts and behaviors related to harm and disasters <u>over the last month</u>. Keep in mind that your experiences might be slightly different than the examples listed above. Please circle the number next to your answer:

1. About how much time have you spent each day thinking about the possibility of harm or disasters and engaging in checking or efforts to get reassurance that such things do not (or did not) occur?

    0   None at all
    1   Less than 1 hour each day
    2   Between 1 and 3 hours each day
    3   Between 3 and 8 hours each day
    4   8 hours or more each day

2. To what extent have you avoided situations so that you did not have to check for danger or worry about possible harm or disasters?

    0   None at all
    1   A little avoidance
    2   A moderate amount of avoidance
    3   A great deal of avoidance
    4   Extreme avoidance of nearly all things

3. When you think about the possibility of harm or disasters, or if you cannot check or get reassurance about these things, how distressed or anxious did you become?

    0   Not at all distressed/anxious
    1   Mildly distressed/anxious
    2   Moderately distressed/anxious
    3   Severely distressed/anxious
    4   Extremely distressed/anxious

4. To what extent has your daily routine (work, school, self-care, social life) been disrupted by thoughts about harm or disasters and excessive checking or asking for reassurance?

    0   No disruption at all.
    1   A little disruption, but I mostly function well.
    2   Many things are disrupted, but I can still manage.
    3   My life is disrupted in many ways and I have trouble managing.
    4   My life is completely disrupted and I cannot function at all.

5. How difficult is it for you to disregard thoughts about possible harm or disasters and refrain from checking or reassurance-seeking behaviors when you try to do so?

    0   Not at all difficult
    1   A little difficult
    2   Moderately difficult
    3   Very difficult
    4   Extremely difficult

Continued →

Category 3: Unacceptable Thoughts

Examples...

-Unpleasant thoughts about sex, immorality, or violence that come to mind against your will.
-Thoughts about doing awful, improper, or embarrassing things that you don't really want to do.
-Repeating an action or following a special routine because of a bad thought.
-Mentally performing an action or saying prayers to get rid of an unwanted or unpleasant thought.
-Avoidance of certain people, places, situations or other triggers of unwanted or unpleasant thoughts

---

The next questions ask about your experiences with unwanted thoughts that come to mind against your will and behaviors designed to deal with these kinds of thoughts <u>over the last month</u>. Keep in mind that your experiences might be slightly different than the examples listed above. Please circle the number next to your answer:

1. About how much time have you spent each day with unwanted unpleasant thoughts and with behavioral or mental actions to deal with them?

   0   None at all
   1   Less than 1 hour each day
   2   Between 1 and 3 hours each day
   3   Between 3 and 8 hours each day
   4   8 hours or more each day

2. To what extent have you been avoiding situations, places, objects and other reminders (e.g., numbers, people) that trigger unwanted or unpleasant thoughts?

   0   None at all
   1   A little avoidance
   2   A moderate amount of avoidance
   3   A great deal of avoidance
   4   Extreme avoidance of nearly all things

3. When unwanted or unpleasant thoughts come to mind against your will how distressed or anxious did you become?

   0   Not at all distressed/anxious
   1   Mildly distressed/anxious
   2   Moderately distressed/anxious
   3   Severely distressed/anxious
   4   Extremely distressed/anxious

4. To what extent has your daily routine (work, school, self-care, social life) been disrupted by unwanted and unpleasant thoughts and efforts to avoid or deal with such thoughts?

   0   No disruption at all.
   1   A little disruption, but I mostly function well.
   2   Many things are disrupted, but I can still manage.
   3   My life is disrupted in many ways and I have trouble managing.
   4   My life is completely disrupted and I cannot function at all.

5. How difficult is it for you to disregard unwanted or unpleasant thoughts and refrain from using behavioral or mental acts to deal with them when you try to do so?

   0   Not at all difficult
   1   A little difficult
   2   Moderately difficult
   3   Very difficult
   4   Extremely difficult

Continued →

Category 4: Concerns about Symmetry, Completeness, and the Need for Things to be "Just Right"

Examples...

-The need for symmetry, evenness, balance, or exactness.
-Feelings that something isn't "just right."
-Repeating a routine action until it feels "just right" or "balanced."
-Counting senseless things (e.g., ceiling tiles, words in a sentence).
-Unnecessarily arranging things in "order."
-Having to say something over and over in the same way until it feels "just right."

The next questions ask about your experiences with feelings that something is not "just right" and behaviors designed to achieve order, symmetry, or balance over the last month. Keep in mind that your experiences might be slightly different than the examples listed above. Please circle the number next to your answer:

1. About how much time have you spent each day with unwanted thoughts about symmetry, order, or balance and with behaviors intended to achieve symmetry, order or balance?

    0   None at all
    1   Less than 1 hour each day
    2   Between 1 and 3 hours each day
    3   Between 3 and 8 hours each day
    4   8 hours or more each day

2. To what extent have you been avoiding situations, places or objects associated with feelings that something is not symmetrical or "just right?"

    0   None at all
    1   A little avoidance
    2   A moderate amount of avoidance
    3   A great deal of avoidance
    4   Extreme avoidance of nearly all things

3. When you have the feeling of something being "not just right," how distressed or anxious did you become?

    0   Not at all distressed/anxious
    1   Mildly distressed/anxious
    2   Moderately distressed/anxious
    3   Severely distressed/anxious
    4   Extremely distressed/anxious

4. To what extent has your daily routine (work, school, self-care, social life) been disrupted by the feeling of things being "not just right," and efforts to put things in order or make them feel right?

    0   No disruption at all.
    1   A little disruption, but I mostly function well.
    2   Many things are disrupted, but I can still manage.
    3   My life is disrupted in many ways and I have trouble managing.
    4   My life is completely disrupted and I cannot function at all.

5. How difficult is it for you to disregard thoughts about the lack of symmetry and order, and refrain from urges to arrange things in order or repeat certain behaviors when you try to do so?

    0   Not at all difficult
    1   A little difficult
    2   Moderately difficult
    3   Very difficult
    4   Extremely difficult

© Jon Abramowitz, 2009

Grading

The DOCS is a 20-item self-report measure of obsessive-compulsive symptoms, with scores ranging from 0–80. It contains four subscales, assessing (a) contamination concerns, (b) symptoms regarding responsibility for harm or mistakes, (c) taboo obsessions, and (d) incompleteness. Subscale scores range from 0–20. The DOCS can be used as a screening measure. A total score of ≥18 is highly suspicious for some form of anxiety disorder and a score of ≥21 is highly suspicious for OCD specifically. In addition, the DOCS can be used at each visit to assess improvement of symptoms with OCD treatment.

A10 Cosmetic Procedures Screening Questionnaire (COPS)

This questionnaire aims to understand how you feel about your appearance prior to a cosmetic procedure. All information will be kept strictly confidential.

Please study this example before completing question 1. In a moment, we will ask you to describe the feature(s) of your body which you dislike or would like to improve. If you want to improve more than one feature, please list all the features in the space provided. Please note, the 1st feature should be the feature you are most concerned about.

This is an example of a woman whose main worry was her nose and who was concerned to a lesser extent by her skin and bottom.

---

1) Features Causing Concern
Please describe the feature(s) of your body, which you dislike or would like to improve.

1st Feature
Nose is too crooked with a bump

2nd Feature

Blemishes and acne scars on face

3rd Feature

Bottom is too big

We will then ask you to draw a pie chart and estimate the percentage of concern allocated to each feature. The person above completed her pie chart like this.

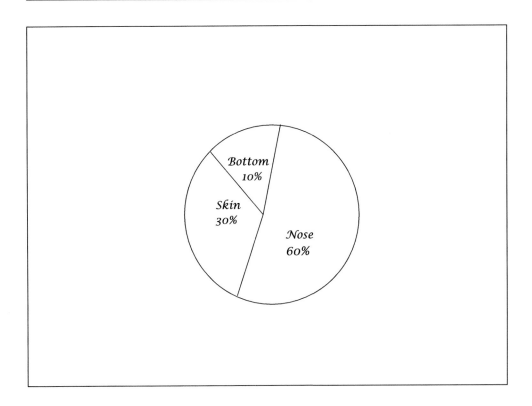

1) **Features Causing Concern**
    Please describe the feature(s) of your body which you dislike or would like to improve.

    1ˢᵗ Feature (feature you are most concerned about)

    _____
    _____

    2nd Feature

    _____
    _____

    3rd Feature

    _____
    _____

    4th Feature

    _____
    _____

    5th Feature

    _____
    _____

Now please draw a pie chart and estimate the percentage of concern allocated to each feature. Please ensure that your percentages add up to 100%!

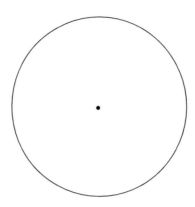

From now on, we will refer to these concerns as your "feature(s)."
Please read the next set of questions below carefully and <u>circle</u> the number that best describes the way that you feel about your feature(s). **Please read the labels carefully to ensure you are circling the number that reflects how you feel because some of the answers are worded in a reverse order.**

2) How often do you **deliberately** check your feature(s)? **Not accidentally catch sight of it.** Please include looking at your feature in a mirror or other reflective surfaces like a shop window or looking at it directly or feeling it with your fingers.

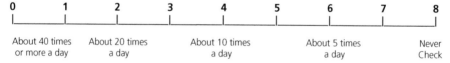

3) How much do you feel your feature(s) is **currently** ugly, unattractive or "not right"?

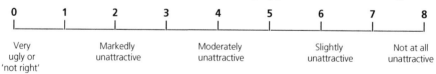

4) How much does your feature(s) **currently** cause you a lot of distress?

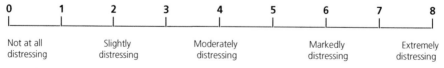

5) How often does your feature(s) **currently** lead you to avoid situations or activities?

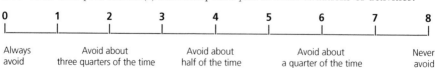

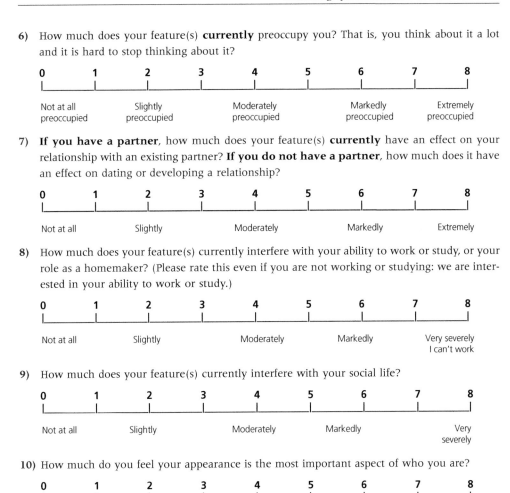

6) How much does your feature(s) **currently** preoccupy you? That is, you think about it a lot and it is hard to stop thinking about it?

```
0       1       2       3       4       5       6       7       8
|_____|_____|_____|_____|_____|_____|_____|_____|
```

Not at all   Slightly   Moderately   Markedly   Extremely
preoccupied   preoccupied   preoccupied   preoccupied   preoccupied

7) **If you have a partner**, how much does your feature(s) **currently** have an effect on your relationship with an existing partner? **If you do not have a partner**, how much does it have an effect on dating or developing a relationship?

```
0       1       2       3       4       5       6       7       8
|_____|_____|_____|_____|_____|_____|_____|_____|
```

Not at all   Slightly   Moderately   Markedly   Extremely

8) How much does your feature(s) currently interfere with your ability to work or study, or your role as a homemaker? (Please rate this even if you are not working or studying: we are interested in your ability to work or study.)

```
0       1       2       3       4       5       6       7       8
|_____|_____|_____|_____|_____|_____|_____|_____|
```

Not at all   Slightly   Moderately   Markedly   Very severely
                                                                                          I can't work

9) How much does your feature(s) currently interfere with your social life?

```
0       1       2       3       4       5       6       7       8
|_____|_____|_____|_____|_____|_____|_____|_____|
```

Not at all   Slightly   Moderately   Markedly   Very
                                                                                          severely

10) How much do you feel your appearance is the most important aspect of who you are?

```
0       1       2       3       4       5       6       7       8
|_____|_____|_____|_____|_____|_____|_____|_____|
```

Not at all   Slightly   Moderately   Mostly   Torally

Source: Veale *et al.*, 2012. Journal of Plastic Reconstructive and Aesthetic Surgery, 65: 530–532. Reproduced with permission of Elsevier.

The score is achieved by summing Q 2–10. Items 2, 3, and 5 are reversed. The total ranges from 0 to 72 with a higher score reflecting greater impairment. Scores above 40 are highly suggestive of BDD.

A11 Screening questionnaire for adults: Do I have BDD?

- **Ask yourself the following questions to determine whether you might have BDD.**
  1. Are you very concerned about the appearance of some part(s) of your body which you consider especially unattractive?
     - ○ Yes
     - ○ No

     If yes: Do these concerns preoccupy you? That is, do you think about them a lot and wish you could worry less?
     - ○ Yes
     - ○ No
  2. How much time do you spend thinking about your defect(s) per day on average? Add up all the time you spend on this.
     a. Less than 1 hour a day
     b. 1–3 hours a day
     c. More than 3 hours a day
  3. Is your main concern with how you look that you aren't thin enough or that you might become too fat?
     - ○ Yes
     - ○ No
  4. What effect has your preoccupation with your appearance had on your life?
     a. Has your defect(s) often caused you a lot of distress, torment, or emotional pain?
        - ○ Yes
        - ○ No
     b. Has your defect(s) often significantly interfered with your social life?
        - ○ Yes
        - ○ No
     c. Has your defect(s) often significantly interfered with your school work, your job, or your ability to function in your role (e.g., as a homemaker)?
        - ○ Yes
        - ○ No
     d. Are there things you avoid because of your defect(s)?
        - ○ Yes
        - ○ No

You're likely to have BDD if you gave the following answers:

Question 1: Yes to both parts
Question 2: Answer b or c
Question 3: While a "yes" answer may indicate that BDD is present, it is possible that an eating disorder is a more accurate diagnosis
Question 4: Yes to any of the questions.

Please note that the above questions are intended to screen for BDD, not diagnose it; the answers indicated above can suggest that BDD is present but can't necessarily give a definitive diagnosis.

Source: Understanding Body Dysmorphic Disorder, Katharine A. Phillips. Reproduced with permission of Oxford University Press.

A12 The Massachusetts General Hospital Hairpulling Scale

Instructions: For each question, pick the one statement in that group which best describes your behaviors and/or feelings over the past week. If you have been having ups and downs, try to estimate an average for the past week. Be sure to read all the statements in each group before making your choice.

For the next three questions, rate only the urges to pull your hair.

1. **Frequency of urges.** On an average day, how often did you feel the urge to pull your hair?
   0 This week I felt no urges to pull my hair.
   1 This week I felt an **occasional** urge to pull my hair.
   2 This week I felt an urge to pull my hair **often**.
   3 This week I felt an urge to pull my hair **very often**.
   4 This week I felt **near constant** urges to pull my hair.

2. **Intensity of urges.** On an average day, how intense or "strong" were the urges to pull your hair?
   0 This week I did not feel any urges to pull my hair.
   1 This week I felt **mild** urges to pull my hair.
   2 This week I felt **moderate** urges to pull my hair.
   3 This week I felt **severe** urges to pull my hair.
   4 This week I felt **extreme** urges to pull my hair.

3. **Ability to control the urges.** On an average day, how much control do you have over the urges to pull your hair?
   0 This week I could **always** control the urges, or I did not feel any urges to pull my hair.
   1 This week I was always able to distract myself from the urges to pull my hair **most of the time**.
   2 This week I was able to distract myself from the urges to pull my hair **some of the time**.
   3 This week I was able to distract myself from the urges to pull my hair **rarely**.
   4 This week I was **never** able to distract myself from the urges to pull my hair.

For the next three questions, rate only the actual hairpulling.

4. **Frequency of hairpulling.** On an average day, how often did you actually pull your hair?
   0 This week I did not pull my hair.
   1 This week I pulled my hair **occasionally**.
   2 This week I pulled my hair **often**.

3 This week I pulled my hair **very often**.
   4 This week I pulled my hair so often it felt like I was **always** doing it.

5. **Attempts to resist hairpulling.** On an average day, how often did you make an attempt to stop yourself from actually pulling your hair?
   0 This week I felt no urges to pull my hair.
   1 This week I tried to resist the urge to pull my hair **almost all of the time**.
   2 This week I tried to resist the urge to pull my hair **some of the time**.
   3 This week I tried to resist the urge to pull my hair **rarely**.
   4 This week I **never** tried to resist the urge to pull my hair.

6. **Control over hairpulling.** On an average day, How often were you successful at actually stopping yourself from pulling your hair?
   0 This week I did not pull my hair.
   1 This week I was able to resist pulling my hair **almost all of the time**.
   2 This week I was able to resist pulling my hair **most of the time**.
   3 This week I was able to resist pulling my hair **some of the time**.
   4 This week I was **rarely** able to resist pulling my hair.

For the last question, rate the consequences of your hairpulling.

7. **Associated distress.** Hairpulling can make some people feel moody, "on edge," or sad. During the past week, how uncomfortable did your hairpulling make you feel?
   0 This week I did not feel uncomfortable about my hairpulling.
   1 This week I felt **vaguely uncomfortable** about my hairpulling.
   2 This week I felt **noticeably uncomfortable** about my hairpulling.
   3 This week I felt **significantly uncomfortable** about my hairpulling.
   4 This week I felt **intensely uncomfortable** about my hairpulling.

Scoring the Massachusetts General Hospital (MGH) Hairpulling Scale

The MGH Hairpulling Scale is a 7-item measure of hair pulling symptoms, with scores ranging from 0–28. Each item is scored on a 5-point scale from 0 = no symptoms to 4 = severe symptoms. Higher scores indicate a higher severity of hairpulling. The Hairpulling Scale can be used at each visit to assess improvement of symptoms with treatment.

Source: Keuthen *et al.*, 2001 Psychother Psychosomat 1995; 64: 141–145. Reproduced with permission of Karger.

Citation: Keuthen NJ, O'Sullivan RL, Ricciardi JN, *et al*. The Massachusetts General Hospital (MGH) Hairpulling Scale: 1. Development and Factor Analyses. *Psychother Psychosomat* 1995; 64: 141–145

A13 The Skin Picking Scale (SPS)

Instructions: For each item, pick the one answer which best describes the past week. If you have been having ups and downs, try to estimate an average for the past week. Please be sure to read all answers in each group before making your choice.

1. FREQUENCY OF URGES How often do you feel the urge to pick your skin?	0 = No urges 1 = Mild, occasionally experience urges to skin pick, less than 1 hr/day 2 = Moderate, often experience urges to skin pick, 1–3 hrs/day 3 = Severe, very often experience urges to skin pick, greater than 3 and up to 8 hrs/day 4 = Extreme, constantly or almost always have an urge to skin pick
2. INTENSITY OF URGES How intense or "strong" are the urges to pick your skin?	0 = Minimal or none 1 = Mild 2 = Moderate 3 = Severe 4 = Extreme
3. TIME SPENT ENGAGED IN SKIN PICKING How much time do you spend picking your skin? How frequently does it occur? How much longer than most people does it take you to complete routine activities because of your picking?	0 = None 1 = Mild, spend less than 1 hr/day picking my skin, or occasional skin picking. 2 = Moderate, spend 1–3 hrs/day picking my skin, or frequent skin picking. 3 = Severe, spend more than 3 and up to 8 hrs/day picking my skin, or very frequent skin picking. 4 = Extreme, spend more than 8 hrs/day picking my skin, or near constant skin picking.
4. INTERFERENCE DUE TO SKIN PICKING How much does your skin picking interfere with your social or work (or role) functioning? (If currently not working determine how much your performance would be affected if you were employed.)	0 = None 1 = Mild, slight interference with social or occupational activities but overall performance not impaired. 2 = Moderate, definite interference with social or occupational performance, but still manageable. 3 = Severe, causes substantial impairment in social or occupational performance. 4 = Extreme, incapacitating.
5. DISTRESS ASSOCIATED WITH SKIN PICKING How much distress do you experience as a result of your skin picking? How would you feel if prevented from picking your skin? How anxious would you become?	0 = None 1 = Mild, only slightly anxious if skin picking prevented, or only slight anxiety during skin picking. 2 = Moderate, anxiety would mount but remain manageable if skin picking prevented, or anxiety increases to manageable levels during skin picking. 3 = Severe, prominent and very disturbing increase in anxiety if skin picking is interrupted, or prominent and very disturbing increase in anxiety during skin picking. 4 = Extreme, incapacitating anxiety from any intervention aimed at modifying activity, or incapacitating anxiety develops during skin picking.
6. AVOIDANCE Have you been avoiding doing anything, going any place, or being with anyone because of your skin picking? If yes, then how much do you avoid?	0 = None 1 = Mild, occasional avoidance in social or work settings. 2 = Moderate, frequent avoidance in social or work settings 3 = Severe, very frequent avoidance in social or work settings. 4 = Extreme, avoid all social and work settings as a result of the skin picking.

Source: Keuthen *et al.* J Psychosom Res 2001; 50: 337–41. Adapted with permission of Elsevier.

The Skin Picking Scale (SPS) is a 6-item measure of skin picking symptoms, with scores ranging from 0–24. The SPS can be used as a screening measure. A score of ≥7 is highly suspicious for a skin picking disorder. In addition, the SPS can be used at each visit to assess improvement of symptoms with treatment.

A14 The Skin Cancer Index

The following questions ask about your views on skin cancer or its treatment and how it may affect you socially, at work, or at home, and other areas of concern. For each of the following, please indicate how much your skin cancer affects your life by circling the number in the **one** box that most closely matches how you feel at the present time.

During the past month, how much have you . . .	Very much	Quite a bit	Moderately	A little bit	Not at all
1. Worried your skin cancer will spread to another part of your body?	1	2	3	4	5
2. Felt anxious about your skin cancer?	1	2	3	4	5
3. Worried that family members may also develop skin cancer?	1	2	3	4	5
4. Worried about the cause of skin cancer?	1	2	3	4	5
5. Felt frustrated about your skin cancer?	1	2	3	4	5
6. Worried that your tumour may become a more serious type of skin cancer?	1	2	3	4	5
7. Worried about new skin cancers occurring in the future?	1	2	3	4	5
8. Felt uncomfortable about meeting new people?	1	2	3	4	5
9. Felt concerned that your skin cancer may worry friends or family?	1	2	3	4	5
10. Worried about the length of time before you can go out in public?	1	2	3	4	5
11. Felt bothered by people's questions related to your skin cancer?	1	2	3	4	5
12. Felt embarrassed by your skin cancer?	1	2	3	4	5
13. Worried about how large the scar will be?	1	2	3	4	5
14. Thought about how skin cancer affects your attractiveness?	1	2	3	4	5
15. Thought about how noticeable the scar will be to others?	1	2	3	4	5
Score total:					

Source: Rhee *et al.* Laryngoscope 2007; 117: 399–405. Reproduced with permission of LWW.

Scoring the Skin Cancer Index

The Skin Cancer Index (SCI) is a 15-item instrument to determine patients' quality of life (QoL) with skin cancer. It has three distinct subscales: emotion, social, and appearance. Standardized scores range from 0 to 100, with higher scores reflecting better QoL.

A15 The Distress Thermometer for skin cancer

Getting the diagnosis of skin cancer and treating skin cancer can be very stressful. Use this distress thermometer to measure your stress levels every day. Then fill out the *Weekly Stress Management Journal* below to keep track.

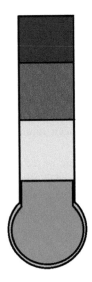

10 Completely overwhelmed/burnout

9 Overwhelmed

8 Losing control

7 Starting to lose control

6 Moderate to severe distress

5 Moderately distressed

4 Mild to moderate distress

3 Mildly distressed

2 A little uneasy

1 Relaxed

0 Completely relaxed and calm

DATE	Level of stress	Thoughts and feelings
Sun		
Mon		
Tues		
Wed		
Thurs		
Fri		
Sat		

A16 Alcohol Use Disorders Identification Test (AUDIT)

Developed to identify current problem drinking in primary care settings.

A weighted score of 8 or more for men up to age 60 or 4 or more for women, adolescents, and men over the age of 60 is considered a positive screening result.

1. How often do you have a drink containing alcohol?
2. How many drinks containing alcohol do you have on a typical day when you are drinking?
3. How often do you have six or more drinks on one occasion?
4. How often during the last year have you found that you were not able to stop drinking once you had started?
5. How often during the last year have you failed to do what was normally expected of you because of drinking?
6. How often during the last year have you needed a first drink in the morning to get yourself going after a heavy drinking session?
7. How often during the last year have you had a feeling of guilt or remorse after drinking?
8. How often during the last year have you been unable to remember what happened the night before because of your drinking?
9. Have you or someone else been injured because of your drinking?
10. Has a relative, friend, doctor, or other healthcare worker been concerned about your drinking or suggested you cut down?

Scoring

Question 1: Never (0), monthly or less (1), 2–4 times a month (2), 2–3 times a week (3), 4 or more times a week (4)

Question 2: 1 or 2 (0), 3 or 4 (1), 5 or 6 (2), 7–9 (3), 10 or more (4)

Questions 3–8: Never (0), less than monthly (1), monthly (2), weekly (3), daily or almost daily (4)

Questions 9 and 10: 2 points for yes, but not in the last year; 4 points for yes, during the last year

Saunders JB *et al.* Development of the Alcohol Use Disorders Identification Test (AUDIT): WHO Collaborative Project on Early Detection of Persons with Harmful Alcohol Consumption–II. *Addiction* 1993; 88: 791–804.

Babor TF *et al.* AUD IT: The Alcohol Use Disorders Identification Test: Guidelines for Use in Primary Health Care. Geneva, Switzerland: World Health Organization, 2001.

The AUDIT is available in questionnaire format as above or in interview form. Both can be downloaded in a manual together with information on development of the measure and its use: AUDIT: The Alcohol Use Identification Test, Guidelines for Use in Primary Care, Thomas F. Babor, John C. Higgins-Biddle, John B. Saunders, Maristela G. Monteiro Second Edition. WHO Department of Mental Health and Substance Dependence. This publication can be downloaded at: http://www.who.int/substance_abuse/activities/sbi/en/

A17 Alcohol, Smoking and Substance Involvement Screening Test (ASSIST)

The full version of this questionnaire together with the patient response cards and feedback cards for the patient are available via the WHO website at http://www.who.int/substance_abuse/activities/assist_v3_english.pdf

The full ASSIST package consists of three WHO publications:
- The Alcohol, Smoking and Substance involvement Screening Test (ASSIST): manual for use in primary care
- The ASSIST-linked brief intervention for hazardous and harmful substance use: a manual for use in primary care
- Self-help strategies for cutting down or stopping substance use: a guide
  All of these are available at http://www.who.int/substance_abuse/activities/assist/en/index.html

Source: www.who.int. Reproduced with permission from WHO.

Index

Note:
  Abbreviations:
    CBT – cognitive-behavioural therapy
    MEMS – medication electronic monitoring system
    OCRDs – obsessive-compulsive and related disorders
    PHQ – Patient Health Questionnaire
  Figures in *italics*, tables in **bold,** boxes indicated with
  "b".

Practical Psychodermatology, First Edition. Anthony Bewley, Ruth E. Taylor, Jason S. Reichenberg and Michelle Magid.
© 2014 John Wiley & Sons, Ltd. Published 2014 by John Wiley & Sons, Ltd.

Printed and bound by CPI Group (UK) Ltd, Croydon, CR0 4YY

16/04/2025

14658503-0001

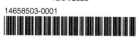